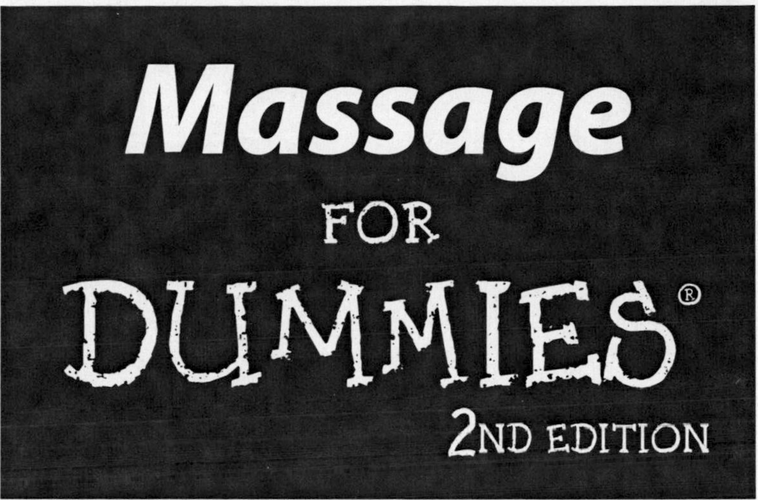

by Steve Capellini, LMT, and
Michel Van Welden, PT, NT

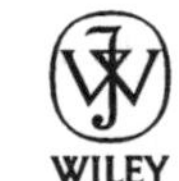

John Wiley & Sons, Inc.

Massage For Dummies®, 2nd Edition

Published by
John Wiley & Sons, Inc.
909 Third Avenue
New York, NY 10022
www.wiley.com

For general information on our other products and services, please contact our Customer Care Department within the U.S. at 877-762-2974, outside the U.S. at 317-572-3993, or fax 317-572-4002.

For technical support, please visit www.wiley.com/techsupport.

Wiley publishes in a variety of print and electronic formats and by print-on-demand. Some material included with standard print versions of this book may not be included in e-books or in print-on-demand. If this book refers to media such as a CD or DVD that is not included in the version you purchased, you may download this material at http://booksupport.wiley.com. For more information about Wiley products, visit www.wiley.com.

Library of Congress Control Number: 2010925698

ISBN 978-0-470-58738-6 (pbk); ISBN 978-0-470-64273-3 (ebk); ISBN 978-0-470-64274-0 (ebk); ISBN 978-0-470-64275-7 (ebk)

Manufactured in the United States of America

10 9 8 7 6 5 4 3

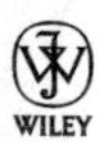

About the Authors

Steve Capellini: You may be thinking to yourself, "What makes him so special that he should write this book on massage?" Perhaps what most specifically qualifies me is the inordinate amount of time, amounting to many thousands of hours, that I've spent cooped up alone in a room with just one other person, touching them all over their bodies and getting paid for it.

What could be more fun? Or weirder? I hope I've got the communication skills to get across to you the reasons why an otherwise sane human being would spend such a large percentage of his life in such a strange manner.

And in addition, to give you an idea of some more specific qualifications, here's a rough chronology of my life in touch:

1977: Received first massage ever, from high school girlfriend Grace, and knew that something important had just transpired.

1983: Attended 108-hour massage class in Los Angeles and became certified. Had to take V.D. test at local health clinic in order to receive license (a local prostitution ordinance).

1984: Massaged members of the cast and crew of a movie being filmed about Ernest Hemingway in Pamplona, Spain, during the famous running of the bulls. Yes, I ran.

1985: First regular massage job, at a spa in Florida, giving 25-minute full body oil rubdowns to cigar-smoking "good ole boys" for $4 an hour.

1986: Rethought career choice. Started working at a friend's landscaping company.

1987: Was called in to work at a new spa in Miami, the Doral. Massaged Dr. Ruth Westheimer, who gave me the "secret" of aphrodisiacs.

1988: Became supervisor of the massage and spa treatments department at the Doral, in charge of 40 therapists.

1989: Became a traveling spa trainer, hiring staff and overseeing openings of spas in Vermont, Jamaica, on cruise ships, and more.

1992: Started teaching workshops to massage therapists and business owners. Massaged Red Cross volunteers and army personnel in aftermath of Hurricane Andrew.

1997: Began publishing books on massage and spas.

1998: First child born. Taught him how to massage Mommy and Daddy by the age of three.

2002: Second child born. Taught him how to massage also. He and his big brother began making extra cash massaging Mommy and Daddy.

2003: Became a media spokesperson for Glade, Lands End, Vaseline, California Avocados and others, going on TV shows to tell people how great it is to use certain products to do spa treatments at home.

2005: Began writing large, comprehensive book about spa therapies for massage therapists.

2009: Finished writing large, comprehensive book about spa therapies for massage therapists.

2010: Family continues to grow and children continue to massage Mommy and Daddy. Start working as expert witness in trials concerning lawsuits against spas and massage therapists. Begin writing memoir: *Touchy Subjects*.

Michel Van Welden, PT, NT, received his training at the Physical Therapy Institute of Paris, specializing in orthopedic and neurological rehabilitation, as well as sports medicine and the treatment of burn victims.

For 26 years, he practiced both in hospitals and in his own private clinic. Working hand in hand (no pun intended) with plastic surgeons, he helped develop Plastic Physical Therapy, which increases the positive results of plastic surgery procedures. He also assembled a procedural manual and produced a video about lymphatic drainage and has taught his technique to therapists throughout France and around the world.

Since arriving in the United States, he has become an "expert on the skin" who in May 1998 substantiated the first derivative claim ever approved by the FDA for the treatment of cellulite using a patented massage device. All the other stuff you see on infomercials about cellulite is a lot of malarkey.

Michel is also a wild and crazy outdoorsman. He has run to the top of Mount Kilamanjaro seven times. He also became the record holder for long distance running along the Great Wall of China, covering 1,500 miles, half of the wall's length. His greatest achievement in the sports field, though, was in helping dozens of other people discover their own potentials by leading fitness trips to the Great Wall, Kilamanjaro, the Andes peaks, and other destinations.

Mr. Van Welden is married and is the father of two children and one grandchild. He lives in Miami, Florida and is the proud owner of a medical device distribution company. He can be contacted by email at `massagefordummies@me.com`.

Dedication

From Steve: I dedicate this book to the coolest massage partner ever, Brandon Sunthorn Capellini.

Authors' Acknowledgments

From Steve: I thank Atchana, my darling partner and wife, who receives fewer massages from me than she deserves because I'm so busy writing all the time. The rest of my family is equally supportive and enthusiastic, too: Mom and Dad, Tina, Bala and Adi, Jim and Lalitha, Rob, Suzanne, Chris, Ari, and Nicole. And, of course, the Thai side of the family: Lek, Pat, Rangsan, Tina, Rolando and Umpun, in memorium. And the father-in-law I never knew, Sunthorn Chuaindhara; he lives on in our hearts.

I appreciate my co-author Michel Van Welden for his help and for being so dedicated to his worldwide massage research.

I'm very grateful to agent Carol Susan Roth, who believed I was right for this project and made it all possible through her dedication and hard work, and to Lori Huneke for introducing us.

All the folks at Wiley have been a pleasure to work with, including Chrissy Guthrie, Tracy Boggier, and Alicia South. I thank my friend and co-author, Michel Van Welden, and my buddy, Yanik Chauvin, photographer extraordinaire, who provided the pictures; and, of course, the models, Jason Barger and Linda Vongkhamphra, who were featured in the first edition as well, plus Fernando Spitaliere, Laura Esquival, Annamaria Salley, Barbara Rozel, Jackie Ferrerosa, Alexis Somoano, Desiree Barger, Richard Obregon, the lovely Jessica Yu, and cute little Cade Akai.

Also, there are so many friends and clients from the massage and spa world who've helped with this book: Jai Varadaraj for all her help from India; Lynda Solien-Wolfe for her guerilla massage marketing and the great *Massage For Dummies* chair; Don Payne; John Fanuzzi; Carole Spellman; Ed Wilson; Iris Burman; Dan and Telka Ulrich; Pat Weinman; Harvey and Phyllis Sandler; Dave Kennedy; Amory Rowe; the Dail family up in Maine for their unparalleled hospitality; and especially Nancy Dail for her technical review of this book.

From Michel: For my Mom, for all that she did for me, including going through sciatica pain to show me the way of my future. Thanks.

To all the patients who knocked on my door to receive a massage and ended up sweating in Africa, China, or Bolivia.

To Steve Capellini, for not thinking that all French are arrogant, carrying their baguettes and bottles of wine everywhere they go, and for offering me the pleasure of sharing the success of this book.

To Elizabeth, my loving wife, for her unconditional support and her great Mexican cuisine.

To Sebastien (my son) and Kim (my granddaughter), for all the support they bring to their too-often-gone-away Dad.

To Jocelyne, who taught me how to speak to pigs about massage and convince them that the guy with the white coat and a strong French accent was not the butcher.

To Dr. James Watson, plastic surgeon at UCLA, and Dr. David Adcok, plastic surgeon at Vanderbilt University, for all the hours spent together in the lab and in the Plastic Surgery Department trying to understand a nonsurgical technique.

To Tami Booth for giving me this extraordinary opportunity — to be published in the United States. And to Carol Susan Roth for making it possible.

Publisher's Acknowledgments

We're proud of this book; please send us your comments at `http://dummies.custhelp.com`. For other comments, please contact our Customer Care Department within the U.S. at 877-762-2974, outside the U.S. at 317-572-3993, or fax 317-572-4002.

Some of the people who helped bring this book to market include the following:

Acquisitions, Editorial, and Media Development

Senior Project Editor: Christina Guthrie (Previous Edition: Tim Gallan)

Acquisitions Editor: Tracy Boggier

Copy Editor: Megan Knoll

Assistant Editor: Erin Calligan Mooney

Senior Editorial Assistant: David Lutton

Technical Editor: Susan E. Baggarly, NCTM

Editorial Manager: Christine Meloy Beck

Editorial Assistants: Jennette ElNaggar and Rachelle Amick

Art Coordinator: Alicia B. South

Cover Photos: © iStock

Cartoons: Rich Tennant (`www.the5thwave.com`)

Composition Services

Project Coordinator: Kristie Rees

Layout and Graphics: SDJumper

Special Art: Interior photography by Yanik Chauvin

Proofreaders: Leeann Harney, Melanie Hoffman

Indexer: Sherry Massey

Publishing and Editorial for Consumer Dummies

Kathleen Nebenhaus, Vice President and Executive Publisher

David Palmer, Associate Publisher

Kristin Ferguson-Wagstaffe, Product Development Director

Publishing for Technology Dummies

Andy Cummings, Vice President and Publisher

Composition Services

Debbie Stailey, Director of Composition Services

Contents at a Glance

Table of Contents

Introduction

For those who've already discovered it, massage is just about the niftiest thing on the planet. Better than chocolate. Better than pizza. It's a great way to feel better, look better, treat people better, and treat yourself better, too. It's 100 percent good for you, with no artificial additives or ingredients, and it's easy to do. In fact, one of the best things about massage is that you don't need a lot of fancy expensive equipment in order to get one or give one. All you really need to get started is a human body. Got one? Great! Then you're ready to go.

About This Book

First, let me introduce myself and explain what qualifies me to teach you about this subject in the first place. I've been massaging people for a living since I was 23 years old. That's well over 15,000 massages. I've trained other massage therapists around the world at resorts, in spas, in workshops, and in massage schools, and I've written a few other books on the subject. But there's something more to it than that. If all I were offering you was technical experience, analytical knowledge, and rah-rah enthusiasm, I wouldn't blame you for approaching this book with indifference or even boredom. Yet another book about the beauties and wonders of massage strokes and maneuvers? Wax on, wax off. Yawn.

What I hope to offer you is more than technique, more than know-how, even more than increased pleasure and greater health in your everyday life. What I try to get across in the pages that follow is a new way to be. I've transformed my own life into an ongoing, unfolding massage adventure and would be most sincerely honored to act as your guide along a similar journey of inner and outer exploration. There's a big, wild world out there, and there's an even bigger, wilder world inside your own body and mind. Massage is an excellent vehicle through which to explore both.

In this book, you find lots of ways to make massage a part of your day-to-day activities so that it becomes as natural as brushing your teeth, driving your car, or peeling the stickers off sale items you buy as Christmas presents. *Massage For Dummies,* 2nd Edition, offers you all the techniques you need to begin doing great massages. You pick up the same moves professional massage practitioners use, and you even get to speak some of their lingo. By the time you're done reading, you can be confident in your ability to massage others safely and create a lot of enjoyment for yourself and your lucky partners.

And in order to help you accomplish this goal, I've enlisted the help of a pretty impressive character, my co-author, Michel Van Welden. He's a physical therapist and naturopathic therapist who's traveled the world teaching other therapists and physicians about massage. An expert on physiology and the skin, he has been personally responsible for getting the U.S. Food and Drug Administration to sit up and pay serious attention to the effects of certain kinds of massage. The way he accomplished this feat was through several highly complex laboratory experiments studying (I'm not making this up) the effects of massage on pigs. I defer to Michel's clinical expertise on many crucial issues, and my hope is that his scientific knowledge sets your mind at ease regarding the effectiveness and safety of massage. Throughout your average, everyday paragraphs in this book, though, it's me, Steve, serving as your guide. Together, Michel and I have created a book that goes beyond any other of its kind to offer you everything you need to know to change your life from a dull, drab, non-massage existence into an exciting massage adventure.

Conventions Used in This Book

Allow me to take a moment to point out and explain a few conventions that I used when writing this book. As you read through it, keep the following in mind:

- Whenever I introduce a new term or piece of jargon, I *italicize* it and then provide a brief definition.
- Web sites and e-mail addresses appear in `monofont` to help them stand out.
- Keywords in lists and key sentences in numbered steps appear in **boldface.**
- I try to vary the genders of the folks in my examples as much as possible, but if you notice that I refer to females more often, that's just because women are more likely to get massages than men.
- When I use the term "your partner," I'm usually referring to nonprofessionals massaging each other.

What You're Not to Read

Although I'd love it if you read every word of this book from cover to cover, you certainly don't have to. If you're pressed for time or just want to get down to business, feel free to skip any text that's marked with a Technical Stuff icon. Also, *sidebars* (you'll see these gray-shaded boxes throughout the book) contain fun and interesting info, but they don't contain any essential information, so feel free to skip them as well.

Foolish Assumptions

As I state earlier in this Introduction, this book is for anyone with a body, which should qualify almost every single reader. Disembodied spirits and poltergeists may find it difficult to get the correct amount of friction necessary to perform effective massage maneuvers and should therefore abstain. Certain people in particular will quickly discover the most obvious benefits in reading these pages; you know who you are, and this book is especially for you if

- You've ever wanted to touch another person with grace, compassion, and caring.
- You want to share a new level of communication with the people you're close to.
- You want to increase your well-being and reduce many types of pain.
- You have a desire to enhance various aspects of your life, including athletic performance, job efficiency, and even your love life.
- You have a handicap of some kind and want to discover how massage is the therapy of choice for many people with physical limitations.
- You want to pursue this adventure more seriously and are perhaps thinking about becoming a massage pro yourself.
- You think knowing how to give a good massage may be a neat way to get more dates.

The world is filled with millions of people who have already started their own massage adventures. In fact, according to the American Massage Therapy Association, almost a quarter of adult Americans (24 percent) had a massage at least once in the last 12 months. Millions more have exchanged massages on a nonprofessional basis with friends and family. Insurance companies are starting to reimburse for it, doctors are including it in their practices, and practically every hair salon in every city is turning into a day spa and offering massage to clients. It's everywhere, and yet, if you're like the majority of people, you still haven't received a massage, and you have quite a few questions about how it works and what it can do for you. If that's the case, this is the book for you.

How This Book Is Organized

Here are the subjects that you find spread out before your eager eyes and fingers as you use this book:

Part I: Discovering Massage

In this part, you find the background information you need to understand how the massage techniques actually work and where they came from in the first place. You can discover all kinds of interesting things about your skin and what's beneath it, for example, and what it is about massage that helps your whole body feel better. If you're up to the task, you can even play that all-time favorite, the Bony Landmark Game, which is loads of fun for the whole family.

Part II: The Art of Receiving Massage

What, there's an art to receiving too, you ask? You mean I can't just lie there like a blob and let someone else do all the work? That's correct. Massage, in this respect, is like the tango, and you know what they say about the tango. In this part, you develop the fine art of tuning in, which allows you to fully enjoy the benefits and pleasures that await you with massage. I describe how you can invite healthy pleasure into your life, choose the right style of massage for you and your body, choose a good massage therapist, and start receiving massages just like the pros do, with all the trimmings like proper breathing, meditative awareness, and other advanced techniques for basically blissing out.

Part III: The Art of Giving Massage

This part is the meat of the book, so to speak, with all the pretty pictures that you may be tempted to flip to immediately and never draw your attention away from again. Resist this temptation, oh hedonistic reader! In fact, go ahead right now (if you haven't already) and flip forward to the photos and then come back after a couple of minutes. Go ahead. I can wait.

There, satisfied? Now promise that you'll look through the other important sections of Part III as well. Make no mistake about it: To give a good massage requires some effort and energy, and you want to prepare mentally beforehand so you don't burn yourself out. You may also discover vital information about when and how not to massage people, including yourself.

Part IV: Massage for Every Body

In the fourth part, you can take your pick from a smorgasbord of offerings, reading through the chapters that intrigue you in whichever order you choose. Whether you're an athlete, a pregnant woman, a world traveler, or whatever, you're sure to pick up a ton of useful info here that you can use to integrate massage into your life. Plus, I give you quick massage tips to ease your own stress at work.

Part V: The Part of Tens

The last part contains lists of ten quick ways you can improve your life with massage, including suggestions for great places to take massage classes and outstanding locations to receive incredible massages.

Icons Used in This Book

Throughout this book, I place lots of little round things in the margins, calling your attention to various details in the text. These pictures are called icons, and I have included some particularly pertinent ones for people learning the ropes of the massage world:

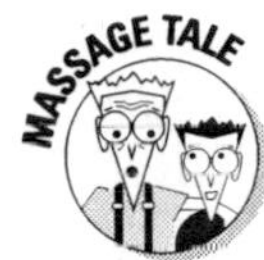

The Massage Tale icon lets you know about a real-life massage story from an actual person in the adjacent paragraph. These stories may leave you happy, misty-eyed, or thoughtful, depending on the subject matter, but they all go to prove how powerful an influence massage can be in your life.

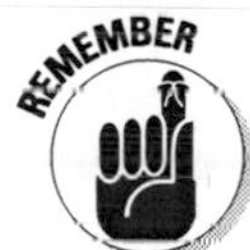

Information flagged with this icon is worth remembering (makes sense, huh?), so be sure not to skip these tidbits.

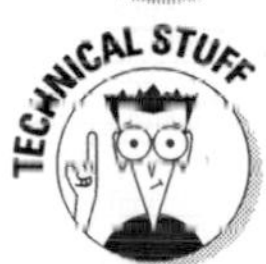

This icon points out information that goes a little beyond strictly need-to-know. Reading it enhances your understanding and appreciation of massage, but if you decide to skip it, you'll still do just fine.

The Tip icon clues you in right away to the presence of some especially important information. Perhaps I reveal a secret technique for massaging your way into Harvard Business School, for example. Perhaps not. You have to check the tip to be sure. At the very least, you may find some quick and easy pointers to make your reading experience as pleasurable as possible.

The practice of massage isn't without its potential dangers. For example, once, after receiving three massages in one day as part of my job interviewing therapists for positions at a new spa, I turned into a human noodle and kept banging my knees into furniture. Seriously, though, you have to watch out for certain things when practicing massage and various reasons why you shouldn't offer massage in certain circumstances (what we professionals call *contraindications*). You can catch them right away when you see this icon.

Where to Go from Here

By now you're probably saying, "All right, Steve. You've convinced me. My muscles are sore and I'm ready to get going. How do I get started with this whole massage thing anyway?"

The best way to use this book is to choose the subject that interests you most and then jump right in at that point. You may be eager to start giving a massage right away, in which case, you can zoom ahead to Part III. I highly encourage you to read all the material in the sections leading up to the how-to stuff, however, instead of simply flipping through the photographs and list of instructions. The attitudes and intentions with which you approach massage are, after all, what make the biggest difference in terms of what you get out of it.

For those of you who like to approach your reading in a systematic fashion, you'll find that each part of the book builds upon the one before it in what is, I hope, a logical manner, so that by the end, you can come away knowing just about as much as you'd ever want to know about massage. Unless of course you start pursuing it as a passion and profession in your life as I have, in which case, the learning never ends.

Massage, ultimately, is a way to share with others and to express yourself in a direct, hands-on way, and I hope this book plays a big part in helping you discover this. If you want to share some thoughts about what you learn on your own massage adventure, you can visit me on the Web at `www.royaltreatment.com` and send e-mail to `steve@royaltreatment.com`. I'll be most pleased to hear how your journey is going.

Part I
Discovering Massage

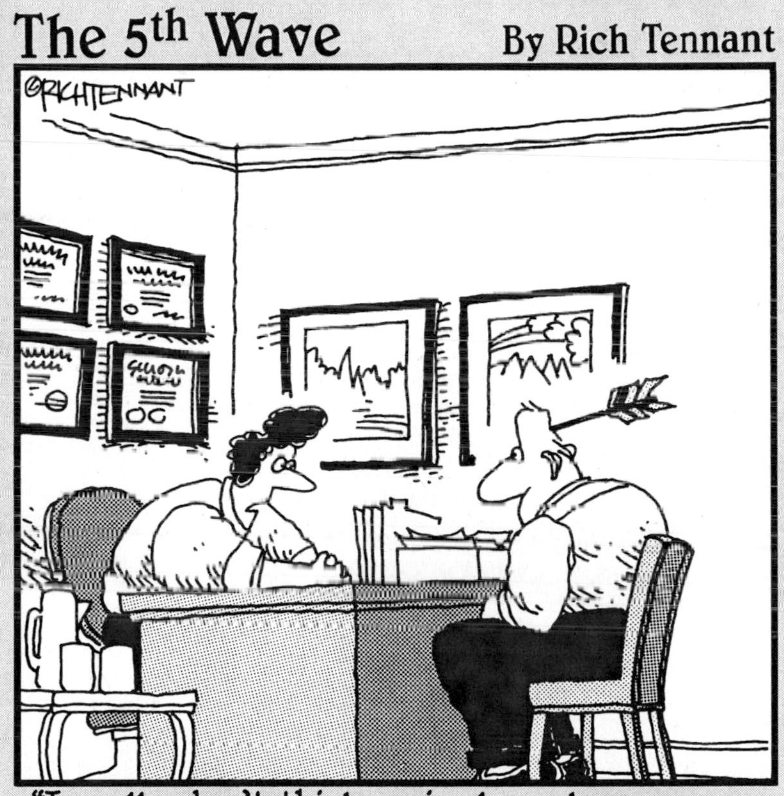

"I really don't think a simple neck massage is going to get rid of your headaches."

In this part . . .

As you explore this first part of the book, you may begin to get a sense that you've been overlooking something big, almost as if you'd failed to see an elephant living in your backyard.

Don't feel bad. You're in the majority. Most people have no clue about the rich tradition that massage has to offer, and some who think they do know only the misconceptions that swarm around the whole issue of massage.

Luckily, this first part of the book eliminates such concerns. The dazzling display of information in the first three chapters will leave you with a jaw-agape appreciation for the tremendous benefits massage can have for you, your family, and your friends.

Whether you're already somewhat familiar with massage and are raring to go, or you're a trembling neophyte slightly intimidated by the very concept of touching another person or being touched, Part I quickly ushers you into a new world filled with the millions who already know and enjoy the many benefits of massage. Welcome to the club.

Chapter 1

Not Just a Rub: How Massage Can Improve Your Life

In This Chapter

- Introducing the benefits of massage
- Running through the various types of massage and how they help you

What does massage really do for you anyway? Sure, receiving one feels incredible, and watching beautiful people massaging each other on how-to videos looks nice, but what's going on beneath the surface? Is it worth it to actually fork over your hard-earned cash to have someone rub your skin for an hour? Should you spend your precious time and energy learning how to give a good massage yourself? Is massage really effective, or is it just an unnecessary, flashy indulgence, like fish eggs on toast?

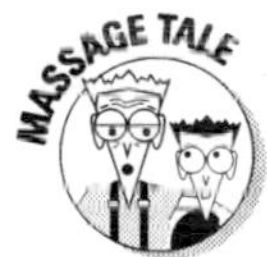

Well, being a massage junkie myself, I can't imagine why anybody *wouldn't* want to get a massage anytime, anyplace, for any reason or no reason at all. For me, massage has just always seemed like such an obviously good thing to do, starting way back in 11th grade when Grace came over to visit at my parent's house one afternoon, and nobody else was home. Being a typical 17-year-old, I was hoping that we were soon going to engage in some good old-fashioned hanky-panky, and when Grace told me to loosen my belt and lie down on the carpet, I began singing Handel's Messiah silently to myself.

Grace touched me then on the small of my back, and I'll never forget the sensation. "This is a massage technique that somebody taught me," she said. "How does it feel?"

"Ah, it feels, um, kind of, uh, unbelievable!" I said, and *unbelievable* was exactly the right word. Grace was doing something clearly nonsexual, and I couldn't believe that anything nonsexual could feel so good, that there was a way to be so intimate with somebody and yet not get in trouble with her father if he were to find out about it. In short, I couldn't believe that something that wasn't illegal, immoral, or fattening could be so sumptuously pleasurable.

I asked Grace to keep doing what she was doing, and as she did so, I began devising, right there with my face buried in my parent's green shag carpeting, a future lifestyle that included the absolutely highest number of massages possible.

This early experience pointed out a fundamental truth about massage therapy that those people who judge it without trying it often miss: There is a difference between sex and massage therapy. There, I said it, right here in Chapter 1, and I'm glad. Some people out there will forever mix the two up, which does a disservice to everybody else, especially those people who have shied away from massage over the years because of a perceived less-than-pristine image.

I discovered, in that youthful, eye-opening experience, that massage does indeed feel unbelievable, and that discovery was a great place to begin. Now, years later, after studying and teaching massage and experiencing the myriad facets of massage in both the United States and other countries, I've been introduced to other, deeper reasons for including it in my life, reasons with profound implications for improved health, well-being, and even longevity.

In this chapter (and throughout this book), I share these reasons with you. I also introduce you to various types of massage and finally provide you with a fun, quick activity to get you started on your massage journey.

Appreciating the Basic Benefits of Massage

If I were to go into some of the stories about how massage has helped people change their lives, heal themselves, become rich and famous, and so on, you probably wouldn't believe me right away, because, after all, I'm still in Chapter 1. So I'm going to start out slowly and offer you some of the simplest, everyday ways that massage can help you, some of which still may come as a surprise to you.

Here, then, not ranked in any particular order, are some basic benefits of massage that perhaps didn't pop straight into your head the first time you thought about it. Massage

- Helps relieve muscular spasm and tension
- Raises immune efficiency
- Improves circulation
- Promotes the healing of tissues

- Increases healthy functioning of the skin
- Engenders profound relaxation
- Offers emotional reassurance
- Improves appearance

The following sections take these points one at a time and let you get comfortable with them.

Helps relieve muscular spasm and tension

As you can see in Figure 1-1, muscles that are relaxed and happy are definitely physically different than muscles that are tensed up due to stress, overuse, injury, and more. The limp rope in the figure is your muscle. The knotted rope is your muscle on stress.

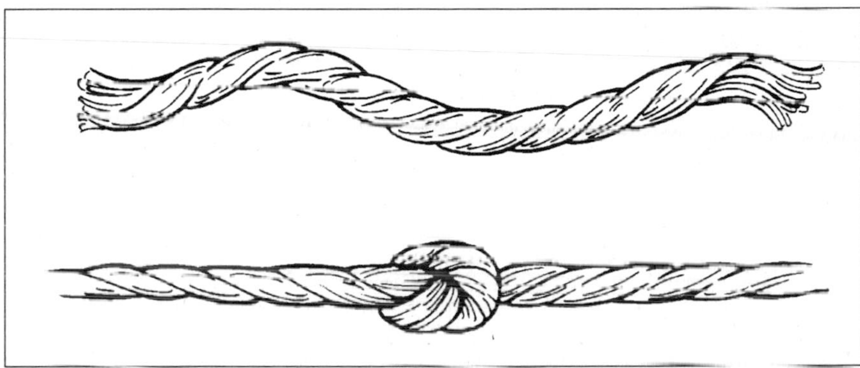

Figure 1-1: Ropes representing stressed and unstressed muscles.

But there's more to it than that, believe it or not. Regardless of how wickedly clever my rope analogy is, the human body is much more complex. In fact, it's so complex that nobody has completely figured it out yet, even though countless researchers have spent a lifetime trying to do so. A whole bunch of really interesting things about the body have been discovered, however, along with how it responds to various types of stimuli, including massage.

For example, one of the most direct effects of massage is to help loosen the tension you experience as knots, kinks, and spasms in your muscles. Massage achieves this goal in a number of ways:

- The application of pressure creates awareness of tension in a particular area, and the person receiving the massage can then begin to consciously release that tension.
- Through the application of friction to the area, a thermodynamic effect takes place, warming and softening tight, hard connective tissue.
- Stimulating trigger points soothes the local nerves, allowing a release of contractions.

Raises immune efficiency

Did you know that you have a vast system of vessels running through your body, roughly parallel to your circulatory system, and that this system is filled with a fluid that is responsible for carrying away and eliminating many of the organisms, bacteria, viruses, and other microscopic bad guys that may otherwise attack you? Yes, it's true. This setup is the lymph system, otherwise known as the Canadian Mounties of your body.

Your lymph system has nodes at various strategically located areas throughout your body, and these nodes have the job of capturing the invaders and processing them before eventual expulsion through your excretory system. Now, you may be wondering, how the heck does this lymph fluid get pumped through my body anyway? Funny you should ask. I've devised a test to discern your knowledge on that very subject. Don't worry, this is just a one-question quiz, so don't let your anxiety levels rise too high over it. Here it goes:

Question: How does the body pump the critically important lymph fluid through its lymph vessels, keeping your inner ocean clean and healthy?

a. The heart pumps the lymph, just like it pumps the blood, even though the heart isn't directly connected to the lymph system and this answer can't possibly be true.

b. The centrifugal force from riding various carnival rides is the best way to get the lymph fluid moving.

c. Fear caused by sudden, unexpected physical proximity to vampires or werewolves causes the lymph vessels to contract, circulating the fluid.

d. Movement, muscular contraction, and massage therapy are the ways lymph fluid is most effectively moved through the body because the lymph system has no pump of its own, such as the heart.

Right! The answer is d. By helping your body circulate this lymph fluid, massage aids in the elimination of noxious invaders (toxins) from your body.

There are other factors at play, too, in massage's effectiveness as an immune booster. Studies in orphanages have shown that infants and children deprived of touch experience stunted growth, both emotionally and physically. Further study showed that touch promotes the release of human growth hormone (HGH), which is essential to our development. If a child doesn't receive sufficient touch, his or her development is stunted, and susceptibility to disease increases, with potentially catastrophic results. Many of the untouched children in orphanages have died for lack of simple contact.

Improves circulation

The cigar-smoking octogenarians who frequented old-fashioned health spas used to give "It's good for the circulation!" as their reason for receiving massage. And they were right.

Students in massage school are taught to always massage in the direction of circulation — toward the heart — whenever they're applying enough pressure to move the blood underneath the skin. The reason is that your veins have little one-way valves in them that keep blood from going back in the wrong direction. So obviously, pushing the blood back against these valves, potentially harming them, isn't a good idea. In fact, when these valves don't work properly on their own, the blood seeps backward and pools up, causing the appearance of varicose veins, which are a *contraindication* (condition making massage unadvisable). But I'm skipping to Chapter 10. Sorry about that.

You have the idea: Some massage movements physically push the blood around in its vessels and can therefore, when done properly, push it in the right direction, improving circulation.

Massage also draws more blood to the surface of the body and into areas of relatively poorer circulation, thus bringing with it much-needed oxygen and other nutrients for the tissues.

Promotes the healing of tissues

This benefit is primarily a result of those in the preceding two sections. By helping to bring nutrient-rich blood into areas that are recovering from any type of problem and by helping to cleanse these same areas of toxins (by stimulating the lymph system), massage promotes quicker healing.

Also, certain types of massage stretch and soften tissues in traumatized areas, helping them regain natural elasticity and strength faster.

But beware: You definitely don't want to rush straight in and massage your cousin John's swollen knee after his recent surgery unless you've been trained in bona-fide massage classes and know what you're doing.

Increases healthy functioning of the skin

The skin is where massage has its most pronounced effects. In fact, I've devoted much of Chapter 3 to it. So let me just say here that massage includes several actions that leave the skin silky, vibrant, and fully functioning in both directions. By that I mean it promotes the shedding of dead cells while also encouraging the absorption of moisture, nutrients, vitamins, and other vital elements, especially with the aid of massage creams, oils, and lotions created for just that purpose.

In this sense, massage helps the skin "breathe." Just as your lungs breathe both in and out, inhaling and exhaling, healthy skin must breathe in both directions, too, and massage can help with that.

Offers emotional reassurance

In a famous experiment conducted by some truly sadistic researchers, some unfortunate little monkeys were brought up in cages with surrogate mothers. Each monkey had two mothers in the cage with him. One was a rag doll and the other was a hard wire shell. The uncomfortable wire mother had a nipple with real milk coming out, but the rag doll mother had no nipples and no milk. The researchers shocked the monkeys and then sat back with smug-researcher-expressions on their faces to see what would happen. In every case, when they were desperate for comfort and safety, the monkeys scampered straight over to rag-doll mommy, regardless of the fact that she had never provided any other kind of food or sustenance beyond the fact of being soft and cuddly. The researchers were able to conclude, with a good degree of confidence, that tactile sensations are the most important factors involved with emotional comforting.

These findings bring up an important realization as far as humans are concerned, too: Almost every person alive, when shocked, would rather squeeze a rag doll than a hard wire shell with a nipple attached. This bit of information, I've found, makes a fascinating ice-breaker at cocktail parties. Massage, by offering a sustained, intentional, caring form of tactile stimulation, is one of the best ways to impart emotional reassurance, and emotional reassurance just may be the number one need of humans in the 21st century. Modern urban dwellers are all a bunch of shocked monkeys searching for Mom, basically. And massage is the ultimate rag doll.

Engenders profound relaxation

Dr. Herbert Benson of Harvard wrote in *The Relaxation Response* (Avon Books) that by repeating certain breathing and concentration exercises, people can greatly reduce their levels of stress. Massage, by its very nature, induces a similar response. It's a mini-vacation that you can take right there inside your own body. No need to buy expensive plane tickets or submit yourself to the hassles of taxi rides and hotel rooms. Just close your eyes and let someone else send you to your own virtual Tahiti.

If you receive a massage and don't allow yourself to relax, it's the same thing as going to Tahiti and not enjoying the scenery, the warmth, the water, or the colorful little umbrellas in the cocktails. In other words, it's up to you. Nobody can force you to relax while receiving a massage, just as no one can force you to enjoy the South Pacific, but you have to be kind of crazy not to.

Improves appearance

The combination of all the preceding benefits leaves just about anybody who receives them looking better than they did before they started, and in that way, massage can improve the appearance of even the most stubbornly unattractive person. You know the type: the man with the big crease down the middle of his forehead, or the woman with her mouth pulled taut like she just chewed an entire lemon. Most of what people deem unattractive is simply poor attitude, and the people with the strangest looking faces and bodies can still be very attractive, especially if they're

- Tension-free
- Healthy
- Flushed with the rosy glow of good circulation
- Quickly recovering from any painful conditions
- Covered with silky "breathing" skin
- Confident and emotionally assured
- Profoundly relaxed

Who can resist a person like this?

Exploring the Massage Menu

There are literally hundreds of types of massage practiced around the world, many of them with wonderfully evocative names like tui-na and Lomilomi. This isn't the section in which I'm going to explain each of those massages to you, but you can find a fairly extensive explanation of several major styles in Chapter 4. Instead, what I'm doing here is explaining the generic types of massage, broken down into categories based on the observable effects they can have in your own life.

Think of this section like the menu in a restaurant. Each category (breakfast, lunch, dinner) consists of distinctly different dishes, and yet the foods used to prepare the dishes can be the same. So the same eggs used to make your omelet at breakfast can be used in your egg salad at lunch or your dessert after dinner. It's the same with the following categories of massage. Any particular massage technique can be used to create various effects.

Relaxation massage

This category may be the most familiar to those who haven't delved into the world of massage before. In essence, the purpose of the relaxation massage is to relax. Relaxation massage is particularly helpful in these instances:

- For stress relief, when the daily grind is just too much and the simple act of lying down and having someone pay solicitous attention to you for an hour is enough to make a big difference
- For pampering, which is fine as long as you don't feel guilty about it

Sports massage

Just ask the world-class athletes who travel with their own personal massage therapists. They can tell you what a difference a massage can make. Many Olympians and high-level players in all sports are true believers, but they aren't the only ones who use massage as part of their training. Even amateur athletes and weekend warriors incorporate it whenever they can: pre-event, post-event, and for ongoing training.

Rehabilitative massage

This type of massage helps the body repair itself. Many people have found that it was the key factor in helping them heal quickly and get back to normal activity levels as soon as possible after injuries and surgery.

Doctors like massage, too

Doctors, in case you haven't noticed, have really gotten aboard the massage bandwagon over the past several years. You seldom hear of any physicians questioning the validity of massage or its ability to help people in many situations. In fact, more and more hospitals have been incorporating massage into their programs, some with stellar results.

The prestigious Mayo Clinic in Minnesota has implemented a Complimentary and Integrative Medicine Program that features massage therapy. The director of the program, Brent Bauer, MD, is a firm believer in the importance of massage, having spearheaded several successful massage-oriented studies in the hospital. One such study involved giving cardiac patients a series of massages after their surgeries. People came from far and wide to sign up for this program, and the massage seemed to help in their healing — on average, they were able to leave the hospital earlier than those patients who weren't part of the program. Dr. Bauer ran into an unanticipated problem, however. Many patients who improved dramatically and were able to leave the hospital early refused to do so. The reason? They didn't want to miss out on the massages that were still owed to them as part of the program!

In France, where my co-author Michel Van Welden received his training, physicians look at massage in a wholly different light. "What we do is respected as part of the medical model all across Europe," says Michel. "Physicians there have no qualms about referring particular cases to massage therapists. In fact, the word we use in France for massage therapist is *kinesiotherapeut,* which really signifies a combination of massage therapist, physical therapist, and holistic practitioner who utilizes a number of healing tools, such as aromatherapy and herbology. There are 25,000 of them in France, which is an area the size of Texas. Most of them have their own clinics, and they are very highly regarded by physicians and patients alike."

Esthetic massage

Folks all want to look as good as they can, and massage can help. Through a combination of several of the benefits I mention earlier in this chapter, massage softens your skin and gives you a healthy glow. It can also improve the appearance of certain skin irregularities such as cellulite, with varying degrees of efficacy. People include massage in their beauty regimen for its ability to promote a youthful appearance and as an auxiliary treatment to enhance the effects of other beautifying procedures, such as plastic surgery and facials.

Energy-balancing massage

If massage were a map of the world, energy-balancing would be China. Yes, that's how big it is. Because energy is invisible, it's easily dismissed as unimportant, as far as our bodies go. But for a moment, imagine your body without energy. That's right: limp as a cooked noodle, flat as a pancake, blah as all get-out. Several of the massage styles I go over in Chapter 4 are based on an understanding of the body's energy systems, focusing on how to balance and enhance your inner invisible energy.

Massage for increased awareness

Most people inhabit their bodies without giving it much thought. They walk, sit, and lie around in them on automatic pilot, relying on the old patterns and habits they picked up in childhood. Sometimes, they're negatively influenced by injuries and other traumas that turn these unconscious habits into potentially debilitating conditions. They feel stuck in certain postures and can't get out. A massage can help you become aware of how you're holding onto certain patterns of tension and thus let you break them, and it can help you gain self-confidence through releasing old, negative body images.

Spiritually oriented massage

Depending on your frame of mind, any massage can be a spiritual experience, regardless of whether you receive it in an ancient Asian temple or the treatment room of your local health club. All you need are two people focused on awareness, breathing, releasing, and compassion. This spiritual aspect of massage can be used in the following ways:

- For meditation, when the sensitive sharing that takes place between two people in a good massage leads you to quiet your mind and remember some of the more important things in life.
- By ministers, nuns, and other clergy members who use this laying on of hands as a means to express compassion and in some cases to invoke healing.
- By practitioners of Eastern traditions such as Taoism and Buddhism. Buddhist monks in Thailand, for example, often learn the art of massage and practice it in their temples.

Massage for emotional growth

Allowing yourself to be touched with caring, therapeutic intentions takes a high degree of maturity. Several types of massage have been developed to access psychological issues and bring them to light. This situation is especially true in cases of past emotional trauma involving abuse and negative body image.

Massage for sensual pleasure

This type of massage can be performed by any two consenting adults who have a relationship of respect and trust between them. It's especially useful for long-term couples seeking new and exciting activities to spice up their lives and for short-term couples looking for ways to slow themselves down and enjoy the moment rather than rush through to you-know-what.

Massage for non-humans

Believe it or not, special courses offer to teach people how to massage animals. As anyone who's ever scratched behind the ear of an appreciative pet can tell you, they love it. Certain animals in particular have been the lucky recipients of massage:

- Horses, especially race and show horses that are each worth more than the gross national product of the average third-world country
- Dogs and cats and other "people with fur" that people live with on an intimate basis

Your Very First Massage Touch

Humans are sensitive creatures, and when you give something as personal as a massage to someone else, you're making yourself vulnerable to his judgment. What if he doesn't like your technique? What if he doesn't like *you?*

When you give of yourself through massage, it's natural to be afraid of what people may think and to wonder, secretly, if you're doing it *right* or if you're *good enough.*

I think you should forget all about that stuff. Your massage abilities are not something to be proud of or ashamed of. Your abilities are something you should share. As long as you tune in and become sensitive to your partner, you can give a good massage. The idea is not to focus on *being* good, but to focus on *doing* good. If you do these things, you never have time to worry about whether you're good or not. As long as your heart is into what you're doing, you're guaranteed to do it the *right* way.

Regardless of what I've just said, you may be nervous about getting your hands on somebody else and actually doing a whole massage. It's intimidating, right? In order to quell those fears right here in the first chapter, you're going to get your hands, ahem, oily, and do one little massage move on the most public, non-threatening, often-touched part of anyone's body, the hand. Don't worry — it's easy:

1. **Place a dime-sized dab of massage oil, cream, or lotion in one hand and rub your hands together vigorously to warm the lotion up.**
2. **Gradually bring both of your hands into contact on either side of your partner's outstretched hand and hold them there for a moment, just feeling the warmth.**
3. **Slowly start to rub — squeeze the fingers, press the palms, and rub your thumbs over the wrist.**
4. **Ask your partner how the movements feel.**

   Does he want more pressure? Less? Does a certain spot feel particularly good? Get used to the give-and-take that is an important part of every good massage.
5. **Keep massaging the hand for at least five minutes; when you're done, slowly bring your hands away.**

   The number one complaint most people have about massage is that it ends too soon, so don't shortchange your partner. You can apply a warm, damp washcloth for an extra added relaxing effect at the end.
6. **Ask your partner to compare the way his massaged and non-massaged hands feel.**

   Both of you may be amazed!

See, that wasn't so scary, was it? That's just the tip of the iceberg. The chapters that follow give you all sorts of information to help you add to this basic technique.

Chapter 2

A Brief History of Touch

In This Chapter

- Tracking the high points of historical massage
- Looking at massage in today's world
- Gazing into massage's crystal ball

This chapter is supposed to extol the virtues of certain Greek physicians who developed massage a couple thousand years ago and then move on to the beginning of the 20th century and talk about a certain Swedish man who was the father of modern Western massage. And then the chapter should chronicle the . . . ZZZZZZZZZZ.

Was that the sound of your head smacking the table? Are you already getting so bored that you're about to fling this book against the nearest wall in desperation? "Why can't he tell me something fascinating and different?"

Okay, hold on! I'm going to make this chapter a teeny bit different from the history chapters in most massage books, the ones that treat the chronology of massage like the dry academic stuff you find in history texts. What could be more unlike the vibrant flesh-and-bones reality of a subject as physical as massage? So, instead of a lot of facts and figures, I'm going to winnow down the essence of this great science and art of massage into a few pithy historical moments. History, or at least massage history, should be fun as well as informative, so settle back as this chapter presents stories from the lives of great massage pioneers, including, yes, even a certain Swedish man. But it's not all history; in this chapter, I also discuss today's massage landscape and how massage may continue to evolve in the future.

Dramatic Moments in Massage History

For your benefit and enlightenment, this section recreates dramatic scenes from various important massage periods throughout history. Much of what follows has been garnished with a large dose of creative license, but rest assured that the information is based on historical fact. Only the boring parts have been deleted to protect the innocent reader.

Great Greeks go nude

Imagine the Greek sun burning in a clear, blue sky. Below, in the outdoor *gymnazein,* dozens of naked athletes are exercising, each of them so tanned and muscled and healthy that they look like, well, Greek gods. Why naked, you ask? The word *gymnasium* itself comes from the Greek *gymnazein,* which means "to exercise naked," from *gymnos,* naked. Those fun-loving Greeks, I tell ya.

At any rate, the sun is beating down, all these naked Greeks are running around outdoing each other in feats of fitness, and old Asclepius is over there in the trainer's corner, ready and waiting each time another Adonis comes running up with a torn Achilles tendon or sore lower back. The natural thing, of course, is to offer massage, along with other herbs and remedies. Supposedly, Asclepius became so proficient at this healing that he could even raise the dead. As a reward, Zeus struck him down with a thunderbolt and killed him.

This tale brings us to one of the very earliest philosophical lessons tied to the practice of massage: If you like to massage naked Greek athletes, try to keep it a secret.

Shaman Bob: Hands-on healer

Thousands of years ago, beneath the primeval rainforest canopies of the vast Amazon jungle in what is now part of Brazil, an old shaman squatted down by a river, twisting the leaves and stems of a hardy vine between his worn fingers. The shaman's name was unintelligible to modern ears, so I'll call him Bob. His fingers were working the powerful *ayahuasca* vine, which gave his people visions that helped them to heal. Bob boiled the leaves and stems of the vine in water with other plants, making a thick syrupy tea that he brought with him back into the village.

It was night. The rainforest canopy above was filled with the screeching sounds of life. Arranging the members of the tribe in a circle around a fire he had built, Bob gave them each sips of the tea, and they began to twirl, dance, and sing traditional songs. Some of them (the ones who needed healing the most), fell into a trance, and Bob approached them.

As the others watched, Bob appeared to literally reach into each person's body with his fingers. Then his fingers would flutter up toward the dark sky above the fire. He would touch them, brush them off, shake their limbs, staying in almost constant contact, and everyone could see (with the help of the ayahuasca) what Bob always saw: blurry spots where each person's body was weak and demons of darkness clinging to a shoulder.

Although Bob used powerful herbs and jungle plants, his primary tool was touch. The difference between a casual touch from another tribe member and an intentional, focused touch from Bob was sometimes the difference between life and death. His touch healed, and everyone knew it.

The Tao of massage

The enigmatic Chinese word *Tao* confuses many people. For one thing, why is the word spelled T-a-o when it's pronounced "Dow"? And for another thing, what's it supposed to mean anyway? Does it have anything to do with the New York Stock Exchange?

Many people have heard of the Tao of Pooh, physics, or flower arranging, and if you ever read one of those far out books on Eastern philosophy published in the 1970s — the kind printed on organic-oatmeal-type paper — you probably remember the phrase "The Tao that can be spoken of is not the true Tao." So how are you supposed to talk about it?

Regardless of the fact that you apparently can't talk about the Tao, you can still talk about massage, which is exactly what an early Chinese Taoist did around 5,000 years ago. He wrote a book called the *Con Fou of Tao-Tse* (Cun Fooh of Dow Zee) that described the use of medicinal plants, exercises, and a system of massage for the treatment of disease. Because it was one of the first books ever written on any subject, the Con Fou really goes to show you just how ancient and important this whole subject of massage is after all.

A Greek man with a mission

Asclepius (as-*klee*-pee-uhs), son of Apollo (the Greek god of healing), may have been an actual Greek man who lived around 1200 BC, but just as likely he was a mythological figment of the Greek imagination. At any rate, he was credited with being the first Westerner to combine exercise with massage. He also founded the world's first gymnasium.

The Middle Ages

Nobody massaged anybody else (or was even allowed to touch much) during the Middle Ages, which almost wiped out Western civilization. Luckily, a few hardy souls decided, despite vigorous opposition, to sneak off and touch each other in barns, stables, and other hidden places whenever possible, thus assuring the continuation of the human race and allowing people a chance to practice rudimentary massage techniques at the same time. Needless to say, the Middle Ages weren't a good time to be a professional massage therapist.

The Hypocritical oath

You may wonder why doctors have to take a hypocritical oath after they finish medical school and before they begin practicing. After all, you trust your physician with your life; why would you want him or her to be a hypocrite?

The answer is simple: They're not taking a hypocritical oath, but rather the Hippocratic Oath, which means that it was first uttered by none other than that great Greek physician himself, Hippocrates (460–380 BC). In the very first line of this oath, Hippocrates swears by Apollo and Asclepius to uphold the virtues of his healing art, to not seduce women (or men) in the households he visits as a physician, and to abstain from mischief of all kinds.

Hippocrates also spoke about massage movements, saying that "hard rubbing binds, much rubbing causes parts to waste, and moderate rubbing makes them grow." He recommended massage for many conditions. So, the man who penned the words that physicians around the world utter to this day was a practitioner of massage. Go figure.

The Swedish scenario

In most places in the Western world today, when you ask for a massage you receive one form or another of Swedish massage. And so, you may ask, why is it called Swedish massage? Here are some of the typical answers people have given to that question:

- People in Sweden were the only ones liberal enough to allow massage to be named after them.
- The Swedish director Ingmar Bergman liked to receive massage after a hard day on the movie set, and so they named the technique after him.
- Nobody knows why it's called Swedish massage, but everyone agrees it sounds better than Lithuanian massage or Uruguayan massage.

Actually, Swedish massage is named after a Swedish physiologist and fencing master by the name of Per Henrik Ling (1776–1839), who developed a system of medical gymnastics that included the moves now used in basic massage. He eventually became known as the father of physical therapy.

Decline of massage in the 20th century

Due to the sudden, powerful influence of technology in the medical world, massage faded from favor during the early and mid-1900s. Also, the earlier popularity of massage induced some people to try to make a profit from it illicitly. Around the turn of the century, several schools in Great Britain, for example, were turning out poorly trained practitioners, some of whom ended up acting as prostitutes, which was a big downfall for massage. Since the days of Hippocrates, and even further back into the ancient history of China and India, massage had been accepted as a healthy pastime by a sizeable number of people. Now, things were different.

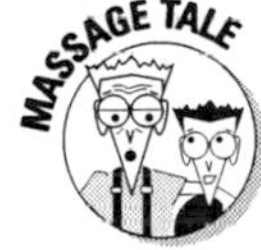

Throughout the mid-1900s, many massage therapists in the United States worked in a YMCA or a Turkish bath house and weren't expected to do much more than pummel their victims (er, clients) with some extraordinarily vigorous maneuvers, usually meant to purge the recipient of excess alcohol and fatty acids ingested the night before. In fact, some spa towns, such as Hot Springs, Arkansas, had massage facilities that were open on Sunday mornings especially for this purpose. The upstanding men of the community came in early to have the effects of Saturday night's revelry pounded and sweated out of them by hardy massage practitioners.

Massaging Cain and Abel

Perhaps the discord in the massage world can be traced back to the pair of American brothers who were responsible for bringing massage to the United States from Sweden — Charles and George Taylor. The Taylor brothers shared similar interests, obviously; they both became doctors, went to Europe to learn these new techniques, and wanted to spend their lives helping other people. But, unfortunately, they just couldn't seem to get along themselves. They opened a clinic together when they came back to New York in the 1850s, but within a year they dissolved it and went their own ways.

"It's *my* technique for helping other people feel better," said Charles, adjusting his bowler hat atop his head.

"No way, it's *my* technique for helping other people feel better," replied George, adjusting his identical bowler cap.

"Mine."

"Mine."

And thus started a problem that has persisted to this day, with various massage innovators and practitioners teaching that their way is the best way. George and Charles Taylor were the Cain and Abel of the modern massage world. And, even though massage as a whole is a glorious way to help people feel better on many levels, it has broken up into sects, with the proponents of certain techniques loudly proclaiming theirs as the best. This book, I hope, helps you cut through all that so that you can gain an appreciation for massage as a whole.

Freud and massage

Sigmund Freud, the inventor of modern psychoanalysis, used massage with his patients. Early on, when Freud wanted to calm and reassure his clients that he was on their side, he used massage maneuvers primarily on their hands. Unfortunately, Freud left massage behind as he further developed his psychoanalytic techniques, perhaps out of a fear that he wouldn't be able to know what was really working, the talking or the touching. But he was greatly in favor of it from the start. In the modern world, many psychologists are rediscovering the power of massage and incorporating it into their practices with body-centered psychotherapy and somatic therapies.

Hippies save massage from extinction

Overall, things weren't going so well for massage in the United States in the first half of the 20th century. And the same was true, for the most part, in Europe. Only people with hangovers wanted massage. Of course, on a worldwide level, massage in many areas still retained the same untainted prestige it had enjoyed for centuries. But even the most remote areas were clamoring for things new — vibrating massagers rather than actual massages, for instance — and as technological revolution swept the planet, it left people high and dry as far as contact goes. The human species was literally getting out of touch.

As always, when society swings too far in one direction, a mounting momentum tends to bring it back toward equilibrium. Somewhere in the 1960s, people began to tire of the soulless sway of machines and technology in their lives and reacted against it. These revolutionaries were hippies, or flower children, and they spread out from San Francisco to cover much of the world, toting with them tie-dyed T-shirts, prayer beads, big black vinyl discs called albums, and homemade massage tables.

Massage Today

Through the years, massage has had a serious case of multiple personalities. Every time you look at it, you're never sure exactly what you're going to see. A Greek physician massaging athletes? A Swedish physiotherapist creating movements to help ease common suffering? A shaman purging evil spirits? A healer sending spiritual vibrations through her fingers during a massage at a spectacular seaside retreat? The following sections give you the scoop on the current state of massage therapy and research.

So many choices

Massage is enjoying such a large renaissance that at times the market may appear glutted with too many massage therapists. An alternative newspaper in Asheville, North Carolina, printed a cartoon summarizing the plight of that city's abundance of highly trained, underemployed massage therapists. The cartoon showed an out-of-work therapist standing at a corner holding up a sign: "Will massage for food."

So where does that leave you as you head out the door today, tomorrow, or next week to go seeking your own massage experiences? Well, you certainly have a lot more choices, which I further explain in Chapter 4. You also have a lot more massage therapists to choose from — somewhere around 300,000 massage therapists and massage therapy students in the United States alone.

Although you do have more choices than ever, I think the assumption that the world is getting anywhere near a critical mass of massage practitioners is mistaken. There are just too many people around these days to massage — nearly 7 billion of them as of 2010 — and the population continues to expand rapidly.

What you can expect in terms of massage in the future is an ever-increasing number of choices, kind of like you find in those designer coffee shops. Whereas before the choice used to be simple — regular or decaf? — now you're faced with an overwhelming array of mochas, frappes, lattes, and on and on.

Touch research

To keep up with all the rapid changes and to document the effectiveness of massage in the midst of all its changes, somebody had to start some serious research into the matter, and that's just what the folks at the Touch Research Institute do.

The Touch Research Institute was founded in Miami in 1992 to study the effects of touch on human beings. Whereas the senses of smell, hearing, sight, and taste have all had their institutes and studies for decades, poor little orphan touch was neglected until the 1990s. Rather than an operating room or a clinic, the institute's studies are conducted in softly lit chambers with flute music playing in the background. And the subjects, instead of undergoing cutting-edge medical technologies, receive the age-old techniques of massage therapy.

Perhaps touch was neglected because it's just so obvious. When you think about it, nothing involves *no* touch; your body is a large antenna feeling everything as it happens to you. The other senses all involve touch in one way or another, too; molecules of various kinds hit you in the taste buds, the optical nerves, the ear drums, and the nasal passages, which set off the sensations that make the senses work.

A massage pilgrimage to Esalen

The pioneering work done at Esalen helped keep massage alive and well after its decline in the early and mid-1900s. Esalen, located in Big Sur, California (a couple of hours south of San Francisco), was founded by Michael Murphy in 1962, and some of the best massage teachers and researchers in the world have taught and worked there. The result of their efforts has been a shifting of the entire paradigm on which massage is built. No longer simply a remedial form of "gymnastics" to restore movement and ease pain, massage has become a way to increase awareness and sometimes even access the spirit.

If you're passionate about learning what massage can be on this spirit-enhancing level, you may want to make a trip to this massage-Mecca yourself. Wherever you are in the world, if you're a massage lover, making your own massage pilgrimage to Esalen will benefit your spirit! Check out `www.esalen.org` for more.

Esalen's location itself is spectacular, perched upon steep cliffs overhanging the Pacific Ocean, where hot springs flow from the mountainside directly into a series of pools adjacent to the massage area. Nudity alert: Esalen is clothing optional, and nudity is common. Think of it as a great way to get used to viewing the grand masterpiece of the human body.

Two international Touch Research Institutes have opened, one in the Philippines and one in France, which points toward a globalization of studies on massage. How can they get away with testing massage like that, you ask? How can people just lie around feeling good and then call it research? First of all, they don't call it massage, but rather Tactile Kinesthetic Stimulation, which translated means "massage that someone can receive a medical research grant for." And the studies include extensive psychological tests, blood analysis, *double-blind* tests (tests in which neither the participants nor the researchers know which subjects have a particular disease or condition and which don't), and a large amount of paperwork. So it's not just a big vacation.

Some of the studies that have been done at the Touch Research Institute include the following groups:

- **HIV patients:** Serotonin and killer T-cells increased due to the massage.
- **Premature infants:** Massaged infants gained weight more quickly and left the hospital an average of six days earlier than non-massaged infants, at an average savings of $3,000.
- **Depressed teenage mothers:** Massage helped them gain self-confidence and provided a way for them to connect with their infants.
- **Children with post-traumatic shock syndrome after hurricanes:** Massage offered psychological reassurance that the world could be a safe place again.

The Future of Massage

John Naisbitt's book *Megatrends* (Warner Books) discusses the problems people face as society heads into an increasingly technological world. Naisbitt says that as people get more high-tech, they have to become equally high-touch as well. Massage, of course, is one obvious answer to this dilemma.

Following are examples of some high-touch trends that show every sign of continuing into the future as massage integrates more and more into society's high-tech lifestyle:

- **Diplomacy:** Massage therapists already travel around the world as ambassadors of compassion. This trend will continue as hands-on techniques evolve and cross-cultural communication develops further.
- **Performance:** More and more performers, athletes, and high-profile individuals will discover the value and relevance of massage. Almost every professional sports team, for example, has a massage therapist on staff, which creates a trickle-down effect as fans and the general public become increasingly aware of massage through the team's example.
- **Affordability:** As the world gradually shifts from a manufacturing-based economy to an information- and services-based economy, the demand for massage will continue to grow. Employers and insurance companies will be increasingly willing to pay for massage services, which will benefit the bottom line by reducing absenteeism, stress-related injury, and so on. Companies like Massage Envy have sprouted up, charging lower-than-typical rates of $39 for massage and attracting an entirely new audience in recent years.
- **Increased sophistication:** Massage techniques (some of which have been around for centuries) will become more and more sophisticated as practitioners from various schools cross-train and add new skills to their repertoires.

Chapter 3

Your Skin and What's Beneath It: What You're Touching When You Massage Somebody

In This Chapter

- Recognizing your skin's connection to your brain
- Looking at your multidimensional skin
- Exploring your skin's various roles
- Treating your body as three-dimensional entity
- Noting the organ systems

"We touch heaven when we lay our hand on a human body."

—Novalis (pen name of Fredrich von Hardenberg)

Skin is the essence of what makes humans human. How do I know, you ask? I saw it in a *Star Trek* movie, so it must be true. In the movie, a wily alien treated Data the android to a taste of being human by grafting a swatch of flesh to his mechanical arm. He already had a brain and a fully functioning body, but the one thing he lacked was sensation. He was just a machine until he had this little patch of skin attached to him, and with it, he became human.

The essence of being human is the ability to feel. "But," you may respond, "I feel things in my mind and with my nerves, too, not just my skin. And besides, can I really trust *Star Trek* as a source of anatomical knowledge?" Well, guess what? In this case, the writers of *Star Trek* happened to be right on the money. Your skin, your nerves, and your mind are really just different layers of the same thing. This chapter leads you through the skin and all those wonderful structures beneath it that you touch when you perform massage.

Thinking with Your Skin

In his book *Job's Body* (Station Hill), Deane Juhan, a researcher into the effectiveness of massage and other touch therapies, says, "Depending upon how you look at it, the skin is the outer surface of the brain, or the brain is the deepest layer of the skin."

This assertion, though it may seem absurd initially, can be proven quite easily if you look closely at the development of the embryo. As you know, you start out as a little clump of cells deep in your mother's womb. In the very first days after conception, these cells begin to divide into three distinct layers that later become your body. The *endoderm* layer of cells eventually forms your internal organs, the *mesoderm* forms the muscles and connective tissues, and the *ectoderm* forms the nervous system and the skin.

As the ectoderm cells develop, they gradually turn into your brain, spinal cord, nerves, and skin, which are really all one unit. "Nowhere along the line can I draw a sharp distinction between a periphery which purely responds as opposed to a central nervous system which purely thinks," writes Juhan. In other words, your skin "thinks" as well as feels, and your brain "feels" as well as thinks. It's all one thing. And it starts at a very early age. In fact, at six weeks and less than an inch long, the little embryo can already "feel" light stroking on its upper lip, which causes a withdrawal reaction.

Just take a look at some of these amazing details about your outer brain (otherwise known as your skin):

- You have more than 3 million cells in a patch of skin about the size of a bottle cap.
- Your skin contains 2 to 5 million sweat glands and about 2 million pores.
- Your skin is your largest organ system: 2,500 square centimeters in newborns and approximately 19,000 square centimeters (19 square feet) in an adult male.
- An adult male's skin weighs approximately 8 pounds.
- Your skin gets strength and form from collagen, which comprises 70 percent of your skin's dry weight.
- You have approximately 640,000 sensory receptors embedded in your skin.
- Your skin ranges in thickness from 1/10 of a millimeter on the eyelids to 3 or 4 millimeters on the soles and palms.
- Your skin becomes softer in summer and denser in winter.

Little skin, lotta feeling

Do you know why little tots seem so extraordinarily sensitive when it comes to touch? Children up to three years old have a total of 80 specialized sensory receptors called Meissner's corpuscles per square millimeter of skin, as opposed to 20 in a young adult and 4 in old age. That's why babies are so overwhelmed by tickles and touches — they feel more than adults do. Check out Chapter 17 for more on Meissner's corpuscles.

Because you have so many sensory receptors in your skin (pain cells are the most plentiful, followed by a variety of pressure sensors, cold sensors, and warmth sensors), it's no wonder you can be so "touchy" if you're "rubbed the wrong way." And no wonder that a caring, calming massage can be so soothing.

In his book *Touching: The Human Significance of the Skin,* Ashley Montagu offers many pearls of wisdom, such as "To shut off any one of the senses is to reduce the dimensions of our reality, and to the extent that that occurs we lose touch with it; we become imprisoned in a world of impersonal words, sans touch, sans taste, sans flavor. The one-dimensionality of the word becomes a substitute for the richness of the multi-dimensionality of the senses, and our world grows crass, flat, and arid in consequence."

Sadly, he's right. People end up ignoring most of what they feel, and as they get less and less in touch with themselves, they become more and more hectic, filling their days with frantic activity rather than just enjoying the sensation-filled miracle of being alive. I think getting more massages would definitely help them get back in touch with themselves and the world around them through the simple act of paying more attention to their skin.

Layering It On: Understanding Skin's Layering

Your skin, like every other part of your body, is a living, growing, changing thing. In fact, you have an entirely new outer layer of skin every 27 days, which means you're an awful lot like snakes, lizards, and other animals who leave their skins behind periodically. You just shed your skin one skin cell at a time, so it's not so obvious.

The *epidermis,* the outer portion of your skin that keeps replenishing itself and flaking off, is made up of several layers. The bottommost layer keeps reproducing new skin cells, which are then pushed toward the upper layers, collectively known as the *horny zone.* It's called the horny zone because the cells there are hardened, like horns. And another thing about them: They're dead.

So, what you're really seeing when you look at somebody's skin is a whole bunch of dead, hardened cells that are about to fall off. In fact, exfoliation, a particular type of spa treatment that I explain further in Chapter 7, assists the skin in this process.

Beneath the epidermis lies the *dermis,* which is filled with fat cells, blood and lymph vessels, oil glands, sweat glands, nerve endings, and hair follicles. The dermis also helps to bind the outer layers of the skin to the *subcutaneous* (which means "beneath the skin") tissues below. In this area, you find some very important cells called *fibroblasts,* which are responsible for producing connective tissues. You owe a great debt of gratitude to your fibroblasts, especially after you break your skin in some way, because these specialized cells are responsible for rushing to the area and filling it with connective fibers, mending you back together. Massage can also affect these fibroblasts to enhance the appearance of your skin.

Getting the Skinny on Your Personal Border Guard

Throughout your life, your skin defines the intimate boundaries of your existence. Skin is the millimeters-thin line that separates you from the rest of reality and allows you to perceive that reality. Here are the six major functions of your own personal border guard, the skin:

- Protection
- Absorption
- Secretion and excretion
- Heat regulation
- Respiration
- Sensation

Protection

Whenever anyone tries to pass over the border from Spain to France, he is stopped by the border guards (usually men in sadly decorative hats, with sour expressions on their faces). The same basic action happens with your body. Your skin says "Stop and present your papers" to anything big and obvious trying to get inside of it, such as steak knives, harmful bacteria, #2 pencils, and so on. Having the men in the sad little hats there to protect you is a very good thing — I'm sure you can appreciate that when you think about what kind of chaos would ensue were millions of Spaniards to suddenly turn up in your pancreas.

Absorption

Once in a while, you want to allow some people across the border to spend those tourist dollars and improve the economy, right? Your skin can do the same thing through a process called *absorption.* Your skin can absorb certain cosmetic products, chemicals, drugs, and water in small amounts. Unfortunately, certain items aren't beneficial to your body, such as toxins and pesticides. Your skin is equally capable of allowing these terrorists to cross the border, which means you should stay on guard regarding the products you come into contact with.

The importance of getting licked

Have you ever watched a cat give birth? Directly afterwards, mama cat begins licking her babies all over, with a special concentration in the genital area. The same is true for dogs. And horses. And cows. And aardvarks, antelopes, and giraffes. In fact, every species of mammal with the exception of man lick their young immediately after birth.

At first, you may assume that this licking is to clean off the gooey stuff plastered all over the newborn's body. That's partially true, but far more important than the cleaning is the licking itself, the touch of tongue to flesh or fur.

I was in my first massage therapy class, in California, when the instructor stated that massaging a newborn baby's *perineum* (the area between the genitals and anus) with a warm, moist cloth was a good idea to simulate the action of licking engaged in by other animals. In other words, he was advising us to metaphorically lick the baby's butt.

At the moment, and for several years afterwards, I thought this California massage instructor was a little too out-there for his own good. But now, after discovering the importance of this type of stimulation in every other species of mammal, it makes perfect sense. This critical form of early contact jump-starts the newborn's gastrointestinal tract and is perhaps the most primal type of "massage" that we humans can offer our young.

You can recreate the natural sensations of licking for your newborn by taking a baby wipe or moist towel and rubbing it gently over the skin in this important area a couple of times a day for the first few months of life, starting on day one.

If you don't touch me, I'll die

Touch is literally a matter of life and death. The philosopher Bertrand Russell noted the importance of touch, saying, "Not only our geometry and our physics, but our whole conception of what exists outside us, is based on the sense of touch." For this reason, it's urgently important that infants and small children receive an abundant supply of human contact.

In the early 1900s, Dr. Henry Dwight Chapin reported that when orphaned babies were routinely put in homes and left to wither away with essentially zero human contact, a startling 99 percent of them died within one year of admission. Those who survived suffered signs of retardation and maladjustment.

To say that the world would truly be a better place if more people received massage — especially as part of their developmental years — isn't an exaggeration. Touch is a vital part of human growth, for individuals and for the entire community.

Excretion and secretion

Your skin can also get rid of toxic elements, like exiling unwanted characters from the country. This process is called *excretion,* and it's handled by those ruffians, the sweat glands. You have several million of these glands, and they eliminate waste products through perspiration.

In addition to excreting, your skin secretes as well, issuing forth an oily substance called *sebum* that coats the skin and helps preserve moisture. Secretion is a good thing, because the skin is about 50 to 70 percent moisture, and you don't want it to dry out.

Heat regulation

Your skin is constantly monitoring the temperature in the environment and helping to maintain your body's internal temperature at an even 98.6 degrees Fahrenheit (37 degrees Celsius) through adjustments of blood vessels and sweat glands, which dilate or contract in response to heat and cold.

Respiration

Oxygen comes in through the pores of the skin, and carbon dioxide goes out, just like in the lungs, but on a smaller scale. If you've seen the classic James Bond movie *Goldfinger,* you may remember the famous opening scene, which featured a woman painted completely gold and then left on a hotel room bed in Miami Beach. In the movie, she died because her skin couldn't "breathe," and a similar fate can happen to you in real life if all of your pores are suddenly blocked.

Pig massage for health and beauty

Even the U.S. Food and Drug Administration (FDA) has become convinced that massage offers undeniable results. My co-author, Michel Van Welden, has worked extensively with the FDA and has substantiated some claims for the effectiveness of massage. Following are some of his findings:

- Scientific evidence points to the fact that massage can positively impact skin tone.
- Pigs love massage.

It's true. In a series of experiments at Vanderbilt University and UCLA, Michel worked with a team of ace physicians administering a series of massage experiments on some very special subjects: Flopsy, Zeus, and Peewee, three Yorkshire pigs.

The three pigs were chosen for their high moral character and love of luxurious spa treatments. No, actually they were chosen because pigs (even though you may not like to admit it) have remarkably similar skin to humans. Twice a week for 13 weeks, the three brave little oinkers received deeply stimulating massages, after which researchers found that

- This type of massage stimulates fibroblasts, which produce collagen.
- An increase in collagen fibers can improve the elasticity and youthful appearance of the skin.
- Massage helps relieve the stress of having your house blown down by a wolf. (Okay, I made that one up.)

So, the next time you see a particularly relaxed-looking sow sauntering down the street, you can bet she's just come from an appointment with her massage therapist.

Sensation

If skin were basically just nature's way of keeping what's inside of our bodies in and what's outside out, life wouldn't be nearly as much fun as it is. Providing you with a rich, complex variety of sensations is by far the most personally gratifying of the skin's functions, which is something you develop an even greater appreciation for as you practice the techniques in the other chapters of this book.

Touching with Awareness: Minding What's under the Skin

Most people would prefer to leave the interior of the human body a mystery, like the ingredients in a Hostess Twinkie. You're better off just enjoying it, they figure, and not asking too many questions. This attitude works fine for most applications in life, such as walking around, going to the movies, eating pizza, and so forth, but after you decide to massage somebody, you benefit by knowing a little about human anatomy.

Here's why:

- You become aware of certain areas that are delicate or sensitive and should therefore be avoided (see Chapter 10 for more information on this issue).
- You develop an idea of what's going on internally when someone complains about specific aches and pains.
- You discover how certain strokes on the surface are acting on deeper structures, such as the circulatory system, the lymph system, and more.
- You come to understand how your touch is affecting the body as a whole.

In this section, I help give you a very basic understanding of what you're touching not just on the surface of the body but also into its depths.

Wow, that's deep: Remembering to treat the body as a three-dimensional object

Perhaps the most fundamental misconception people have as they first set out to massage somebody is that the human body is a two-dimensional object rather than a three-dimensional object. How is that possible, you say? Everyone knows humans aren't flat. Right?

Well, that's true, but everyone knows that a lake is three-dimensional, too, having depth as well as width and breadth, and yet when most people think of a lake, they think of the surface of the lake, the visible area of water surrounded on all sides by the shore.

And in a similar way, even though you know there's depth inside you, too, containing all the unfathomable mysteries of tissue and bone, you may still habitually concern yourself with the surface because that's what you see.

The problem with this two-dimensional way of thinking is obvious if you consider what would happen if you were to attempt to walk out to the middle of the lake. Quite quickly, you'd understand about the lake's three-dimensionality. The same applies when you wade out onto the seemingly two-dimensional surface of a person's body as you give her a massage. The mysterious liquid depths beneath the skin suddenly surge up around your fingers, and if you don't know how to swim, you drown.

You can give a nice, pleasant rubdown without knowing a thing about what you're doing — the mere tactile stimulation of skin-to-skin has positive therapeutic effects. But to give a good massage, one that makes people say "wow, that was incredible," you have to do a little more than just rubbing. But that's one of the reasons you bought this book, right?

Discovering how to feel: Palpation

For a moment, imagine you have a bas-relief map of the world before you in which all the landmarks are raised from the surface. Now imagine an opaque layer of rubber covering the whole thing. Reaching down and touching this smooth surface, can you tell where your fingers are just by feeling? Where's California? Where's the tip of South America? Where's the protruding peninsula of Iberia? Can you determine what it is you're feeling, even without seeing it?

Now think of the human body as that covered-up map that you're trying to identify by feeling its contours. This type of feeling-with-a-purpose is called *palpation*. Many professional massage people use palpation to determine what type of massage they're going to give to an individual, based on the way the person's body feels compared to the norm. You can get very sensitive fingers by practicing this technique, and in this section, I lead you through an exercise to help you start that sensitization process.

Proof that you're three-dimensional

Here's a way to prove scientifically that you're indeed a three-dimensional being and that all kinds of secrets exist below the surface of your skin. You only need two things to do this experiment: your hand and a flat surface such as a table or desk.

First, turn your hand palm-downward and hold it over the table a few inches high. Then reach down with just your fingertips to touch the surface, bending your middle finger and folding it under your hand until the first two knuckles are flat on the table. Good.

Now lift your other fingers up and away from the table top one at a time while leaving your middle finger firmly planted. Go ahead and do this right along with me as you're reading if you want. First try the thumb; it lifts downright easily, doesn't it? Way up high. Next try the index finger; not quite as impressive as the thumb but still definitely off the table. Try the pinkie finger; you see how it lifts up about the same or higher than the index finger? And lastly, try the ring finger. Go ahead. I'll wait. What's wrong? Come on! Lift it up already. Can't do it?

You may have tried this experiment before; somebody showed it to me when I was in high school, but it wasn't until I was studying anatomy as part of massage training that I understood what's happening.

Why can't you lift your ring finger? The secret is this: Buried within the depths of your forearm are four tiny little muscles — one lifts your index finger, one lifts your pinkie finger, and one lifts your thumb. But you have just one muscle that lifts both the ring finger and the middle finger, and so when one of them is held down, the other one can't lift up. Go ahead, try it with the ring finger on the table rather than the middle finger. Same result, right?

This example is just to show the effects of your three-dimensional depths on your two-dimensional surface. It's important to remember this when you're getting ready to massage someone, and I remind you to "think 3-D" in the chapters in Part III.

Getting a feeling for palpation

Try this exercise to begin sensitizing your fingers to the various textures, shapes, and landmarks you find beneath the skin:

1. **Sitting in a chair with your back straight, turn your head to the right, as if you're trying to look back over your right shoulder.**
2. **Reach up with your right hand and, using just the fingertips, feel gently along the front left side of your neck until you locate the long band of vertical muscle stretching from your collarbone up to the side of your head just below your left ear.**

   This muscle is called the *sternocleidomastoid muscle* and is illustrated in Figure 3-1.
3. **Walk your fingertips up and down this muscle, feeling for where it connects near the center of your collarbone (the origin) and up along the base of your skull (the insertion).**

   Do certain parts feel tighter than others? Is part of the muscle thinner than another?

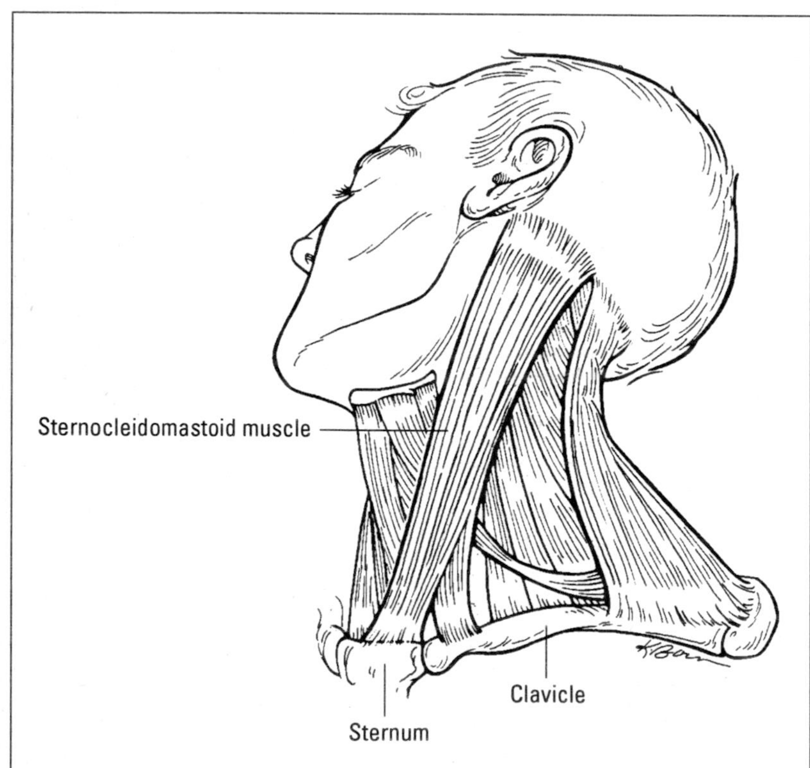

Figure 3-1: Turning your head to one side exposes your sternocleidomastoid muscle.

4. **Grasp the muscle between your fingertips as if you were going to pluck it like a guitar string.**

   Be careful not to dig your fingers into the sensitive front part of your neck.

5. **Still grasping the muscle, slowly bring your head back to center, feeling the softening in the muscle between your fingers as you do so.**

   Repeat this step several times, back and forth. This repetition gives you a feel for how muscle fibers contract and relax in order to make you move. Without contracting and relaxing muscle fibers, you would be a big, unmovable blob. Not good.

6. **Walk your fingers down to the base of this muscle and then onto the collarbone.** How does the bone feel different than the muscle? In what ways is it the same?

7. **Walk your fingers up the sternocleidomastoid and then off this muscle and onto the top of your shoulder.** Use a little pressure to feel along the length of the muscle that runs from shoulder to neck. Where does it feel harder? Where does it feel softer? Do you notice any knots or bands of harder tissue within the more pliable surrounding area?

   Notice whether you find any points that feel tenderer when you touch them, and whether these tender points correspond to the "knots."

Take several minutes to do this process. Get a feeling for feeling. Let your fingers become familiar with all the permutations of texture, density, and tone that you can find just below the surface of the skin.

Bony landmarks

You have at least 47 *bony landmarks* (specific areas on the skeleton that you can feel from above the skin) throughout your body. Now, before you go making any crude comments about bony landmarks, let me assure you that this term is indeed what professionals everywhere call them. They have compelling names, such as *xiphoid process, occipital protuberance,* and *greater tuberosity of the humerus*. I'm going to use laymen's terms, though, and expose you to a few of these landmarks as part of a game. That's right, it's time to play . . . the bony landmark game!

The game is simple: I describe a particular landmark (see Figure 3-2) for you in terms that you can understand and give you directions on how to locate it through palpation. Then, all you have to do is supply the common, everyday term used to describe this landmark. It's important that you actually do the palpation, not just read the words, because the process is what familiarizes you with the terrain you massage in other chapters.

Ready?

1. You can find this landmark by holding one hand out in front of you with your palm facing you. Using the fingertips of your other hand, notice that you have two bones in the forearm, one on the pinkie finger side (the ulna), and one on the thumb side (the radius). Follow the bone on the pinkie finger side all the way from your wrist to its extreme other end. You find a bump there called the *olecranon process,* otherwise known as the ________.
2. Cross one of your feet up and rest it on the other knee so you can examine it. Then feel with both hands along the shinbone (tibia) in the front of your lower leg. Follow it down all the way to your foot and see what happens to it. Feel how it curves back toward you and ends up in a bump at the top of your foot? This spot is the *medial malleolus,* or ________.
3. With your fingers, trace down the top of your foot and then back under the foot in the opposite direction from your toes onto the *calcaneus,* or ________.
4. Now sit up straight. Reach down along one side of your body until your hand almost slips underneath you. Right at that point you should feel a bony knob at the top of the longest bone in the body. That's the *greater trochanter of the femur,* which is otherwise known as the ________.
5. Walk your fingers back up along the side of your body about 6 to 8 inches until you hit the next bony landmark, a sharp ridge that sticks out that you can follow along toward the front of your body for a few inches. This landmark is the *iliac crest,* also known as the ________.
6. Reaching your hands up to your face, locate your chin and then feel back along the lower ridge toward your ear. It curves up here, forming the *ramus of the mandible,* otherwise known as the point at the angle of the ________.
7. You need a partner for this one. Have her lie facedown on a comfortable surface with her back exposed and then gently lift her arm, bend it at the elbow, and place her hand on her lower back. Let her upper arm rest down along her side. By doing this movement, you cause a big bump to appear on her upper back. Feel along the edges of this triangular-shaped bone called the scapula, otherwise known as the ________.

   Answers: 1. elbow, 2. inner ankle bone, 3. heel, 4. thighbone, 5. hipbone, 6. jawbone, 7. shoulder blade.

Sensitive fingers come in handy

Your fingertips have the largest concentration of sensory receptors of any part of your body. This feature is quite convenient for giving massages, which requires a real sensitivity to the person you're touching.

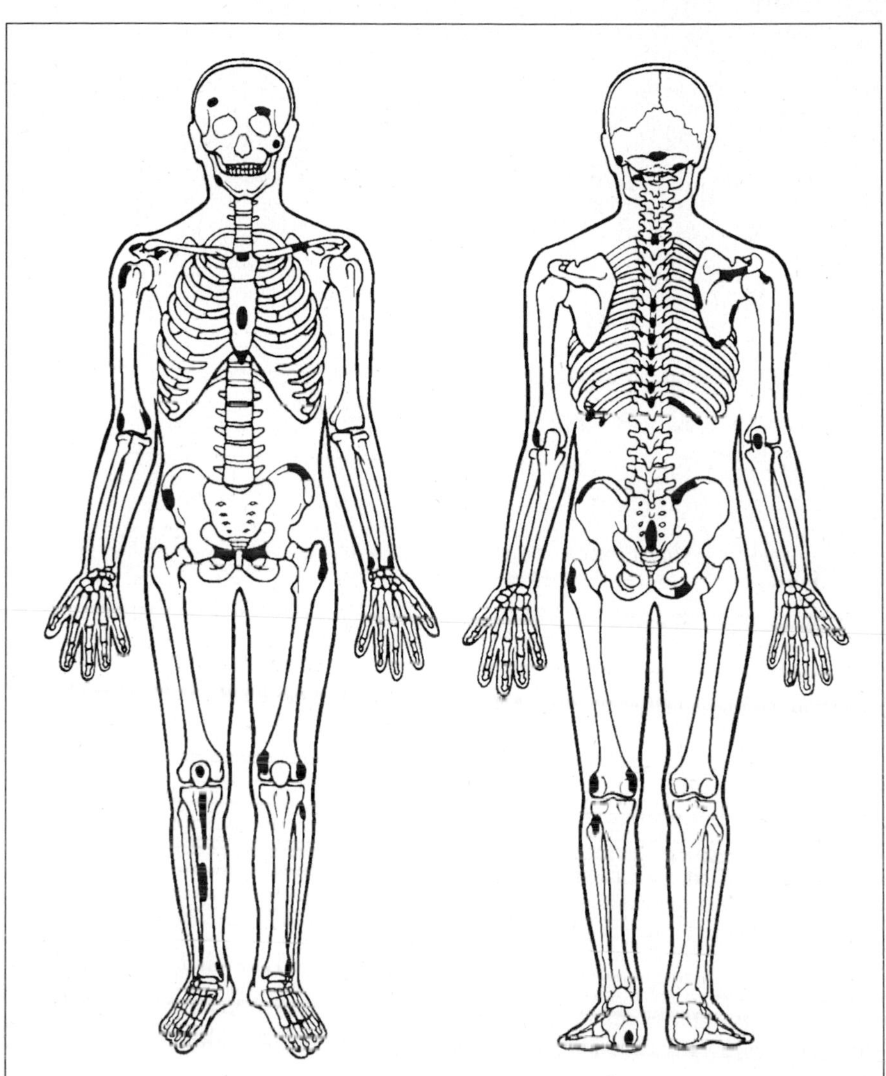

Figure 3-2: Some common bony landmarks.

These spots are just a few of the many landmarks you can palpate, and this game is meant to get you comfortable with the fact that you can actually feel and affect the structures of anatomy without being a scientist or doctor. When you practice hands-on massage, remember this fact and use your knowledge to guide you through your partner's body.

Cartilage, ligaments, and tendons

Many people find themselves confusedly referring to various connective tissue structures between the muscles and bones as *tendons, ligaments,* or *cartilage* without really knowing what the heck they're talking about. Now, I know you're not one of those people, but just in case you have a friend who's guilty of such anatomical faux pas, here's the skinny to set you straight:

- *Cartilage* gives shape to external features like the nose and ears and is also found between bones as a cushion at the joints. (Vertebral discs are made from cartilage, for example.)
- *Ligaments* connect bone to bone.
- *Tendons* connect muscle to bone.

Soft tissues

After you know how to familiarize yourself with bony landmarks (see the preceding section), you're probably wondering about all the other parts of your body that aren't bony landmarks. After all, you're not going to be massaging bones. The soft tissue is what you have in your hands most of the time, and by *soft tissue,* I mean muscles, mostly, and a little bit of connective tissue as well.

Muscles comprise 40 to 60 percent of your total body weight, depending upon your gender and physical condition, and you have over 600 of them, large and small. Each one is compartmentalized in a sheath of *fascia,* which sets it apart and helps it function as a distinct unit, although the truth is that you never use just one muscle to perform any given action. They're always working in groups to create movement. The slightest movement of the most mundane part of your anatomy (your left knee, for example) requires the precisely timed and perfectly executed synchronization of many muscles.

Muscle tissue itself is largely *insensate,* meaning if someone were to cut, jab, or even burn you directly on an exposed muscle, you quite likely wouldn't feel much at all. Your muscles don't so much feel massage as they experience massage as it retrains them how to be more relaxed in stillness and fluid in movement. In other words, muscles learn, and massage teaches.

Remembering Other Body Systems

Don't get the idea that it's just the skin, muscles, and bones that count when it comes time to massage somebody. You also deal with a few other anatomical systems that are strongly affected by your touch as well. These include the

- Circulatory system
- Nervous system

- Digestive system
- Respiratory system

The next few sections take a brief look at these systems and discuss how they're important when you give or receive a massage.

Circulatory system

The heart is constantly pumping your blood (about 11 pints of it in a 160-pound adult) out through your arteries and into each and every tiny little cell of your body, carrying the nutrients and oxygen that make it possible for you to stay alive. Then the blood travels back to your heart through the veins. On this return trip, the blood has to pass through a series of one-way valves that keep it from accidentally heading back in the wrong direction.

Massage strokes have a direct effect on the flow of blood in the veins, so keep in mind that when you massage someone, your strokes should always be in the direction of venous flow. You wouldn't want to accidentally push the blood back through these valves and therefore weaken them. When a number of the valves weaken and stop working efficiently, blood can pool up visibly and form varicose veins.

As much as half of all your blood is in your skin at any given moment, which accounts for that rosy glow certain people have, and also for the less healthy appearance of varicose veins and other problems. Massage works powerfully on your circulatory system, and for this reason you should always be aware of how your hands are affecting it.

Massage also affects that other circulating fluid referred to in Chapter 1, the lymph. In fact, an entire system of massage called *manual lymphatic drainage* assists the movement of the lymph because, as you may know from Chapter 1, lymph has no heart of its own to pump it along.

Nervous system

As a busy person in the 21st century, you don't have any time to fiddle around reminding your heart to beat, your lungs to breathe, and so on. Luckily, your *autonomic nervous system* takes care of all that for you. This system is further broken down into the sympathetic and parasympathetic nervous systems. The sympathetic nerves prepare your body for action, and the parasympathetic nerves calm you down. Massage is a great way to stimulate the parasympathetic nervous system, thereby lowering the pulse, slowing breathing, and in general, chilling you out.

The largest and longest nerve in the body is the *sciatic,* which many people are painfully familiar with. It runs from the base of your spine down the back of your leg, and when any of its length becomes pinched or trapped between muscles, bones, and connective tissues, it can cause the condition known as *sciatica*. That's the way all nerves work; you don't want to get in their way or get them irritated. Massage can help soften the muscles and other soft tissue that surround nerves and sometimes entrap them.

You also have specialized nerves called proprioceptors that tell you where your body is in space, giving you your sense of depth, position, and movement. Without them, you'd be internally blind, and by making you more aware of them, massage can help you "see" yourself in a new way from the inside out.

Chapter 6 has some exercises to get you in touch with your proprioceptors.

Digestive system

Your digestive system is a tube approximately five times as long as you are tall (see Figure 3-3). From input to output, your food travels about 30 feet. This tube, along with several digestive organs, has the magical ability to transform whatever enters it into a very special substance known as "you." Massage can beneficially stimulate this process if you're familiar with the various twists and turns this tube follows through your body, especially over the large intestine. Just remember to follow the general direction of the large intestine when massaging the abdomen.

Respiratory system

Breathing is an extremely important activity for human beings, as can be attested to by the millions of people around the world who have stopped breathing and suffered serious side-effects, even death. Massage is an excellent opportunity to engage in some full, deep breathing, as described in Chapter 6. This breathing reconnects you with the source of life and fills your blood with fresh oxygen, which is important because the first place your blood goes when it leaves your heart is the lungs.

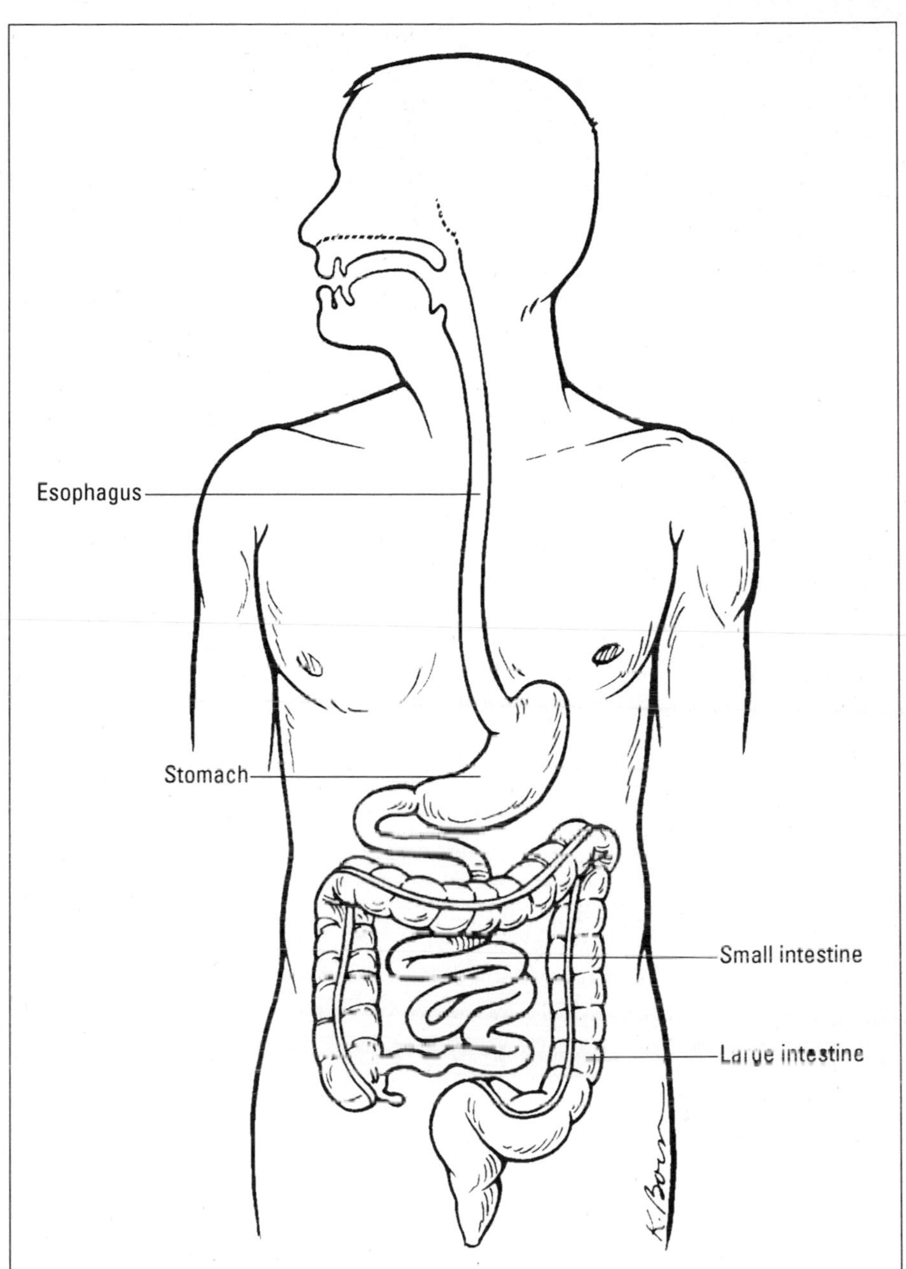

Figure 3-3: The digestive system.

The mind-body connection

Did you ever wonder what the heck people were talking about when they used the term "mind-body connection"? Is it part of the nervous system you weren't told about in school? Did you think maybe there was a tube or special cable of some kind that linked your mind and your body, and that you were the only one who hadn't been shown where it was? Well, don't worry; you're not alone. Typical incorrect notions about what the mind-body connection is include the following:

- That sinking feeling you get when your mind realizes your body did something it shouldn't have
- Nerves
- The neck

Actually, the mind-body connection is simply awareness. It's an awareness that permeates way down into every cell of your body, as compared to the awareness of your brain alone. It's the entire You consciously affecting every other part of you.

This whole mind/body split problem developed gradually over many centuries and wasn't really caused by any one individual, but many scholars have pointed to the French philosopher and mathematician René Descartes as having had the greatest influence. He's the one who coined that famous Latin phrase *"Cogito, ergo sum,"* which means "I think, therefore I am." That was in 1637. Well, pretty much ever since then people have been assuming that only specific types of electrical activity inside their skulls proved they indeed existed. What's glossed over in the history books is that Descartes never received a great massage from an expert therapist. If he had, he certainly would have modified his statement a bit, to something like *"Cogito et sentio, ergo sum.":* "I think and I feel, therefore I am."

Part II
The Art of Receiving Massage

The 5th Wave
By Rich Tennant
©RICHTENNANT
This feels wonderful! What do you call this type of massage?
Screwing the lightbulb.

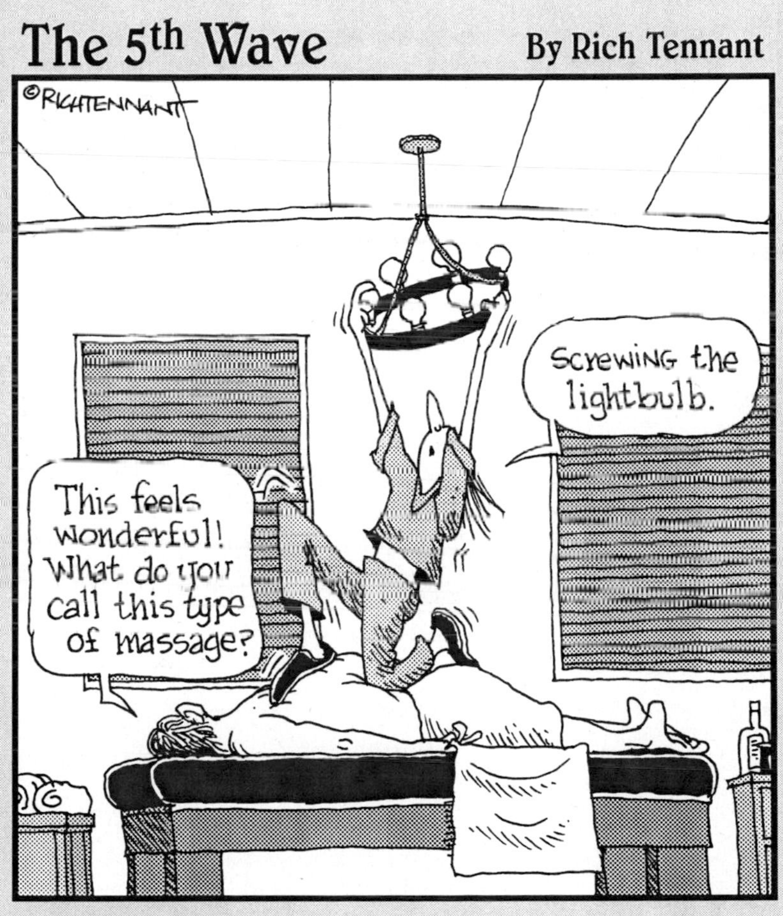

In this part . . .

Okay, I can hear you scoffing now: the art of receiving massage? That's like the art of getting rained on. You really don't have to try very hard; just step outside and get wet. Anyone can do it. Receiving massage? Nothin' to it. Right? Wrong.

Receiving massage is more like dancing your part in a very intricate pas-de-deux, such as the tango (which, interestingly, means "I touch" in Latin). Both activities, at their best, are extremely interactive. During the tango, if you just stand there and don't do anything, you're going to make your partner look pretty bad. Similarly, when you receive a massage, you've got to communicate with your partner, through both verbal and nonverbal means, in order to get the most out of the experience.

A good massage is a two-way street, equal parts proper giving and informed receiving. That's the focus of this part of the book, which begins with Massage 101 and then graduates just four chapters later to receiving a massage (or a luxurious spa treatment) like a real pro. I know, it's tough, but somebody's gotta do it. Along the way, you master the tricky intricacies of massage vocabulary, discover the ten rules for receiving a massage, and get the scoop on the most popular massage and spa techniques. I also discuss how to enjoy the pleasures of massage without guilt, offer techniques for getting the most out of your very first professional massage, and lots more.

Chapter 4

Making Massage Part of Your Life: A Massage Road Map

In This Chapter

- Eliminating guilt over massage
- Choosing the right style of massage for you
- Locating and developing a relationship with a massage therapist
- Understanding some massage jargon

When you first begin to discover massage, you undoubtedly encounter some strange new words and concepts that may confuse you at first. Have no fear! This chapter is your own personal travel guide to navigating the sometimes puzzling new terrain in the world of massage. Here you find out how to accept the pleasures of massage into your life and how to choose the type of massage that's right for you. You even find an English–Massage dictionary at the end of the chapter that can help you speak the language of massage with other people.

Recognizing Massage as Healthy Pleasure

Many people just can't seem to understand that massage is anything more than indulgence, luxury, and pampering, so they pass on it. Some people turn their noses up at its pleasures as if it were a waste of time. Others shy away from the experience, calling it expensive and extravagant as if massage were a waste of money.

The underlying reasons for both these attitudes are guilt and fear. Many people simply have trouble justifying paying for something that feels as good as massage or having another human pay such lavish attention to them for an entire hour. Plus, they may just be afraid of something new.

This guilt is truly unfortunate and completely unnecessary, because massage is 100 percent good for you. In fact, it has all of the pleasures of many illegal, immoral, or fattening things without any of the negative side effects. That's right, there's not a single thing wrong with massage.

Massage

- Is calorie- and fat-free
- Won't rot your teeth
- Is impossible to overdose on

Well, okay, massage does have one catch: It can be addictive. After you taste good massage, you're going to want more — lots more. But that's not necessarily a bad thing. You can receive a massage every day for the rest of your life with absolutely no negative side effects.

In fact, beloved entertainer Bob Hope received a massage almost every day of his life for over 50 years until he passed away at the very ripe old age of 100. (You think massage may have helped with that longevity? It couldn't hurt!) He dragged a number of massage therapists all over the globe with him while he was off entertaining the troops and making his movies. I had the opportunity to massage him once myself. Because of all the massage he'd received over the years, his skin was smooth and supple, and his muscles were amazingly well toned, even though he was pushing 90 at the time.

Of course, you may not have the time or money for a massage every day. But time or money isn't what's most likely to stop you in the first place. It's your attitude.

Reducing the stress and tension in your life is a very good reason for wanting to get a massage. You don't need any more justification than that.

So Little Time, So Many Massages: Knowing What You Want to Ask For

Okay, so you're filled with enthusiasm to go out and experience your first massage; you pick up the phone, call a massage school or clinic in your area, and ask to book an appointment. (See Chapter 5 for details on booking an appointment).

"What kind of bodywork do you prefer?" asks the receptionist.

"Bodywork?"

"Yes. Massage."

"Oh. Just something that feels good," you say.

"Of course. But we offer several modalities. Would you prefer the Swedish, the sports massage, the deep tissue, the Hellerwork, the Aston Kinetics, the Thai massage, or the neuromuscular session?"

"Ah, let me get back to you on that," you say, and you hang up, ready to slip quietly back into your non-massage lifestyle before you even begin.

Don't let this scenario happen to you! Now that you've decided to get a massage, the last thing you want is to get confused by the vast array of choices available and end up not receiving any kind of massage at all.

Be forewarned, this section is just an overview of the types of massage available. For now, I just want to familiarize you with a few of the choices, based on the three main reasons people decide to get a massage:

- To relax
- To feel better
- To improve the body's functioning

Often, your reasons are probably a combination of all three. You may have a little pain in your shoulder you want to ease, but at the same time, you want to lower your overall stress level. The three components of massage dovetail with each other; what helps you relax may lessen your pain, what realigns your body may help you relax, and so on.

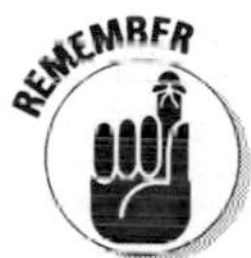

The spiritual aspect of massage is a fourth component, a wild card that can pop up unannounced during any type of massage. This spiritual aspect is the way that you can use massage to attune to your own inner experience and get in touch — literally — with a deeper sense of self. (Head to Chapter 6 for more information on this topic.)

So which is the right style for you? Take a glance at the following categories and become familiar with some of the massage styles associated with each.

Massage for relaxation

Stress and tension are real. The human body has developed through eons of evolution to respond to stress and tension by preparing to either fight the obstacle or run away from it. This fight-or-flight response came in very handy when primitive man confronted the occasional large, dangerous animal. But in modern times, people face a constant, unceasing barrage of tension-inducing stimuli, and it's overloading them. If you live in a large metropolitan area, for instance, you're exposed to the equivalent of several dozen grizzly bears and a pack of ravenous wolves every time you venture out into rush-hour traffic.

If you're interested in relaxing massage, ask for the following:

- **Swedish massage:** This method (what most people envision when they think "massage") includes stroking, kneading, squeezing, rubbing, and so on.
- **Light work:** *Light work* is a generic term for nonintrusive, gentle massage.
- **Relaxation massage:** Another generic term for nice-and-easy massage, *relaxation massage* usually refers to a light form of Swedish massage.
- **Esalen massage:** Developed at the famous Esalen Institute in Big Sur, California, this massage features many long, flowing, gentle strokes.

When in Hawaii . . .

Once, in Hawaii, I was in the mood for a relaxing massage to help relieve jet lag after a long trip. I was working at a spa there, and one of the massage therapists on staff, a native Hawaiian named Wesley Sen, offered to give me a Lomilomi massage.

"Is that relaxing?" I asked as we walked together back to my hotel room.

"Sure, it's relaxing," he said.

"Then why are you carrying that pole with you?"

Sure enough, Wesley was carrying a thick, ten-foot wooden pole in one hand. "It's just for balance," he said. "Don't worry."

Back in my room, Wesley had me lie down on the floor and then proceeded to pray over me in Hawaiian, which sets the mood at the beginning of every true Lomilomi experience. In his prayer, he invited healing forces to be present with us in the room. Then, for the next hour he stood on me, kneeled on me, pressed on me, and tossed my limbs around, all the while skillfully keeping his weight partially supported by the pole, one end of which he pushed against the floor to balance himself.

Wesley wasn't a small guy, so I was amazed that he could perform this entire balancing act, using my body as a tightrope, and never once cause me the slightest discomfort. Afterwards, I was more relaxed than I'd felt in many months; the relaxation penetrated way down into my joints and up my nerves into my brain. Also, a pain I'd been experiencing in my shoulder disappeared, never to return again, and my digestion improved noticeably, too.

Skillful relaxation massage can take you way beyond relaxation, healing what ails you and improving your body's functioning as well. Several massage styles offer relaxation as well as deeply therapeutic results, such as Lomilomi, Trager, and many others.

Plenty of massage styles leave you relaxed, but the Swedish style is the one you're most likely to run into. Swedish massage is kind of like the Visa or MasterCard of massage: It's accepted at millions of establishments around the world. It has many therapeutic benefits also, and some of its more advanced moves can be quite vigorous. (Check out the section "Remodeling your body for fun and profit" later in this chapter for information about deeper massage.) If your intention is simply to chill out and be soothed by soft fingers, make sure to request light, easy pressure during your Swedish massage.

Communicate! Even if you're just trading massage with a friend, you have to let the other person know what you want out of the experience.

Remedial massage

Many people visit their massage therapists for the same reason they visit their doctors — to fix something that's painful. This type of massage is called *remedial massage* or *therapeutic massage* because it serves as a remedy. Several types of massage, including good-old relaxing Swedish massage, can have definite remedial effects, but here's a short list of some styles particularly well-known for their therapeutic benefits.

Of course, only well-trained professionals should attempt to give these types of massage.

If you're interested in remedial massage, ask for the following:

- **Manual lymphatic drainage:** This type of massage helps your body flush toxins, such as pesticides and residual chemicals, by stimulating the flow of lymph in your body. It's a very gentle massage that features light superficial movements on the skin.
- **Touch for health:** This treatment, which helps balance your inner healing energies, isn't really a massage at all because the therapist's hands don't necessarily come into contact with the recipient's body. It was developed by a nurse on the faculty at New York University and has been taught to thousands of healthcare practitioners.
- **Neuromuscular therapy:** This type of massage works on tight muscles that create the deep patterns of tension that can keep you in pain.
- **Craniosacral:** This type of massage adjusts the healthy functioning of your spine and cranium.
- **Deep tissue massage:** This generic term refers to any number of therapies that apply deep pressure and affect the body's connective tissues.

- **Shiatsu:** This massage involves pressure point therapy — to balance the entire body and restore health — on specific points along invisible energy lines in the body called *meridians.*

  Shiatsu is the most well-known of several types of massage that work on the meridians. It can be quite relaxing, but its primary focus is on restoring health and balance, as are other types of massage that work on these energy lines.

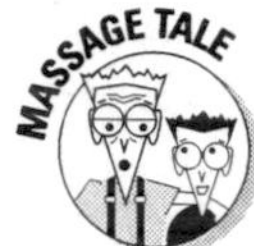

After having a serious car accident, a young man in Ohio began experiencing severe, debilitating pain every day. His doctors told him they had no drugs or surgery that could help him and that he'd have to learn to live with the pain, but his mother refused to accept that. She took him to see a massage therapist who treated the young man for several months by using neuromuscular and craniosacral therapies. The end result was a pain-free young man who has now decided to become a massage therapist himself in order to help other people.

Remodeling your body for fun and profit

Several types of massage have developed over the years that focus on realigning your body, straightening you out, and helping you form a healthier relationship with gravity and a more graceful, efficient way of moving. People often refer to this type of massage as *structural bodywork.* You want to only sign up for one of these massages if you have specific goals in mind (such as improved posture, better athletic performance, and so on), and, of course, you want a highly trained pro to do the work. The movements involved are quite deep, and the experience isn't relaxing in the normal sense of the word, but your massage therapist always keeps your comfort foremost in mind.

If you're interested in structural massage, ask for the following:

- **Rolfing:** The most well-known form of structural bodywork, this type of massage was invented by Ida Rolf. It can be very intense and super deep; the goal of Rolfing is to rearrange the way your connective tissues hold your bones in place — a complete posture adjustment from the inside out.
- **Hellerwork:** A unique development of Rolfing, this type of massage was created by Joseph Heller. It helps to restructure the body's fascia, or connective tissues, into a healthier alignment.

- **Aston Kinetics:** This type of massage is a combination of touch techniques and movement repatterning that helps people move with ease and improve their posture.
- **Myofascial release:** This type of massage is a combination of techniques that unwind and release the chronic tension patterns in deep tissues that can cause many painful conditions.

Locating a Massage Therapist

So you're absolutely convinced that massage would make a truly superb addition to your life, and you're just about ready to pick up that phone (yes, that one right over there), dial one of the contact numbers I give you later in this section, and order up your very first session of "touch take-out." Soon, a chipper and thoroughly professional person will show up at your door carrying a monstrous padded folding table. He or she will open the table in the privacy of your own comfortable dwelling. You'll smile self-confidently, take all your clothes off, and then . . . *wait* a minute!

Did I say, "Take all your clothes off?" Well, by golly, I guess I did. Suddenly, this whole wonderfully abstract concept of massage has become disconcertingly real. And, in spite of your appreciation for the undeniably therapeutic benefits of massage, if that professional stranger were to ring your doorbell right this minute, you may be tempted to say, "Excuse me for a moment, will you? I just have to go get my law degree at Columbia University and then I'll be right with you."

If that sounds like you, don't worry. The information in this section can help make you more comfortable with whoever is massaging you, including someone you already know with whom sharing massage is a new adventure.

Stalking the elusive referral

One time-honored concept used to battle your fear of a stranger in your home is to assure that the person who shows up on your doorstep to give you a massage isn't a stranger. You can accomplish this goal in two ways:

- Give your cousin Billy several thousand dollars and send him through massage school so you can call him later and make an appointment.
- Get a referral.

A six-point mental checklist (to help decide which massage therapist to try)

No matter how qualified and highly recommended a massage therapist is, and no matter what other people say about her, you still must decide whether she's the right massage therapist for you. Remember, you're very likely to share a great deal of yourself with this person (massage therapists are like hairdressers on steroids when it comes to the confiding-in factor). And, because your massage therapist gets to know your body better than anyone else except an intimate partner, you have to be willing to trust her. Sometimes, you have no precise way to gauge which massage therapist is precisely the best fit with your personality, and no amount of analytical deliberation can help you decide who to choose.

That said, try using this quick checklist to judge your own gut reaction to the person you're about to spend a considerable amount of quality time with:

- **Does she immediately make you feel like you're important?**
- **Does she look you right in the eye and fill you with a sense of confidence so that you're already feeling better before she even touches you?**
- **Is she someone you want to emulate as far as calmness and tranquility go?** Like it or not, you may likely look upon your massage therapist as a role model in the relaxation category. A tense, uptight massage therapist isn't setting a good example.
- **Is she *soft* (unobtrusive and non-opinionated) where she needs to be soft and *hard* (unrelenting in her serious desire to see you feel better) where she needs to be hard?**
- **Is she someone you feel an immediate sense of empathy with?** To use a precise scientific term here, do the two of you click?
- **Is she the right sex?** The decision on whether to receive massage from a male or female massage therapist is entirely up to you. Many people have no preference, as long as the massage therapist is competent and strong, but others feel more comfortable with one sex than with the other in a massage setting. Most massage establishments give you a choice when you request a therapist. After you get started with the actual massage, the massage therapist's gender probably won't really matter as much as you may have thought.

The second option is by far the more common choice (but that doesn't mean you should entirely dismiss the concept of financing massage school for friends or family members. The world needs more massage therapists!) The following sections show you some avenues for digging up referrals.

General public referrals

If you don't happen to have a massage therapist in your immediate family, you can still find plenty of helpful folks ready to steer you toward the nearest qualified therapists. Some of the places where you're most likely to get a good referral from include

- Enlightened physicians and chiropractors who are aware of the benefits of massage and who are more than happy to refer you to the ones they work with. In fact, many doctors these days have a massage therapist or two on staff.
- Athlete friends who receive massage as part of their training.
- A co-worker or family member who's had a particularly good experience with the massage therapist he's been using for an extended period of time.
- The "best-of" articles that health and beauty magazines such as *Shape, Self, Glamour,* and so on often feature.
- Your friend Tina, the one who wears the Birkenstock sandals all the time and has that look of blissed-out satisfaction on her face even when she's standing in line at the grocery store checkout counter.

Massage association referrals

One of the best places to get a referral for a therapist you can trust is a professional massage association. In fact, you can collectively refer to the four associations I'm about to give you as "massage central." Among them, you can find the contact information for tens of thousands qualified massage therapists in the United States right at your fingertips.

Drumroll please . . . and the associations are

- To find a massage therapist who is a member of the American Massage Therapy Association (AMTA), the oldest nationwide organization, call 877-905-2700 or visit `www.amtamassage.org`.
- To find the nearest member of Associated Bodywork and Massage Professionals (ABMP), call 800-458-2267 or visit `www.massagetherapy.com/find/`.
- To find a member massage therapist of the International Massage Association (IMA), call 540-351-0800 or visit `www.imagroup.com`.
- For a list of massage therapists who have passed the test given by the National Certification Board for Therapeutic Massage and Bodywork (NCBTMB) and are nationally certified, call 800-296-0664 or visit `www.ncbtmb.org`.

Of course, among those thousands of massage therapists, you're going to find quite a range of skills and offerings, and no one single tried-and-true means lets you prequalify someone. However, you're living in an extremely lucky time, oh fortunate massage recipient, because in the past several years the number of highly skilled and fully trained massage pros has grown at an amazing rate all around the world.

Following is a list of contact numbers for professional massage practitioners in several countries:

- **Australia:** Massage Australia, Sydney, phone (02) 4883 9500
- **France:** French Federation of Masseurs Kinesitherapeutes (FFMKR), Paris, phone 01 44 83 46 00
- **Italy:** Federazione Nazionale dei Collegi dei Massofisioterapisti (F.N.C.M.), Rome, phone 0461 263257
- **U.K.:** The Institute for Complementary Medicine, London, phone 0207 922 7980

If for some reason you can't locate a massage therapist by simply calling one of the numbers listed here, you can pursue several other avenues in quest of massage, which I cover in the following sections.

Checking the ads

Each locale has its own regulations regarding the advertising of massage, and sometimes the regulations vary from city to city. What may be perfectly legal in Los Angeles, for example, may be verboten in Sioux City, Iowa.

Beware those ads featuring massage therapists with huge muscles wearing black leather vests with no shirt underneath and staring straight into the camera with a come-hither look in their eyes. These pictures may be a clue tipping you off to the extra curricular intentions of this particular massage therapist, licensed or not. Then again, they may just be a fashion statement.

Letting your fingers do the walking

In some areas, massage therapists must include an official massage license number as part of any phone book listing for massage. According to Dan Ulrich, past president of the Florida State Massage Therapy Association, the inclusion of the license number in phone book and other ads significantly reduced the amount of unethical massage advertising. Although the license number isn't mandatory everywhere, it's a clue that you're dealing with a therapeutic professional. If you don't see a license number or some other professional credentials listed, call and ask for one. Then again, some not-so-therapeutic massage offers are made occasionally by people who do have a license, so you still have to be cautious.

Getting the most massage for your money

When dealing with your massage therapist, certain tactics can increase happiness for both of you and in the process maximize the value you receive from your experience.

- **Offer to pay up front for a discounted series of massages.** For example, if the massage therapist charges $50 for a massage, offer $400 dollars for ten massages. Often, massage therapists appreciate the immediate cash flow and the guarantee of ongoing business. This arrangement is good for their business and good for your pocketbook.
- **Ask for a massage in exchange for referring a new client to your massage therapist.** She probably appreciates the new customer, and you deserve the recognition.
- **Inquire about rates for longer massage sessions.** Often the price drops proportionally with the length of the massage, and you can receive a 90-minute massage for not too much more than a 60-minute massage. A massage therapist who charges $60 for an hour massage may offer an hour and a half massage for $75 or $80, for example.

Opening the bureau door

You may occasionally run into ads for massage service bureaus that guarantee you a massage within a specified period of time (usually a couple of hours). Bureaus are most useful when you're traveling and have no other means of contacting a massage therapist. You call the bureau's central number, and they send one of the many independent massage therapists on their list out to you at your choice of location. Quite often, these outfits are very up-and-up enterprises run by entrepreneurial massage therapists who have discovered a new way to multiply their effectiveness and their income. At times, though, the quality of the services these bureaus offer can be a little iffy because not all the massage therapists are carefully screened all the time in all the bureaus. So if you're not personally familiar with the service and you haven't received a specific recommendation, you're never sure exactly what you're going to get when you call one of these places.

Going back to school

Wherever you are, one excellent way to get in touch with a massage practitioner is to call a massage school in your area. The United States alone has over 1,000. Look in the phone book under "vocational schools" or "schools, massage therapy." The schools often have a list of graduates in the area that they can recommend, and quite often they offer massage services in a clinic in the school.

Pampering Your Massage Therapist

After you choose a massage therapist (see the preceding section) and begin to develop a working relationship with him, a few endearing personality quirks may begin to surface. Some massage therapists work barefoot, even in the winter, for example. Others hold a giant quartz crystal over your body before the massage. And some tape a bunch of magnets under their massage table to "align your energy" while they work on you. Try not to take your massage therapist's idiosyncrasies too seriously. He's just trying to do the best job he can. It's just that some therapists' methods may seem a little, um, colorful at first. Check out Chapter 6 for advice on letting your massage therapist know what you are and aren't comfortable with. After all, you're the boss.

As a general rule, massage therapists are a finicky and extremely sensitive lot. They're somewhat like purebred cats, and although their job description calls for a great deal of touching, they also need to receive strokes themselves (often to that most delicate muscle, the ego). If you become an expert at scratching behind the ears of your massage therapist's self-image, you can coax a better performance from him, and your relationship will be a happier one all around.

The following are some simple points to remember whenever you're dealing directly with your massage therapist:

- **Always offer encouragement before you criticize:** For example, if your massage therapist is applying a little too much pressure in a particular area, definitely let him know about it, but first say something like, "What you were doing a minute ago felt really great. You can lighten up the pressure a little right now, though."
- **Always, always, always praise the massage your therapist just gave you immediately after you receive it, even if it's the 789th massage you've received from him:** The immediate gratification of this simple act is powerful. It's the same reason all an actress's friends rush backstage after the play to heartily laud her skills. The ego muscle is most delicate directly after the big performance, and for a great massage therapist, every massage is a type of performance.
- **Always communicate clearly about exactly what fee you expect to pay for exactly which services:** Pricing of massage services may be a sensitive issue. Be clear on the answers to the following questions before you begin:
    - If you arrive late for your appointment, do you still receive the full massage? If not, do you still have to pay full price?
    - Does the massage therapist have a cancellation policy?
    - Does your massage therapist reimburse insurance claims?

Tackling Touch Terminology

Massage has its own lingo, much of which can be somewhat confusing or intimidating at first for two main reasons:

- Some massage terminology has origins in the medical field and can sound academically dense.
- Some of the words used are just plain weird.

Truthfully, though, no insider's massage clique is sitting around in cashmere robes at some exclusive country-club spa, ready to snicker at you for not knowing what the word *acupressure* means. Most of the massage words you encounter are the result of cultural influences from around the world, with a medical/scientific reference thrown in now and then.

Massage is all about making you feel comfortable in your own skin, and the last thing you want is to have a language barrier make you feel uncomfortable before you even begin. Words you don't know can make you feel like an outsider, which may have the tragic consequence of keeping you from doing what you really want to do when you get a massage — relax and feel better.

Your goal may be to become one of those knowledgeable clients who enters a massage clinic and requests "a bit of craniosacral for this headache I've had for two days now, and then some Trager in the hip area to loosen my tight psoas, and throw in some trigger point work on my traps, will you?" Or, on the other hand, perhaps this massage mumbo-jumbo seems completely pointless to you, and all you really want to do is lie down and get rubbed. Even if you belong to the latter group, knowing at least a few of the terms that massage therapists (and those who receive massage) commonly employ is helpful.

This section is a primer on massage lingo to help familiarize you with the terms you may run into when you

- Contact a massage professional to inquire about rates, services, and so on
- Visit a massage clinic
- Read journals, magazines, or books in the field
- Attempt to explain massage to a friend
- Ask people to recommend a massage therapist or style for you

Table 4-1 lists several specialized massage words and phrases that at first glance seem deceptively like everyday words and phrases. But don't be deceived. These words, when used in regards to massage, are highly specific and, when used correctly, can lead you to hours and hours of enjoyment, health benefits, and pleasure.

Table 4-1 Massage–English, English–Massage Dictionary

Word	*Non-massage definition*	*Massage definition*
Rolfed	Past-tense of "to throw up on," a variant spelling of "Ralphed"	Deep massage work on connective tissues that realigns the body with gravity.
Bodyworker	Mechanic specializing in repairing cars after accidents	A practitioner of massage or similar hands-on healing techniques.
Structural work	Carpentry, mostly done on house frames	Massage that works on the body's muscles and connective tissues to better align them with gravity.
Spa	Hot tub or Jacuzzi	Health facility where people go to learn holistic practices, eat healthy foods, exercise, and receive massages and spa treatments.
Ayurveda	Misspelling of a famous brand of natural beauty products found in salons	An ancient healing system from India that uses diet, meditation, herbs, and massage to balance the body.
Swedish	Anything from the country of Sweden	The most well-known and widely practiced form of massage in the Western world, consisting of stroking, kneading, applying pressure, stretching, and so on.

Word	***Non-massage definition***	***Massage definition***
Trigger point	The fine, pointed end of a pistol's trigger	A tight, tender spot in a muscle that responds well to massage.
Connective tissues	Facial tissues all linked together in a box	The web of tissue (primarily collagen fibers) that surrounds your every muscle, organ, and bone, holding your body together.
Deep tissue	Tissues stuck deep between the cushions on your couch	A type of massage that targets the deeper layers of muscle and connective tissue.
Energy work	Repairs on the electrical lines of your house	Type of massage that focuses on vital, invisible energies in your body
Adhesion	The sticky mark left on your skin after removing an adhesive bandage	Muscle and connective tissue fibers that are stuck together because of injuries, scars, aging, and lack of movement. Massage can help separate most adhesions, which are sometimes painful, though not usually dangerous.
Drape	Decorative material that hangs in front of a window	Towels, sheets, and so on used to cover a person receiving a massage.
Knots	Things tied in ropes	Tight bands of muscle fibers and connective tissues that massage often softens.
On-site massage	Massage given at construction sites	Seated and clothed massage given in special chairs — usually in offices, in stores, or at special events.

Bon jour, monsieur masseuse

You walk into a health club and sign up for a massage. A big, burly, bodybuilder of a man walks out, shakes your hand in his massive paw, and tells you his name is John.

"Nice to meet you," you say, slightly awed. "How long have you been a masseuse?"

"I'm not a masseuse!" he thunders, causing you to shake in your sneakers. And once again you have that terrible realization that you've flubbed up the whole masseur/masseuse thing.

"Sorry," you stammer, confused and embarrassed, but inside you're also a little mad. How are you supposed to remember the difference between those silly French words, and who made them up in the first place anyway?

Strangely enough, it was a Dutch man, Dr. Johann Mezger (1839–1909), who decided to use French words to describe the movements of massage, and even the word "massage" itself. The words for someone who performs massage therefore come from the French also:

- A *masseur* is a male practitioner of massage.
- A *masseuse* is a female practitioner.

An easy way for you to remember the correct term is to think of *monsieur* — the French word for *Mr.* — which sounds like *masseur.* And an even easier method is to avoid the masseur/masseuse dilemma altogether by using the more modern, non-gender-based term "massage therapist" for males and females alike, which is what most professionals prefer anyway.

Chapter 5

Your First Massage Appointment, Step-by-Step

In This Chapter

- Walking through your first appointment
- Choosing the right massage location for you

Probably the biggest barrier that stops people from ever signing up for their first professional massage is a fear of the unknown. If you have never ventured into a room with a stranger to get rubbed before, you just don't know what to expect, and the thought of becoming vulnerable in any way doesn't inspire you to take the first step.

But think back for just a minute. Do you remember any experience in your entire life that *wasn't* scary the first time you tried it? Go as far back as your first day at kindergarten. That's scary. Getting your first massage is just another step along the road of discovery in your life, and this chapter helps you through it.

Deciding Where to Go to Get Massaged

You have an array of choices when it comes to where you receive a professional massage, ranging from right in your own bedroom all the way up to super luxurious spa resorts on the island of Maui. I personally recommend Maui. Wherever you are, it helps if you know a little bit about each environment and what you can expect when you receive a massage there. That's what this section's all about.

Because of the wide disparity between massage therapists and the environments they create to work in, go check out each environment personally, or at least get a detailed description of it from a friend or online *before* you sign up for your first massage there. That way, you can avoid any surprises that may surface, such as when you make an appointment at your local day spa for a relaxing hour of escape only to find the massage room is directly adjacent to a bank of two dozen noisy hair-drying machines.

Your own home

Getting a professional massage in your own home is great. In fact, some people think it's the crème de la crème of massage experiences. You don't have to drive anywhere. You're in safe, familiar surroundings. And, best of all, afterwards all you have to do is roll over into your own bed or onto your own couch. The massage therapist leaves, and you float off on a wave of bliss in the comfort of your own home. What could be better?

However, there are some downsides to the in-home massage visit. For one thing, you're basically inviting a stranger to set up her business right in your own bedroom or den, which is kind of an invasion of privacy. And another thing — when you're at home, you're surrounded by your own life. Every detail is there to remind you of your pre- and post-massage existence, which may perhaps detract from the "escape" factor of your experience.

Then there are the distractions. If you have children, you can pretty much count on them wanting to crawl up on the massage table with you and "help" the nice massage person do her job. This desire is very endearing of the little tykes, but it's not the straight and narrow road to total relaxation.

Only sign up for an in-home massage if you're comfortable with other people in your private space and you can keep distractions to a minimum.

The massage therapist's home

Many massage therapists have a space set up in their own homes for giving massage. This arrangement can range from a dinky little corner in one end of the living room to an entire suite of offices with a separate entrance. You may like the "personalized" feeling of visiting a massage therapist in her home, where you can take advantage of the relaxing environment she has (hopefully) set up. On the other hand, if you're the type of person who prefers a more clearly defined edge between the personal and professional aspects of your transactions, the massage therapist's home may not be the best choice of location for you.

Also, you have to take into account certain practical details as well, such as whether or not the massage therapist has pets. If you're allergic to cats, and the massage therapist's house is a veritable kitty kennel, you may break out in a rash and not enjoy the massage at all.

A good massage therapist should put the rest of her life on hold while you're in her home, but a few of them have a tendency to attend to their own business while you're there, answering the phone and the doorbell, for instance, which can greatly detract from your experience. You may need to make an extra effort to reinforce that you're the boss (see Chapter 6), even if you're in her home, and that for this hour you're in charge.

Spas

Some of the most beautiful massage environments in the world occur in spas, and you find out more about them in Chapter 7. Grand *destination spas* dot the map all around the world, and you can likely find a *day spa* that you can check out right in your own town.

Although spas are often pleasant and luxurious, keep a couple of things in mind when signing up for a massage in one:

- Massage therapists in spas only keep a percentage of the fee rather than the whole thing, which may lead some of them to give less than their absolute best work.
- Massage therapists in spas are on the clock, and you're likely to get a massage that is exactly 50 minutes long, 80 minutes long, and so on. Good spa therapists can still give you a feeling of timeless bliss within that strict time frame, but it's a little challenging.
- The style of massage given in certain spas is dictated by a lowest-common-denominator mentality, and massage therapists aren't allowed to use their advanced techniques for fear of alienating a clientele who just wants a rubdown.

These warnings notwithstanding, there's no reason to believe you can't receive an incredible massage in a spa. Some of the best massage therapists work in them. Also, if you end up finding a massage therapist you really like, you can ask her whether she also takes private clients outside the spa, which may mean a better deal for her and a better massage for you. Be diplomatic when doing so though, and always ask whether it's okay with management because many spas have a policy against this setup.

Cruise ships

Cruise ships are fun places to get massages, if you don't mind rocking back and forth a little bit while you're on the table. Almost every ship has its own spa, and you can visit for a half-hour or an hour of massage as easily as visiting the midnight buffet (though expect an additional charge for the massage). A massage during your cruise may add to the exotic flavor of your trip, but remember these less-than-exotic points as well:

- **Because floor space and portholes are at a premium on ships, massage rooms onboard are usually smallish quarters with no natural light.** If you're used to ample luxurious massage spaces, you may feel a little claustrophobic in this environment.
- **Shipboard massage therapists are part of a massage assembly line.** Coaxing the best from your massage therapist can be tough because she sees so many people come and go — none of whom are repeat customers.
- **Be aware that most massages onboard include some kind of sales pitch for products at the end.** You aren't required to buy anything, of course, but you may be uncharacteristically prone to make a spontaneous purchase because of your relaxed state of mind. Know before you go that the pitch will likely happen, and make a conscious decision about possible purchases beforehand.
- **Make sure to sign up early — as soon as you come on board — if you're thinking about getting a massage during your cruise because the best time slots fill up fast.** You may want an appointment during a sea day, rather than in port, so you don't have to decide between getting a massage and going ashore to sightsee or shop.

Hotels

Many hotels have their own spas, so all you have to do to book a massage is call the spa desk. For those hotels without a spa, contact the concierge to arrange your appointment.

One note about concierges: They often take a good chunk of the massage therapist's fee for themselves, and they have a stable of ever-ready massage therapists at hand who allow them to do that. So, the quality of therapist isn't always the best. You may be better off placing a call directly to a professional that you find listed under licensed practitioners in one of the online directories listed in Chapter 4. That way you can avoid the fee and perhaps find higher-quality work as well.

All in all, hotel rooms are on the low end of the totem pole as far as receiving massages go. They're impersonal, they're cramped, and they often have that funny hotel-room-smell that no amount of incense or positive thinking can overcome. If you find yourself in a hotel room somewhere with nowhere else to go for your massage, and only a concierge to put your trust in, do what seasoned massage recipients the world over have done for years: enjoy it anyway.

Health clubs

Health clubs are becoming better places to receive massages. In the past, you were likely to wind up in a tiny cinder-block cubicle vibrating with the sounds of music from the aerobics room next door. These days, health-club owners are more aware that their customers want a little nook of tranquility and a well-trained massage therapist. Depending on the place, some of these clubs offer massage therapists a good percentage of the profits, and even a chance to run their own massage business within the confines of the larger club business, so you may very well find some motivated individuals. The massage is often high-quality, especially if you're interested in sports-related therapy. And in a health club you can receive your massage immediately after a strenuous workout and a limb-loosening sauna.

Clinics

Many massage therapists open up their own clinics. The setup is similar to any other professional office, like a chiropractor's, a doctor's, or a dentist's. You walk in the front door into a waiting area with a potted plant, some magazines, chairs, and a reception desk. Behind the desk is a hallway with a few doors opening into rooms. The rooms behind those doors, however, can differ decidedly from other clinics. Depending upon the personality and style of the massage therapist, a massage treatment room can range from white-tiled sterility with anatomical charts on the walls to a softly glowing, plush chamber of warmth filled with the strains of celestial music. Some massage clinics are located in wellness centers that offer other healthy pursuits as well, such as acupuncture, yoga, dance, and T'ai Chi.

One specialty in this area is known as the *sports massage clinic*. The massage therapists in these facilities concentrate on rehabilitating you after an injury. They often work with orthopedic physicians and physical therapists. A trip to this type of no-nonsense massage clinic may feel more like a doctor visit than a spa visit. Check out Chapter 15 for more on sports massage.

Student massage clinics

One excellent deal that many people take advantage of is known as the *student massage clinic.* In this setup, massage students receive part of their training by working on real customers who come into the school, which has a special area set up to receive them. Student massages go for only fraction of the normal cost, usually only ¼ to ⅓ the going rate of a professional massage in the area. More often than not, the students are already quite good at what they do, and dollar for dollar this option is one of the best bargains in massage.

Keep in mind that you may be asked to fill out a detailed feedback form after the massage for training purposes. Also, the student clinics sometimes take place in a big room with curtains separating the massage tables. Quite often, an instructor stops in to observe the student in action. So if you're a super-private individual who doesn't like to have other people around when you're getting a massage, the student clinic is probably not for you. Also, if you have a specific health problem that you want to address with massage, visit a licensed professional. For relaxation and stress relief, though, student massages are often as effective as professional massages because the students are trying extra hard to please you (and pass their coursework at the same time!).

Soaring through Your First Appointment with a Pro

You can use the following seven steps as a guide to help you breeze through your first appointment with confidence and poise, starting before you even arrive and lasting right up until you walk out the door.

Preparation

In order to get the most out of your massage, you have to do a little more planning and preparation than you would to go get, say, a haircut. When you schedule your massage, keep these points in mind:

- **Don't eat a large meal within a couple hours before starting the massage.** You don't want to be lying face down on a belly full of lasagna while somebody is pressing on your back. Light meals and snacks are okay, and a larger meal several hours earlier doesn't affect you.
- **If possible, don't wear a lot of jewelry, which takes a lot of time to take off and put back on again.**

- **Refrain from consuming alcohol before your massage (unless it's a sensual massage — see Chapter 16 — and you're sharing a bottle of bubbly with that special someone to get in the mood).** Although alcohol can help relax you, it also slows your responses and deadens some sensations. You want to be alert and responsive because massage is a two-way dance, and you need to do your part.
- **Make sure to schedule enough time before and after your massage.** You don't want to be rushing to get there and flying out the door when you leave. Hurrying tends to counteract the relaxing effects of the massage itself.
- **Turn off your cellphone during the massage.** This step probably seems obvious, but beeps, buzzes, and rings have interrupted many tranquil, soothing massages.
- **Make sure any childcare details are completely taken care of before you begin so your mind can be at ease during your session.**

No particular time of day is best to receive a massage, but most people have their own personal preference. Some like the morning so they can experience the benefits throughout the day, and others like a massage right before going to bed at night. Whichever your choice is, try to schedule far enough in advance so you get the time you prefer. Many massage therapists are busy, and their prime times fill up early.

Communication

When you arrive at your massage destination, especially for the first time, you need to engage in a little communication with the person who is going to massage you. So of course, speaking the same language as that person is helpful. And I don't mean just the same native tongue, but the same *intention,* too. If what you want out of the experience is fundamentally different than what the massage therapist intends to give, you're headed for trouble.

For example, if you came in for an hour of blissful relaxation and escape from stress but the massage therapist intends on giving you a session of active, muscle-stretching sports therapy, neither one of you is going to have a good time. The best time to confirm your intentions is on the phone, before you meet face-to-face, but you need to reconfirm this understanding with some clear verbal communication after you arrive, as well.

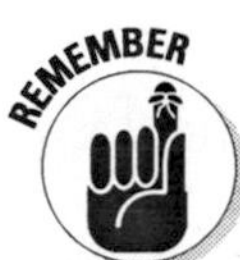

When you finally meet your massage therapist for the first time, she may also require some nonverbal communication in the form of paperwork (such as an intake form) to fill out. "Why do I have to fill out these medical forms if all I want is a simple massage?" you may ask. Well, it's for your own good. Massage affects the entire body, and it's best if your massage therapist knows as much as possible about your health history and any *contraindications* (conditions that may affect the massage, which I cover in Chapter 10). If a massage therapist doesn't ask you to fill out a form, however, it doesn't mean she doesn't care about your health; that's just her style, or the policy of the spa or health club where she works.

Another type of communication you share with your massage therapist is both nonverbal and non-written — body language. As you may imagine, massage therapists become very adept at making their clients feel at ease in a potentially uneasy situation. The little things they do (and don't do) — where they point their eyes or how they manipulate sheets and towels to make you feel protected and respected — are what make the difference. It's the way they just relax and accept you when you make yourself vulnerable by being there.

Besides, they're just as eager to make a good first impression as you are, partly because it's human nature and partly because they want you as a repeat customer!

Getting comfortable

In most massage situations, after you arrive and go through your communication rituals, the next step is undressing and lying down, which can be tricky. It's the moment many people dread, and the one that keeps them from ever getting a "real" massage. The way it works is like this:

1. The massage therapist explains how you're supposed to get up on the massage table, pointing out where your head should be and whether you should be face up or face down.

   If you ask whether you should get completely undressed or not, the stock answer is something to the effect of, "Most people take all their clothes off, but you can get undressed to the level of your comfort." Then she leaves the room. Don't feel intimidated by "most people" who all so bravely get naked for their massages. Whether you want to keep your underwear or some clothes on is up to you, and it's okay either way. Chapter 6 delves into this and other guidelines for enjoying a massage.

   After the massage therapist is out of the room, remember to take your time. Don't worry about getting barged in on, 'cause it ain't gonna happen. She knocks before coming back in, and she usually waits much longer than necessary to make sure you have plenty of time. Take this opportunity to remove jewelry, watches, and anything else that may entangle a finger (wedding bands are okay). You usually find a little table or shelf to hold your belongings and a hook for your clothes. If you have long hair, you may want to tie it back so it doesn't get in the way.

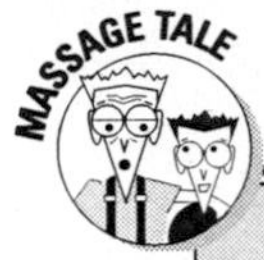

Modesty's overrated

Sometimes no matter how hard you try, all these massage rules go out the window. Like the time I was working at a spa and had the opportunity to massage Dr. Ruth Westheimer. I'll never forget the experience because, for one thing, she threw her robe off before I ever had the chance to leave the room and let her get undressed. Then, full of confidence, she strode to the massage table and tried to climb aboard. I say "tried" because, as it turns out, she was a little too short to reach. I wanted to reach down and give her a boost, but I couldn't figure out how to do it without getting a little too personal with Dr. Ruth, so I averted my eyes as best I could and offered ineffectual words of general encouragement.

Luckily, she knew what to do. "Don't worry!" she chimed. "I've had this problem before!" Then she proceeded to push a chair up next to the massage table, climbed onto the chair and then the table, and I immediately covered her with a sheet in the proper professional fashion.

Visit the bathroom before you lay down on the table, even if you don't think you have to go. Getting a massage with a full bladder takes a lot of the enjoyment out of it.

Lie down on the table in the position you were told and pull the sheet or towel up over your body, completely covering yourself.

2. The massage therapist knocks and asks whether you're ready for her to enter again. When you give the go-ahead, she comes in and then usually washes her hands. She does so for three reasons:
   - To reassure you that her hands are clean.
   - To wash away any dirt or germs she may have contacted since scrubbing them the last time a few minutes earlier.
   - In many areas, the law requires it.
3. She makes sure you're comfortable, checking the room temperature, tucking the towel around your body, and adjusting the lights and music. She may also slip a little pillow or piece of foam rubber beneath your knees, ankles, or head to help support you. These cushions are called *bolsters*, and they really help you feel more comfortable. If you feel a strain or lack of support in any area of your body, just let the massage therapist know.
4. After everything's set, your massage therapist uncovers just the area that she is going to work on. If she plans to massage your neck, she pulls the sheet down to the top of your chest. Massage therapists cover women's breasts, and no one's "private parts" ever get exposed.

Avoiding the bathrobe dance

As a massage therapist working in spas, on many occasions I've entered the massage room to begin a massage only to find my client lying there, face down, rigid with nervousness, with her bathrobe tied super-tight around her waist. Before leaving the room to let her disrobe, I'd instructed her to take her robe off and lie down under the sheet I'd provided, but some clients are too tense to hear those instructions. And so that's when we begin the bathrobe dance.

The *bathrobe dance* is an awkward ordeal that usually lasts about two minutes. While the massage therapist tries to assist as best he can, the client rolls, wriggles, and writhes her way out of the bathrobe while remaining face down and completely covered at all times. The client's rump usually scoots up in the air, arms and legs splay every which way, and her face turns bright red.

Then, after the robe is finally loosened from around her body and her arms are out of the armholes, the massage therapist has to drape a sheet or towel over it before skillfully slipping the robe from underneath. This entire procedure leaves the client even more tense than when she started and more embarrassed than she would have been if she'd simply listened to the instructions.

So, when you go for your first massage, especially if you're nervous, remember to listen closely to your therapist's instructions. It'll make things a lot easier. If you find yourself on the table still wrapped in your robe, make things easy on yourself. Don't wear yourself out before the massage by wrestling with your robe. Instead, say something like, "That was so silly of me," and ask the massage therapist to leave the room again to give you another chance. Then get off the table, slip out of your robe, and lie down beneath the sheet like you were supposed to in the first place.

If you have a towel wrapped around you before the massage, make sure not to lie down directly on the knotted part so that you have to do the "rock-n-roll" to loosen it. Instead, open the towel up and lie straight on the table with the towel still covering your backside.

The first touch

The very first moment of contact between you and the massage therapist can tell you an awful lot about how the rest of the massage is going to feel. Each massage therapist has a personality in her hands that you quickly get to know.

When the massage therapist is closely attuned to you and your body, this moment can be almost sacred. It's an intimate joining-together of your consciousness with the consciousness of another person, which just plain doesn't happen that often in the modern world.

Take advantage of this initial contact by tuning in especially closely to what's happening in your own body. In the same way that you pick up a lot of information about the person who's touching you, she's picking up a lot of information about you. It's a good opportunity for you to concentrate on your breathing and relaxation.

During the massage

During the massage, your massage therapist continues to keep you covered at all times, only exposing those areas that she's working on at the moment. Massage therapists are experts at this technique, called *draping*, and they make you feel completely comfortable, almost as if you were fully dressed during the experience.

Yes, you're comfortable and modestly covered the whole time, but what are you supposed to actually *do* while you're getting a massage? That's the biggest problem many people have, especially type-A people. They figure that getting a massage is just plain boring and that's why they decide not to do it.

Okay, so getting a massage isn't exactly the same as bungee jumping from a hot-air balloon, attending a rock concert, or brokering a multimillion dollar deal in a corporate boardroom. But if you let it, massage can become compelling, even thrilling, in a very internal kind of way. It's like taking a roller coaster ride inside your own skin.

The trick isn't to try to make anything happen, but to just let whatever happens happen. You're not supposed to do anything. Your massage therapist tells you if you have to move a certain way or breathe a certain way or visualize a certain image. Besides that, the less you do the better. Think of massage as a trip to the beach. You're *supposed to* just lie there and do nothing.

"But what if I fall asleep?" you gasp. "Wouldn't that insult the massage therapist?" Not at all. In fact, some massage therapists take it as a compliment that they can get their clients to relax this deeply. However, your creative input to the massage process is just as valuable as the massage therapist's input, so it's better if you stay awake for most of the session. Drifting off at the very end can feel wonderful, but if you snooze through an entire massage, you may be missing some of the most pleasurable moments of your life. Who wants to pay good money for a nap?

If you're the type that can't conceive of an entire hour spent doing nothing, try this technique: Talk to the massage therapist about things that matter, like your health. Most massage people are pretty well versed in the art of taking-care-of-yourself, and you stand a good chance of having a conversation that goes beyond mere chitchat, offering you some real benefits.

Under pressure

So, what's the right amount of pressure to ask for during a massage anyway? Pressure refers to how hard or soft the massage feels, how painful or soothing. Usually, your massage therapist has a lot of experience in this area and can find just the right pressure to suit your particular body type and your level of sensitivity. But sometimes you may want her to change the pressure, and it helps if you know what to ask for.

Don't suffer through a massage that's too soft or too hard just because you're too bashful to say anything about it. You can use this scale from 1 to 10 to communicate your desired pressure level to your massage therapist:

- **1: Light as a feather:** The fingertips merely skim over the surface of the skin to provide stimulation to the nerve endings but exert no pressure onto the body.
- **2 to 3: Very light to light:** Many people prefer this kind of silky, gliding touch, but it drives others crazy because they think the massage therapist isn't getting in there and working the muscles.
- **4 to 6: Moderate to moderately firm:** This range is where most massage takes place. You can definitely feel some pressure, and you know the massage is having some definite physical effects, but never so much that it's annoying.
- **7 to 9: Firm to very firm to deep:** At these levels, you may begin to squirm a little. And you may even say something like, "What are you trying to do, kill me?" Rest assured, the massage therapist isn't trying to kill you. She's just being merciless in her attempt to root out and destroy any tightness she's found. Mercilessness can be a good quality in a massage therapist.
- **10: Profoundly deep massage:** This level reaches to the core of your body's deeper structures, actually altering your posture and inner alignment. This level should be reserved for masochists, people with a high pain tolerance, and those who know what they're doing.

If some sort of distraction pops up, such as a loud noise or a telephone ringing, try not to take it personally. Nobody is out to ruin your massage experience. Instead of letting an interruption spoil things for you, focus instead on the exchange of positive energy between you and the person giving you the massage.

Keep communicating. When appropriate during the massage, give feedback to your massage therapist. Words spoken about the massage help keep you focused on the massage. If at any point you want the massage therapist to change what she's doing, you have a right to let her know. After all, you're paying, and the customer is always right. Let her know what you want, which may include

- **More pressure or less pressure:** You can convey your pressure needs on a scale from 1 to 10 (see the nearby sidebar "Under pressure" for info on the scale).
- **More or less time spent in a particular area:** But be aware that the massage therapist may be using her knowledge to achieve a certain goal, working in the area that's most effective, even if you think it's not directly connected to your problem.
- **A glass of water**
- **A trip to the bathroom**
- **A chance to express your feelings and ask for reassurance, especially if a strong emotion begins to surface during your massage**

Beware of the massage therapist who claims she can only perform "deep" work and then proceeds to pummel your body even after you request lighter pressure. You never need to undergo a painful ordeal in order to experience the relaxation you seek. If the massage is too deep, tell the therapist to back off. If they don't back off, you have every right to end the massage and not pay for the service.

Coming back slowly

Take it easy getting off the table and back into your life — no need to hurry. In fact, most massage therapists suggest that you just lie there and absorb the effects of the massage and the relaxation for a few minutes before getting up again. Unless you're late for something urgent, such as an international plane trip to go receive the Nobel Prize, follow this suggestion. These few minutes can be an exquisite interlude during which your cares and concerns seem a million miles away. Relish them. Stretch out a little. Breathe. Just relax.

Then, when you finally decide to get up, don't be shy about asking for help if you need it, as you may feel a little wobbly at first.

There's a special way to get yourself off a massage table that helps you keep the effects intact. Instead of essentially doing a sit-up and retensing all your muscles in order to get upright again, simply roll onto your side and push gently against the table with both hands while you slowly roll back into a sitting position. Your feet and legs end up hanging over the edge of the table, as you see illustrated in Figure 5-1. Then you can slide your rear end off the table like a buttered pancake.

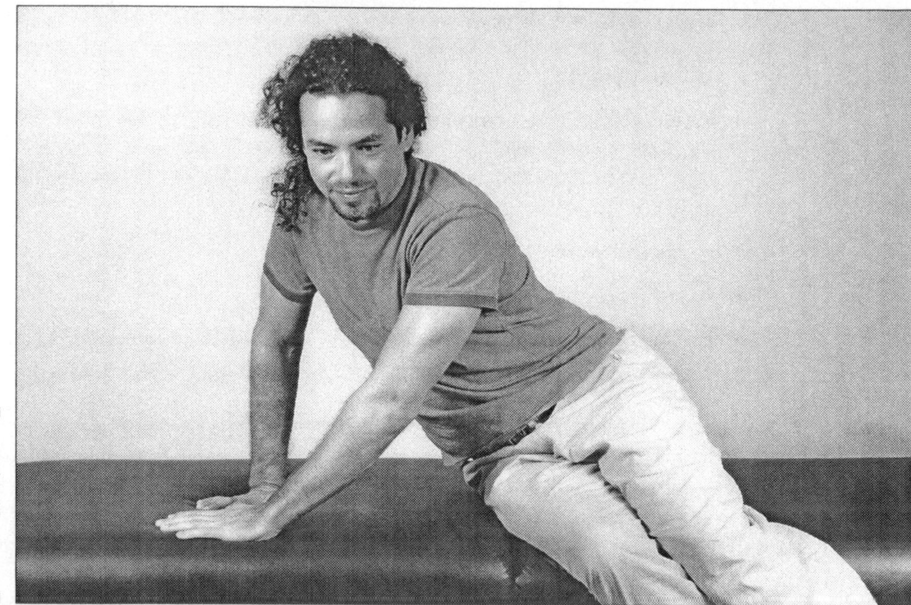

Figure 5-1: The right way to get off a massage table.

Afterglow

When you first step on the floor again, exercise caution because any massage oil that may have been left on the soles of your feet can cause you to slip. Take your time getting dressed, making sure you're not forgetting anything. You don't need to take a shower, because your skin absorbs normal amounts of oil or cream, though you may want to take one if you're going out later. If the massage therapist used excess oil, you can wipe it off with a towel or some rubbing alcohol before putting clothes back on, especially silk garments. Some therapists perform this wipe down themselves at the end of the massage.

Take some time to reorient yourself. Be cautious about driving your car right away as you may feel a bit "disconnected," as if your body were inside of a big box filled with cotton. Before you leave, take the massage therapist's business card, and consider making another appointment so you don't have to worry about it later.

To tip or not to tip

You're all ready to head out the door when suddenly it occurs to you that perhaps you should tip the person who just gave you the massage. Is it appropriate? Would she be insulted if you gave her a tip? Upset if you didn't? The answer is . . . "it depends."

Overcoming the heebie-jeebies

If, even after trying some of the suggestions in this chapter, you're still harboring a tiny bit of fear and loathing about massage somewhere in your subconscious mind, that's all right. I felt the same way, too, the first time I disrobed for a session as a student at the Massage School of Santa Monica many years ago.

It's perfectly natural to feel somewhat anxious at the thought of somebody you don't even know touching you for an extended period of time. And the thought of somebody you do know touching you for a whole hour may even be worse! In the highly sophisticated, jet-setter world of massage therapy, these feelings of anxiety are known by the incredibly technical term *heebie-jeebies.* Unless you grew up in a household where massage was common, the heebie-jeebies may present a problem when you're first getting ready to climb up on a massage table and simply receive.

My advice? Feel the fear and do it anyway. Plunge in and get that massage. Afterwards, if you're like 99.9 percent of all people, you say to yourself, "That wasn't so bad! Why didn't I do this a long time ago?"

It depends upon where you received the massage. Was it a spa? Then a tip is almost always expected, unless the spa has a policy against it. Was it at a sports medicine clinic? Then tips aren't usually part of the procedure. Did you receive the massage at home? A tip is definitely appreciated in this case because the massage therapist went out of her way to provide the service. No massage therapist should make you feel uncomfortable for not tipping, however, so if you forget to tip sometimes or don't feel you can afford it on any particular day, don't sweat it.

Some massage therapists feel tipping for a massage is inappropriate. They want their work to be considered in the same category as any other health-care provider's. You wouldn't tip your chiropractor, your homeopath, or your MD, right?

So how do you know what to do? Tipping ultimately boils down to an understanding with the massage therapist. If you're at all uncertain, simply ask, "Is tipping allowed here?" The customary tip amount in most locations is usually in the $5 to $10 range, or 10 percent of the total bill, more if the massage therapist is working late, went far out of her way, or did an especially good job. And remember, you never *have* to tip for massage. It's not like tipping a waiter, who's making the bulk of his income through gratuities. Massage therapists are usually pretty well paid for what they do. Tips are the icing on the cake for them.

Chapter 6

The Rules for Receiving Massage

In This Chapter

- Tuning in to the experience
- Taking responsibility for your role in a massage

From the day you were born, your body has been hanging around you like a shadow. It never leaves you alone. You wake up in the morning, and your body is there, faithful as a puppy thumping its little tail against your freshly washed bedspread. At first, having a body is a novelty, a fact reflected in the faces of babies and small children. Even the most mundane details about their bodies fill them with delight. "Oh boy, there's my hand again!"

As you mature, however, you become more accustomed to having a body, and it begins to bore you. This boredom usually occurs as young people enter their teenage years. "Oh boy, my hand again, big deal." At this point, they begin to pierce their bodies in various locations and cover them with decorative tattoos. By the time people are full-fledged adults, though, most of them have begun to concentrate on other things, leaving their bodies far behind. The only time they really get connected to their bodies is when they're learning a new skill of some kind, like soccer, or neurosurgery.

The result? Most people take their bodies for granted. One of massage's main objectives is to get you back "into" your body again. A good massage should rekindle your childlike enthusiasm for life.

In order for massage to help you achieve the lofty goal of getting back in touch with yourself, you need to follow certain guidelines, which I just happen to outline in this chapter. At first, some of these rules may seem a little simplistic to you, and others may appear irrelevant. However, I give you my personal guarantee that if you try them out when you're on the receiving end of a massage, you're going to get much more out of the experience.

So, approach these guidelines with an open mind, apply them when you feel that doing so is appropriate during your own massage exchanges, and watch your enjoyment of massage soar to levels beyond your expectations.

Rule 1: Keep Breathing

When you receive a massage from a professional, she may remind you several times in a soft, soothing voice to breathe. And you may be tempted to say right back to her in a not-so-soothing voice, "I'm already breathing, in case you haven't noticed."

Don't be offended. The massage therapist's comments aren't meant to imply that she thinks you're deceased, and she's not trying to insult you for your poor breathing skills. In fact, many massage therapists start each and every massage by having you take a series of deep breaths, regardless of how obviously alive you are to begin with. A massage therapist may tell you to take deep breaths during a massage for the following reasons:

- To help you focus on the sensations you're feeling in your body rather than the internal monologue going on in your mind
- To get you to fill your lungs and thus all your cells with fresh oxygen, enlivening your entire body
- To help you become aware of muscles that you've been holding tense so you can start to relax them

Most people walk around not actually breathing much. People tend to use only a tiny percentage of their lung capacity, just like they use only a tiny percentage of their brain capacity. Proper breathing changes that.

While receiving a massage, focus your mind as fully as possible on the very important act of breathing. Focusing your mind on your breath brings your awareness back to your body quicker than anything else.

Going with the diaphragm's flow

The *diaphragm* is the muscle in your abdomen responsible for keeping you breathing (see Figure 6-1). Most of the time, your diaphragm contracts and relaxes without conscious thought from you, but you can teach yourself to control this activity. In the following section, I give you an exercise that helps you use this muscle more consciously, enabling you to exert more control over your breathing and making it fuller and deeper.

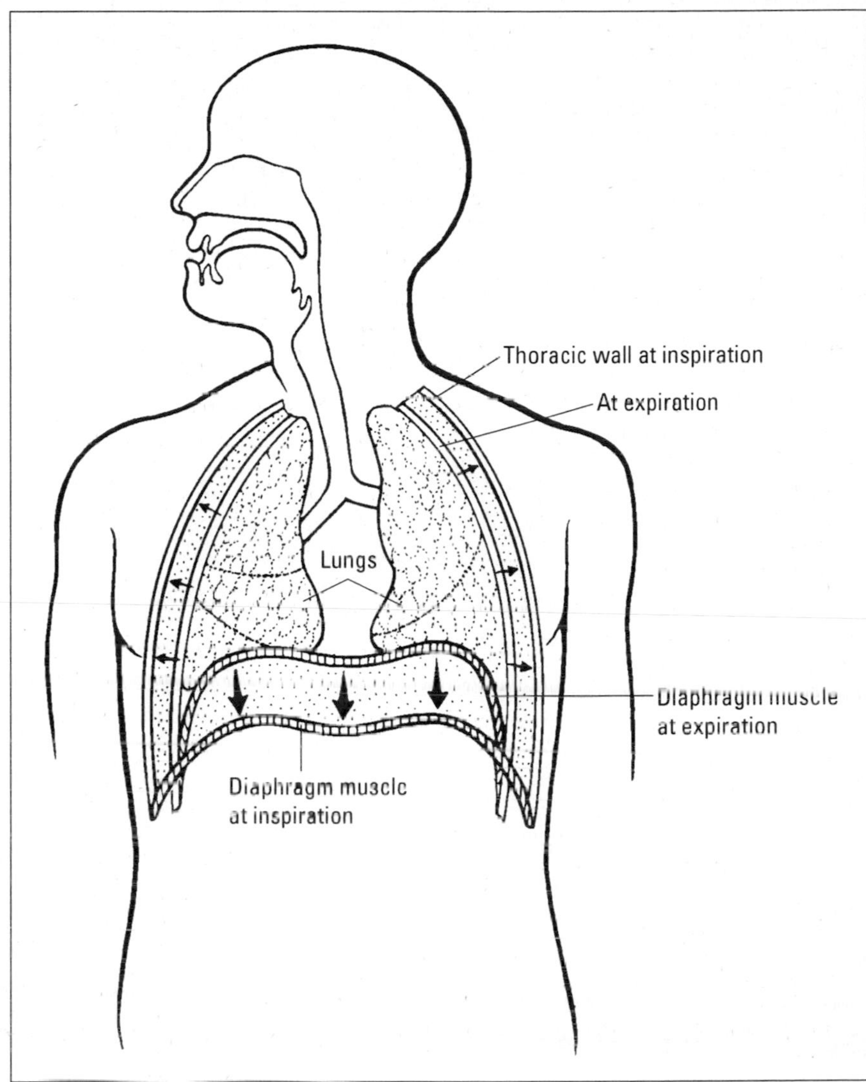

Figure 6-1: The diaphragm and other elements of your respiratory system.

Exercising your breathing muscles

The next time you have the chance, spend a few minutes observing a sleeping — or at least relaxed — infant or toddler breathe. Pay close attention to the abdomen, and you can see the entire area gently lift and lower. This movement is the result of an active, uninhibited diaphragm at work.

Then look down at your own abdomen while you breathe for a few minutes. Notice a difference? Where did all the lifting and lowering go? You still have the same breathing mechanisms you always did; they're not something you grow out of. With each breath you take, you should indeed have a visibly rhythmical, moving body. Somewhere along the line, though, most people stifle themselves into taking shallow, insufficient breaths. This type of breathing is a common reaction to the act of growing older. Don't worry, you're still getting enough oxygen to survive. But, are you getting enough to thrive? By practicing deep breathing during massage, you can literally rejuvenate your body, sending extra-oxygenated blood out all the way to your toes.

The key to breathing properly while getting a massage is to take *whole breaths,* a term that basically means "breathe like a kid." Go ahead and try a whole breath now. Lie down on your back, placing your palms gently on your abdomen, and then begin this four-step process:

1. **Breathe deep and low into your lungs so that your abdomen pushes your hands upward.**

   Make sure that you're not just pushing up with your stomach muscles, but that you're actually expanding the entire abdominal area.

2. **Continue the expansion up into your ribs, allowing them to push outward toward each side.**
3. **When your ribs have expanded out as far as they go, expand them up toward your head, taking the last bit of breath into the area just beneath your collar bones.**
4. **Let the whole thing collapse.**

   You don't need to try to push the air out; just let it flow. When your lungs feel empty and your abdomen is flat once again, you can restart the process.

Rule 2: Stay Loose

As you probably know, one of the main points of getting a massage is to relax. Logically, you may think that you can just give your body to a massage therapist to relax it for you, like giving your car to a mechanic and expecting him to fix it.

Expecting a massage therapist to do all your body's relaxing is giving up responsibility for your own relaxation, and it's a no-no. Staying loose is your responsibility; the massage therapist can help you, but you basically have to do the relaxing yourself.

Untying your own knots

After you receive several massages, you gradually become accustomed to relaxing your own muscles. Eventually you notice that you can do the same thing even when you're not receiving massage, like when you're waiting in line at the grocery store, stuck in traffic, or sitting in a meeting with your boss. "Twang," goes one of your muscle fibers, and you feel it beginning to tighten up. Then, silently, without anyone noticing, you send a mental message to the growing knot, telling it to go away, in the same way that your massage therapist helps you do it during a massage. You can take this side benefit of massage with you wherever you go.

You accomplish relaxation by becoming more aware of what you're feeling in your own body. During the massage, your massage therapist often reminds you to focus on "knots" or tight areas. In those moments, using the power of your own imagination, you can begin to visualize what those knots may look like in your muscles and let go of them.

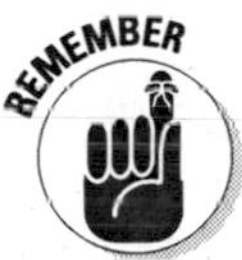

If you're not staying loose by engaging your mind to relax your own muscles, you're missing many of the benefits and effects of the massage.

Rule 3: Let Go

When you receive a massage, especially the first time, you may have a tendency — like just about everyone else in the world — to "help" the person working on you. You may graciously lift your limbs, hold your head up, and twist your body around, all to make things easier for the other person. Although this helping may seem like the friendliest thing to do, you're actually hindering the massage process and making your massage therapist's job more difficult. Relaxing a person who is holding her own arm up in the air as stiff as a flag pole is pretty darn hard.

The technical term for this tendency during massage is *hanging on,* and you want to do exactly the opposite, which is letting go. But what exactly does *letting go* mean?

Specialized nerve cells called *proprioceptors* monitor the position and relative movement of your body while you're getting a massage (check out Chapter 3 for more information). These cells constantly tell you where you are in space, something everybody likes to have a pretty firm control over all of the time, even while asleep. These cells keep you from just rolling right out of bed every night. Through these cells, you're actually holding onto yourself in order to protect yourself, and massage helps tell these cells they can safely relax a little so you can let go.

The limp-arm experiment

You're basically hanging onto yourself for dear life, even the parts of your body that are painful, stiff, or tense. This hanging on is a natural tendency, but to get the most out of a massage, you have to let go. The *limp-arm experiment* is an easy way to begin training yourself to let go. All you need is a partner and someplace comfortable to lie down. Here's how it works:

1. **Lie on your back and have your partner lift your arm up in the air several inches.**
2. **After a few seconds, have your partner let go of your arm without any warning to you.**

   Let your arm drop back down. (Make sure that you're lying on a soft surface.)
3. **Watch to see whether your arm plops back down limp as a noodle, or whether you hold it right where he left it, stiff as a board.**

   What do you have to do to let your arm drop back down? What thought process do you have to go through? What mental image? What body sensation?
4. **Tell your partner to lift your arm a little higher each time.**

   Instead of dropping your arm all the way back down, tell him to catch it in his other hand.
5. **Keep repeating this exercise until your arm completely lets go and your partner can drop it from any height with absolutely no resistance.**

   This ability may come naturally to you the very first time you try to let go, but normally the exercise takes quite a bit of conscious effort. You may not be able to let go until you make several separate attempts on different days. After you master one arm, you can try the other arm, or a leg.

Use this newly formed skill to let go the next time you receive a massage.

About the only time you completely let go of all your holding patterns, tensions, and proprioceptive rigidities is when you're under deep anesthesia. Under anesthesia, people sometimes release the tension they normally think of as built-in through age or heredity, including stooped shoulders, stiff hips, ugly grimaces, and more. When they come out of anesthesia, they reclaim these habitual patterns almost instantaneously. They can't sustain the relaxation because it's unconscious. Massage, conversely, allows people to achieve a conscious relaxation, which can last indefinitely.

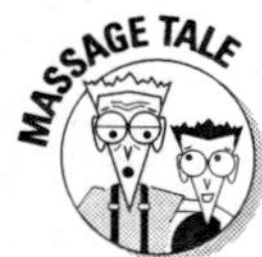

One of my clients suffered for years from debilitating pain due to whiplash. Then one day she received a massage from a woman at Gurney's Inn, a spa in Montauk, New York. After that massage, the pain was almost entirely gone, and it continued to gradually fade away. My client was able to make such a drastic change by letting herself go fully into the healing hands of the massage therapist. When she did, she stopped holding onto the same painful, habitual patterns that had formed in her body since the accident.

Rule 4: Stop Thinking, Start Being

The problem with your mind is that it just works too darn well, thinking and thinking and thinking without stopping all day long from the first moment you wake up until well after your head hits the pillow. This feature is fine during most of your daily activities, but when it comes to getting a massage, too much thinking is definitely a drawback.

Believe it or not, many people get a massage and barely even notice it because they aren't really paying attention to it while it's happening. Instead, an ongoing stream of thoughts keeps them from fully experiencing the massage.

When you're getting a massage, don't think about what you should have done the day before or what you plan to do an hour later. A massage is time to be here now. The sensations you're feeling offer a great opportunity to quiet your mind, focus, and think of nothing else for a little while. In this way, every massage is a potential meditation. Don't get me wrong: relaxing and joking around during a massage is perfectly okay, too, but most people, at least once in a while, can benefit from a massage meditation, which I cover in the "A massage meditation" sidebar later in this chapter.

Rule 5: No Pain, No Gain? No Way!

You may have heard of the massage masochists who don't believe they're receiving a real massage unless they have to grit their teeth to keep from screaming through the whole thing. They're the ones you can hear yelling from behind massage room doors, "More pressure! More pressure!"

This green-beret school of massage is an unfortunate result of the "no-pain, no-gain" mentality that military academies, full-contact sports enthusiasts, and certain daytime-television talk show hosts foster. You don't need to buy into this way of thinking, and you shouldn't let this attitude scare you away from getting a massage.

So, how much pain should you experience during a massage? In my opinion, none. Zero. However, the line is indeed thin between the pleasure you receive during massage and a certain kind of therapeutic pain. Some people like to walk that line while they're getting a massage. If you want to experiment with walking this line yourself, make sure to do so with an experienced professional.

A massage meditation

Meditation, in a nutshell, is the act of focusing your entire attention on just one thing, thus stopping the constant chatter inside your head and experiencing a state of timelessness, contentment, and wholeness. People achieve this state in many ways — through sports, silence, or prayer, for example — and massage is yet another activity that you can use to effectively shut out the rest of the world and tune into your own inner peace. The next time you receive a massage, try this meditation:

1. **Close your eyes and begin to get in touch with your breath as I describe in "Rule 1: Keep Breathing" earlier in this chapter.**

   Before you receive the first touch of the massage, spend several minutes trying to clear your mind of any other thoughts. Concentrate only on your breathing.

2. **When your massage therapist first makes contact, imagine yourself breathing in through that very spot.**

   For example, if she starts by massaging your neck, imagine a stream of fresh oxygen and energy entering through your neck exactly where her fingers are.

3. **On the exhalation, imagine your muscles in that same area becoming softer, warmer, and looser.**

4. **Continue with this awareness, breathing relaxation into each successive point that the massage therapist touches.**

   Eventually, you become aware that the massage therapist is tuning in to your breath as well, and the massage becomes a shared meditation.

5. **Communicate with your massage therapist, both verbally and nonverbally.**

   Together, you can create a special massage mood that helps you focus on your experience, making the massage more like a meditation.

6. **Keep bringing your mind back to the massage.**

   You may realize at various points during the massage that your mind has wandered off on some train of thought. This situation is completely natural and happens even to advanced meditation practitioners. Simply bring your mind gently back to the breath and the relaxation. Don't worry about how good you are at meditation. Head to Stephan Bodian's *Meditation For Dummies,* 2nd Edition (Wiley) for more guidance and tips about meditation.

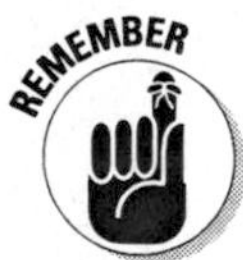

Although certain muscle knots and patterns of tension do respond well to firm, well-focused pressure, you don't necessarily need to experience it for yourself. Harder massage isn't always better massage, and at times the lightest touch can achieve the most profound benefits.

Rule 6: Listen to Your Emotions

Don't be surprised if during a massage one day you suddenly feel like crying your eyes out or laughing hysterically for no reason at all. Massage sometimes has that effect on people. Some of the reasons for this emotional response include the following:

- Certain emotional memories — usually the result of powerful experiences — can resurface when your body is massaged.
- No one has touched you with care, compassion, and gentleness for a very long time. In that case, the experience suddenly overwhelms you with gratitude, bringing forth tears.
- You're a very ticklish person.

As esoteric as the first two explanations may sound, they're entirely plausible. In fact, certain types of massage (for example, Rolfing) are famous for stirring up emotions. The explanation for this emotional component of massage is straightforward — your body and mind have faithfully recorded your every experience, but some of these experiences were so unpleasant that you filed them away in your unconscious and shut down certain feelings in the corresponding part of your body. Massaging the affected areas can bring your awareness back to your body, thus unlocking the memories.

If you encounter one of these emotional peaks yourself during a massage, relax, breathe, and allow it to happen. Remembering that you're safe in your present environment, let your mind drift to whatever images or memories seem to be surfacing. You may find yourself remembering all sorts of things that you hadn't thought of for years, and you can benefit from letting the attendant emotions flow freely through your body without trying to stifle them. Professional massage therapists are accustomed to this type of emotional release and know how to make you feel comfortable while it's happening. You don't need to feel embarrassed by the experience.

If, as occasionally happens, one of these resurfacing memories is particularly traumatic, such as in the case of abuse, do whatever is necessary to comfort yourself. Communicate with the person massaging you, letting her know that you need to sit up again, or get wrapped in a blanket for a feeling of safety. Have some tissues nearby to dry away tears. Later you can decide whether you want to pursue these memories further with the guidance of a psychologist or other counselor.

Rule 7: Blissing Out Is Okay

Sometimes, massage doesn't just make you feel great; it makes you feel ecstatic, rapturous, and filled with bliss. The feeling is visceral. You're lying there one minute relaxing (hopefully concentrating on your breathing — see "Rule 1: Keep Breathing" — but perhaps just going over your grocery list in your head) when KABOOM! It hits you, and suddenly you're just floating there in a syrupy sea of endorphins, not knowing what to do with yourself. I can tell you what to do: Enjoy this feeling while it lasts, because, like every other human experience, it passes.

These experiences are different for everyone, and nobody knows exactly what causes them. They've been responsible for many people changing their entire lives and heading in a new direction, sometimes even into a career as a massage therapist. And people with spiritual inclinations have created entire ministries devoted to the "laying on of hands" after they've been touched in this fashion.

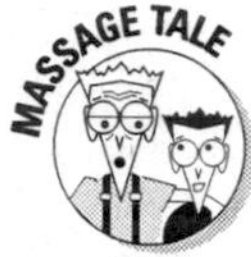

A minister named Zach Thomas from North Carolina once had such a powerful experience receiving a massage that he went on to become a massage therapist himself. At first, his church was opposed to his hands-on work, and Zach had to practice massage privately. Eventually, though, he took his skills and his compassionate touch out to the public, performing massage for dying people in hospices and hospitals. He helped form a group called the National Association of Bodywork in Religious Services (NABRS). Much of the work the members of this association do is for those people who wouldn't otherwise be able to afford it.

The spiritual secret behind massage? Simple: Massage is two people just being together fully in the present moment, which has been the essence of spiritual traditions forever, especially in the East. The mystical traditions of the West have expressed similar sentiments, as noted in the phrase, "Be still and know that I am God." These understandings are mystical in nature, not reserved for any one particular religion.

Think of it this way — massage is one sure-fire way to follow the Golden Rule that exists in almost all cultures and every religion, from the Good Samaritan to the compassionate Buddha. *Do unto others as you would have them do unto you.* Well, who doesn't want to be touched with care and compassion? Who doesn't like others to help them feel better and lighten their load? Massage is compassion turned into action.

Rule 8: It's Cool to Be Nude (Or Not)

Whether you like it or not, you're naked all the time beneath your clothes. You were born nude, just like every other human on the planet. Nudity is natural. However, each culture develops its own peculiar attitudes about nudity, ranging from those who consider it extremely awkward, embarrassing, and inappropriate at all times to those who don't think twice about it, anytime, anywhere, for any reason.

Neither attitude is healthier than the other, they're just different. The key for massage situations is to respect the attitudes of both people at all times. If either the person receiving or giving the massage is uncomfortable with any kind of skin exposure whatsoever, you're much better off to cover that area up and keep it covered than to cause discomfort. This guideline applies to the entire body, even the legs and arms, which most people are comfortable exposing. Although gliding an oiled palm is definitely easier over bare skin than covered skin, massage has other moves besides gliding, and you can give a very good massage to a fully clothed person. Some traditional techniques, such as Thai massage, never require the recipient to disrobe; instead, you receive your massage dressed in loose, comfortable pajamas.

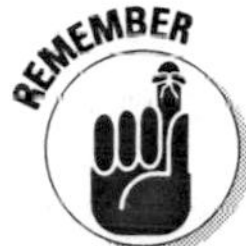

When you receive a massage, you're okay the way you are — nude or totally covered up. Just be comfortable.

Rule 9: You're the Boss

Even though you're lying down with your eyes closed during most massages, you're still in charge. With the slightest word or gesture, you can change the course of the proceedings. Deeper pressure? It's up to you. Slower pace? That's your call, too. Less chitchat? Your decision.

You have complete authority to change anything that may be making you uncomfortable. Requesting a change of music, for example, is perfectly permissible, as is turning the music off altogether. If you want to be covered more modestly, just ask. Whatever you say goes. You can say exactly what you're feeling, even ending the massage at any time, for any reason you want. Period. You always have the option of standing up and saying, "Enough!"

Of course, when you're receiving a massage from a professional massage therapist, listening to his suggestions makes sense. If he thinks you should quiet down and focus on the massage rather than conversation, for example, following his advice is probably a good idea. However, don't mistakenly place yourself in a submissive role just because you're lying down. Even if the other person knows more about massage than you, is older than you, or has a louder personality than you, the bottom line is, when you're receiving a massage, you're the boss.

Rule 10: Be Grateful

During the massage itself, spend some time being grateful for what you're experiencing in the moment. This course is by far the best one to take, instead of the alternatives, which consist of

- Wondering when the massage is going to end
- Plotting the next time you can get a massage
- Planning your next business trip
- Worrying about the world economy

Also, be sure to share your feelings of gratitude with the person who just gave you the massage, being especially vocal about her fantastic skills and techniques. That way, she looks forward to giving you your next massage as much as you look forward to getting it.

Chapter 7

Enjoying the Spa Experience (There and at Home)

In This Chapter

- Understanding spas
- Choosing the right spa
- Looking at fantastic spa treatments

Ever notice how some people seem like they were born with a silver-plated bottle of Evian water in their mouths? They're the corporate bigwig types out there living it up at expensive luxury spas, getting all the massages and fancy body treatments at the public's expense, right? Not!

Spas: More than just a pretty hot tub

Spas aren't, as commonly believed, just a kind of hot tub. Although the word *spa* has become interchangeable with *hot tub,* a spa can also be a really cool place where all kinds of exciting things (like chardonnay grape massages) take place.

Back in the good old days of King Louis' court in France (it may have been Louis XV, or XIV, or perhaps VIP . . . I'm not sure), certain ladies-in-waiting found themselves waiting around so much that they began feeling jaded. "Another typical almond-oil massage from our love slave, Gregory?" said one lady to the next. "How boring."

So, they came up with a new idea. Their servants filled huge vats with smashed chardonnay grapes, and the ladies proceeded to jump in *au naturel* for a total-immersion aromatherapy experience. The sensation was so new, and the positive effects of the grapes on their skin so pronounced, that they decided to make it a tradition.

Thus was born an early version of a spa treatment that can still be experienced today. The Meadowood Spa in Napa Valley, California, for example, offers a treatment based on this theme (ladies-in-waiting not included). The distilled essence of various grapes is infused into body scrubs and massage creams used by the massage therapists there.

Over the past several years, the household income of the average spa-goer has dropped dramatically. Today, spas are for everybody. As more and more *day spas* continue to open everywhere — in big cities and even the smallest towns — the experience of therapeutic luxury is becoming accessible to people from all walks of life. And if you're steadfastly opposed to spending money on yourself in this way, this chapter also contains a few tips and techniques to turn your very own home into a luxury spa almost for free.

Choosing a Spa

Today, whether you plan to immerse yourself in grapes, or to simply try to lose a few pounds and look your best, you can choose from a large array of spas to visit. They range from super-luxurious to down-home rustic. So how do you decide where to go?

First, knowing what kinds of spas you have to pick from helps. Spas fall into three basic categories:

- **Destination spas:** This type is the King Louis kind of spa, the sort of place you go when you want a super special experience. They're called *destination spas* because they're dedicated to the spa experience and nothing else. When people visit them, the spa is their final destination, and they usually stay for several days to a week.
- **Resort spas:** Becoming more and more popular, these spas are an important part of a larger resort. Guests may travel to the resort for other reasons, but many of them take advantage of the spa while they're there.
- **Day spas:** The fast-food joints of the spa world. *Day spas* are places to go to receive spa treatments, massages, and more, and you don't have to travel far or stay overnight to do so.

Several other sub-types of spas exist as well, including cruise ship spas, health club spas, mineral spring spas, medical spas, and even dental spas. About 15,000 spas are spread from coast to coast in the United States, and you can find tens of thousands more around the world.

Choosing a spa that's right for you

Spas range from rugged adventure outposts in the desert to the puffiest pampering palaces on the planet. You have almost unlimited choices when you're deciding where to go, which is great, but the number of choices may also make your decision kind of difficult. So, how do you choose?

Belgium: Home to more than just chocolate

What does the word *spa* really mean, anyway? The meaning derives from a town in modern-day Belgium that has healing hot spring waters bubbling out of the ground. The Romans called this town Spa, perhaps in reference to the Latin words *espa* (meaning "fountain") or *sparsa* (from *spargere,* meaning "to bubble up"). As in many Roman bathing towns, people used the springs for healing and relaxation. Roman centurions, for example, would go there to recuperate after battle.

In 16th century England, people began using springs medicinally in the same manner. One such spring, the Harrogate Tewit Well, was referred to in 1596 by English physician Dr. Timothy Bright as the "English Spaw." In this manner, the term spa began to be used as a general description of a place with healing waters rather than the one specific place in Belgium alone. You can go to Spa, Belgium yourself today and immerse yourself in the waters there.

One note: Many people think the word spa originally derived from an acronym for the Latin words, *Sanitas Per Aqua,* meaning "health through water." This acronym, however, was actually applied much later, when the word spa had already been in use for a long time. Acronyms are a relatively modern invention.

First, decide what's important to you and what you want to accomplish on your spa trip. You can usually break your goals down into a few basic categories: fitness, healing, spirituality, relaxation, or some combination of these.

Next, talk to someone who's been to your prospective spa before, or get the details from a reliable source. Here are three sources that may help you make the right match with a spa:

- Get in touch with Spa Finders travel agency and check out their magazine by calling 800 ALL-SPAS (800-255-7727) or visiting `www.spafinder.com`.
- Pick up the spa travel guide *Fodor's Healthy Escapes* (Fodor's Travel Publications) by Bernard Burt, which lists great spas of all types in many parts of the world.
- The International SPA Association (ISPA) has a Web site, `www.experienceispa.com`, featuring a section that can help you plan your next spa trip. Click "spa-goers" and then "search for a spa."

Some spas, such as the Green Valley spa in St. George, Utah, offer rock climbing on the menu right alongside their massages. Some spas expect you to join in on every exhausting 6-a.m. mountain hike they offer. Others leave you alone to steep in aromatic baths all day. You're sure to find one that meets your needs.

Visiting the spa down the street

These days, you can probably find a day spa available right in your very own neighborhood. Several multimillion dollar day spas have opened recently, but most are smaller operations run by individuals. Some existed first as hair salons that expanded into spa services. Good massage is going on at day spas, because many skilled massage therapists are finding work there.

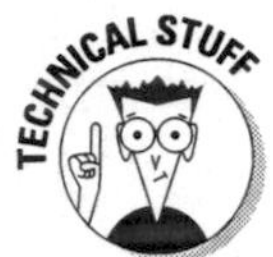

Although the true origins of the term *day spa* are somewhat shrouded in mystery, the term is generally attributed to a business woman and spa owner from Connecticut named Noelle DeCaprio. She started her day spa in 1978 and is credited with being the first person to classify her establishment in this manner.

Want to give your Aunt Minnie in Cleveland a spa surprise for her birthday, but you don't know how to set it up? Just call 1-888-SPA-WISH (888-772-9474) or visit `www.salonwish.com` and order a gift certificate that's good for massages, facials, and other treats at over 4,000 day spas and salons across the United States.

Creating Your Own Spa Treatments

So what do people actually do at spas all day, other than get massages? Believe it or not, they're also in pursuit of improved health. Yes, that's right. And the way they achieve it is to eat spa food, follow a spa exercise program, and receive what are known as *spa treatments,* all of which are good for you in one way or another. Spa treatments include

- Scrubs
- Wraps
- Hydrotherapy
- Facials
- Mud, seaweed, and other messy things

If you don't want to travel to one of the three types of spas to receive these treatments, you can create them at home for yourself and your family. The advantages of this approach are obvious. First, if you're like most people, you live right in your own home, so you don't have to travel far to get there. Also, having your husband, wife, or best friend wrap you in aromatherapy-infused sheets is a lot cheaper than paying a professional wrapper to do it.

For most people, a ten-day spa vacation in Maui is a little out of reach, except perhaps as a once-in-a-lifetime dream vacation. But you can still take advantage of your local day spa a few times a year and create some spa experiences for yourself at home whenever you feel like it. Each type of spa treatment I list in this section includes a version you can try at home, and, as you can see, they're not that difficult.

For the following treatments, you need a very specialized piece of equipment. Don't worry — it's very inexpensive, and it looks amazingly like a simple six-pack cooler (though I like to call it a *spa thermal unit* to impress people). Use it to store the hot moist towels that you need to wipe spa goop off your partner's body.

Scrubs

During their stay at a spa, many people sign up for an *exfoliation*, which is a word that comes from that ancient spa language, Latin. It means "to strip away dead leaves." In other words, it's a fancy name for a body scrub.

Body scrubs are good for you because they slough away dead skin cells, allowing your skin to breathe again and preparing your pores to absorb all those enriching ingredients like massage oils from India and mango bath salts from The Body Shop.

If you don't have the time or patience to create the entire body scrub experience that follows, try using a pair of *scrub gloves*. You can find them in beauty supply stores, drugstores, and gift shops. These textured gloves do the exfoliation for you while you simply rub the skin — no water, soaps, or other ingredients necessary.

Body scrub ingredients

Body scrubs are very easy to do. You need just a few simple ingredients:

- Loofah sponge
- 4 cups of warm water in a bowl
- 4 hot, moist, wrung-out hand towels in a cooler
- Washcloth
- 2 bath towels
- Body wash
- Exfoliant (either store-bought or homemade using the recipe that follows)

The exfoliant itself is quite simple. Mix ½ cup sea salt with approximately 3 tablespoons water a little at a time until you have a batter-like consistency, and then add three drops of your favorite essential oil. Any of the many over-the-counter skin scrubbing products you can buy at the beauty store or department store work quite nicely, too.

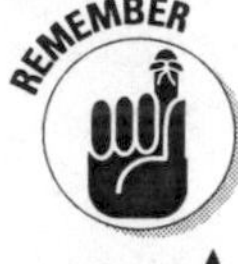

Never use sea salt or body exfoliants on the face. You can purchase exfoliants made specifically for the face in the cosmetics departments of most major department stores.

You may not want to do this treatment on your new $8,000 silk carpet from Turkey because drips and drops of salt and other ingredients may tend to find their way onto whatever surface you're using.

Step-by-step body scrub

The following steps show you how to create a body scrub that's as nice as one you experience at a spa. Just make sure to keep your partner warm because wet bodies cool down fast. You can cover the areas you're not working on with a towel.

1. **With your partner face down on a bath towel, moisten her back and the back of her legs with a washcloth or sponge as in Figure 7-1.**

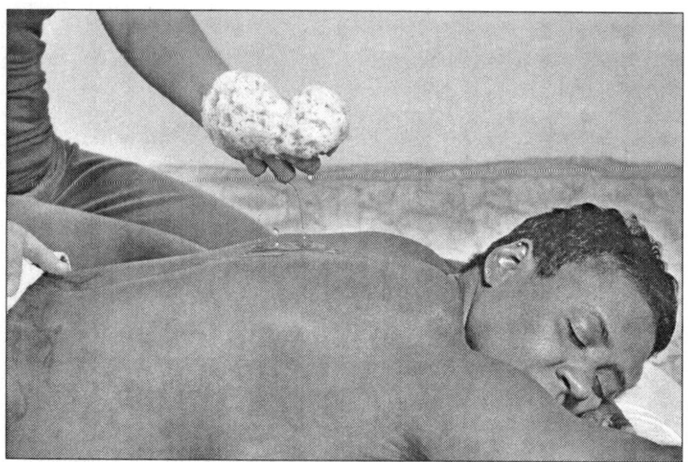

Figure 7-1: Moisten your partner's back.

2. **Place a dab of exfoliant in one palm and use circular movements to scrub your partner's skin as shown in Figure 7-2.**

   Keep replenishing the scrub as you move from one area to another.

3. **Use a hot, moist towel from the cooler to wipe off the exfoliant as Figure 7-3 illustrates.**

4. **Dip the loofah mitt in the bowl of water, squeeze a dab of body wash onto it, and then go back over your partner's skin again with circular movements, as shown in Figure 7-4.**

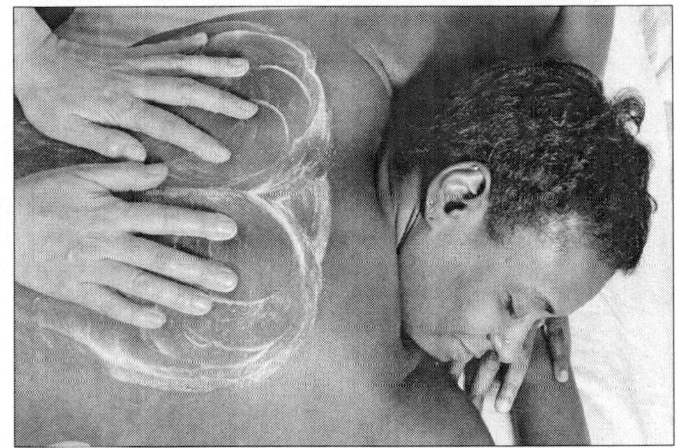

Figure 7-2: Exfoliate your partner with circular hand movements.

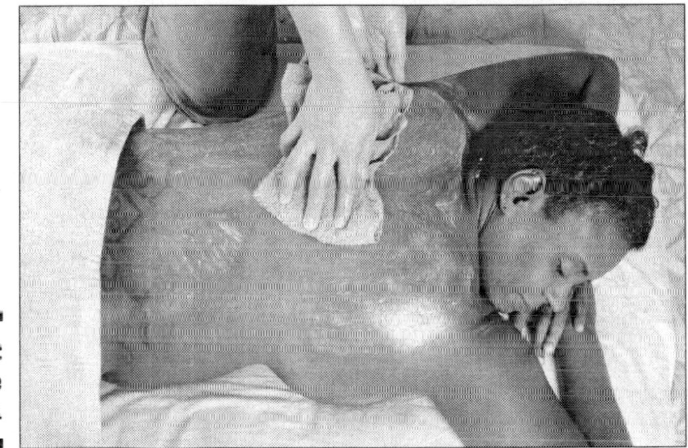

Figure 7-3: Wipe off the exfoliant.

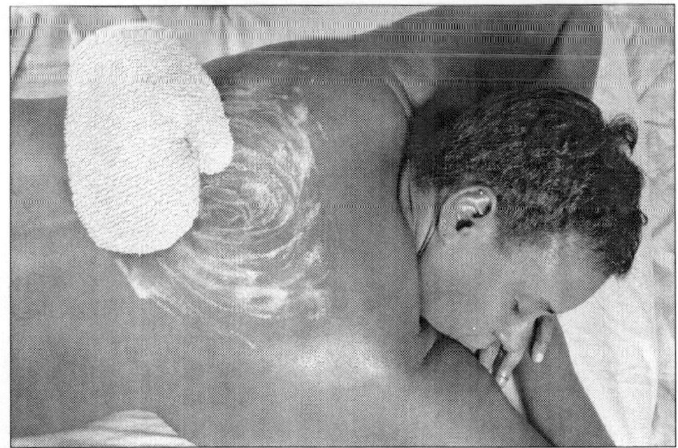

Figure 7-4: Sponge your partner with body wash.

5. **Use your second hand towel to wipe the skin as in Figure 7-5.**
6. **Have your partner turn over; repeat Steps 1 through 5 on the front of her legs, torso, and arms, covering any bits your partner wants with a towel or sheet.**
7. **When you've finished exfoliating the front of the body, apply some massage lotion to the skin as shown in Figure 7-6.**

   You can either do this application of lotion quickly, or you can linger and perform an entire massage, depending upon you and your partner's mood.

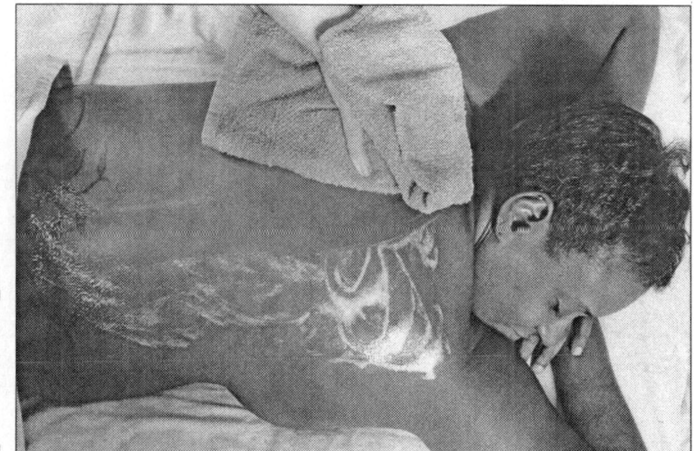

Figure 7-5: Wipe away the body wash.

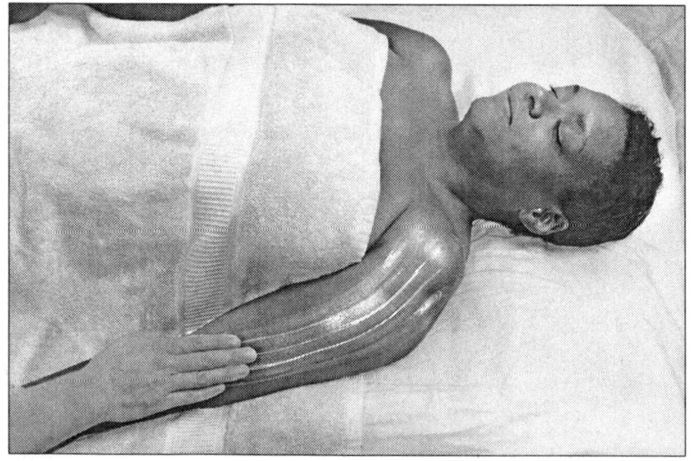

Figure 7-6: Apply massage lotion.

8. **Have your partner turn over once more, replacing the damp bath towel beneath her with a dry one, and apply skin lotion to her back and the backs of her legs.**

   If you used a towel to cover your partner in Step 6, you can reuse that towel here.

9. **Touch your partner's skin (or have somebody else touch it) gingerly, exclaiming, "Ooh, aah, you feel so smooth!"**

Facials

As you may know, the cosmetics industry is big business, with lots of expensive products for you to buy, but all you need in order to give yourself or a partner a very nice face treatment is a little bit of aloe and a ripe papaya. You never knew it could be so easy, did you?

Facial ingredients

You have to have just a few things ready in order to perform a fun and effective facial:

- 3 hot, moist hand towels in your cooler
- Cotton pads
- ½ a ripe papaya (no seeds or skin) mixed thoroughly with 1 teaspoon of aloe vera gel
- Skin cream

Step-by-step facial

Follow the steps in this section to create a relaxing, rejuvenating facial.

1. **Cleanse your partner's face with the cotton pads and remove any makeup.**
2. **Place a hot, moist towel on your partner's face and hold it in place for two minutes, allowing the pores to open.**

   Remember to leave an opening for the mouth and nose if you want your partner to be able to breathe through this procedure.

3. **Remove the towel and apply the papaya/aloe blend in a thin smooth layer over your partner's face, using your fingers as demonstrated in Figure 7-7.**
4. **Place another hot towel over your partner's face to keep the mixture moist.**

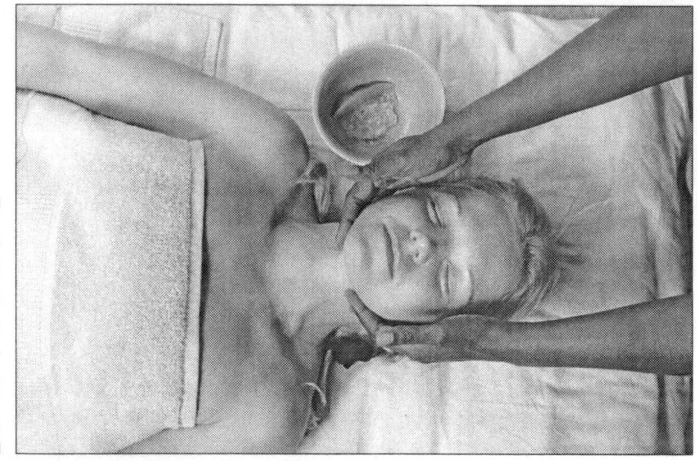

Figure 7-7: Smooth the facial mixture over your partner's face.

5. **Massage your partner's hands while her face is covered as Figure 7-8 demonstrates.**

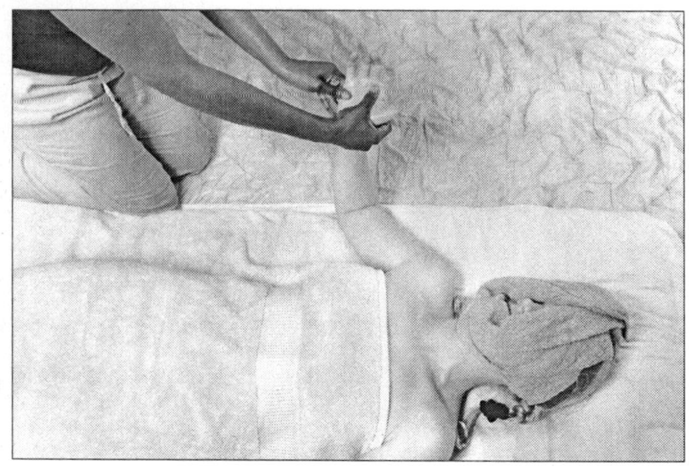

Figure 7-8: Massage your partner's hands.

6. **Exchange the towel for a warm one after a few minutes and continue massaging the hands.**
7. **Remove the towel, wiping off whatever's left of the papaya/aloe mixture with it as shown in Figure 7-9.**
8. **Using a face cream, do the face massage routine from Chapter 12.**

Remember to always stroke upwards when you're giving a facial, like professional estheticians do, so you don't pull down on the delicate collagen fibers that give your skin its tone.

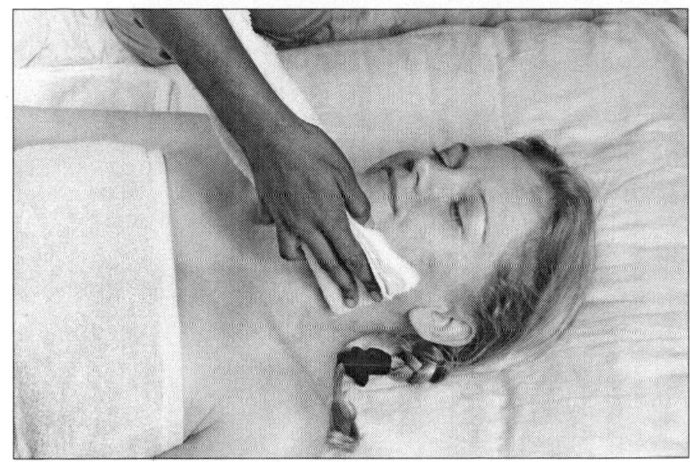

Figure 7-9: Wipe off the facial mixture.

Wraps

Some people think that body wraps are only good for losing inches. And certain wraps *can* help you slip into that red dress that's been hanging in your closet for years. But, as you've probably been told (by everyone except the manufacturers of the wraps), what you're really losing is water weight, which will, unfortunately, come back.

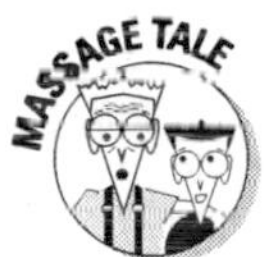

Serious health spas use wraps that detoxify the body, usually known as *herbal wraps.* They work by tricking your body into thinking it has a fever, causing it to purge itself of internal toxins. While working as a wrapper at big spas, I used to routinely unwrap people and find the sheets permeated with the smell of nicotine and other products that the client's body was purging.

My favorite wrap is the herbal wrap because it's the most deeply detoxifying, but I don't describe it for you here because it's quite involved and you should really have the right equipment to perform it. Other types of wraps, like seaweed and mud, for example, can get a little messy. So here I describe the nice 'n' neat aromatherapy wrap for you; it can be quite an enjoyable experience and doesn't create a laundry nightmare for you.

Aromatherapy wrap ingredients

For an aromatherapy wrap, all you need to do is gather up a sheet and a blanket and mix five or six drops of your favorite aromatherapy oil into a few tablespoons of unscented massage cream.

Warming this blend up a little before application is a nice touch.

Aromatherapy wrap step-by-step

To give a great aromatherapy wrap, just follow these easy steps:

1. **Have your partner lie face down on a sheet that is layered above a blanket as shown in Figure 7-10.**

   You can drape her with a towel as shown if she prefers.

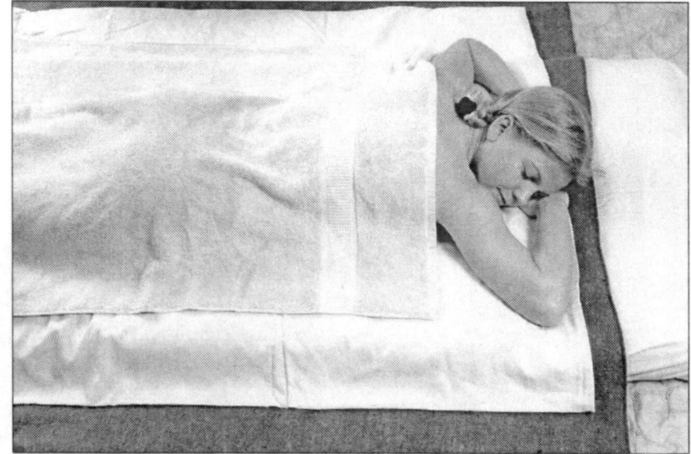

Figure 7-10: Lay your partner on a sheet and blanket.

2. **Rub a couple drops of your chosen essential oils in your palms and then allow your partner to breathe in the aroma for several moments by making a cup near her face as Figure 7-11 illustrates.**

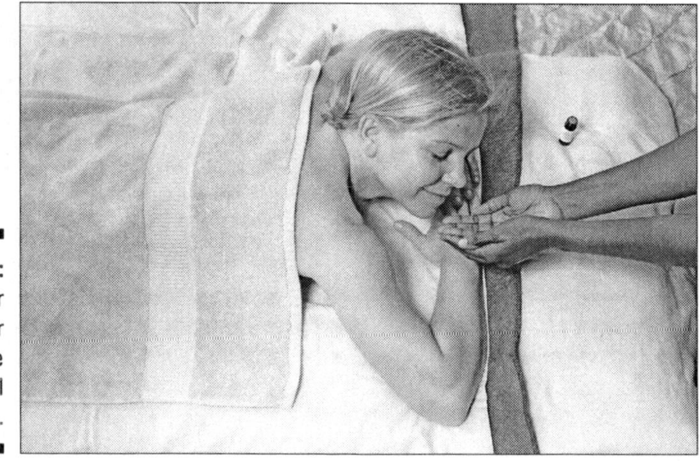

Figure 7-11: Let your partner breathe the essential oils' aroma.

3. **Apply the cream you scented to the back of your partner's legs, using light gliding movements as shown in Figure 7-12a, and then to her back as shown in Figure 7-12b.**

   This step lasts about 15 minutes.

4. **Have your partner turn over; begin applying the cream to her feet and legs, using light, hypnotically slow techniques as shown in Figure 7-13.**

5. **Cover your partner's legs with a sheet as you complete application and then apply the cream to her torso and arms as Figure 7-14 demonstrates.**

6. **Sit at the head of the table and apply the cream to your partner's shoulders, neck, and face as in Figure 7-15.**

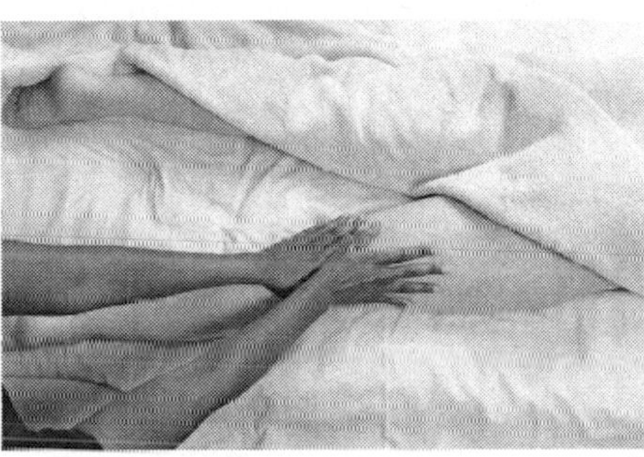

a

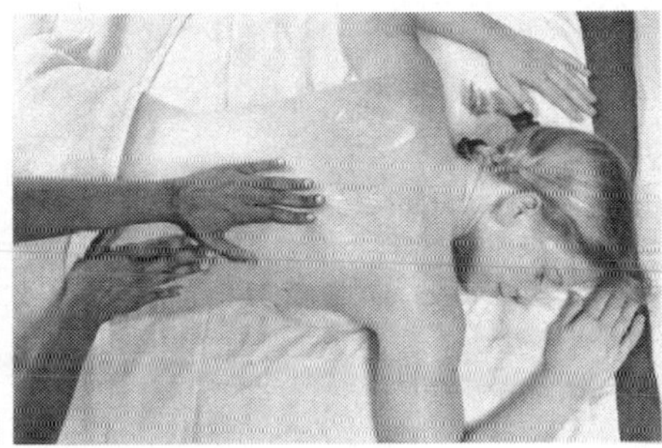

b

Figure 7-12: Apply massage cream to your partner's legs and back.

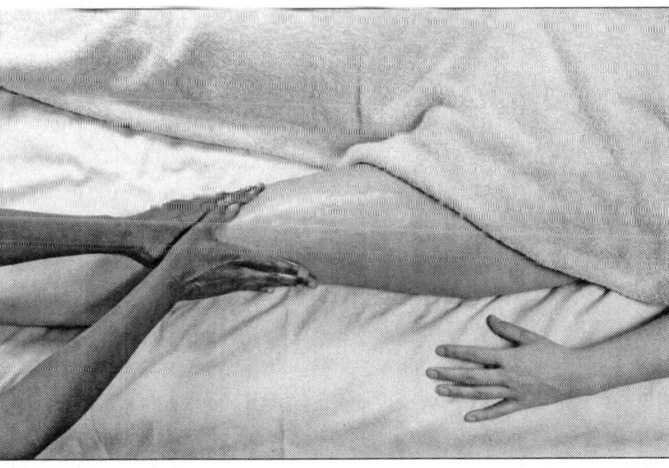

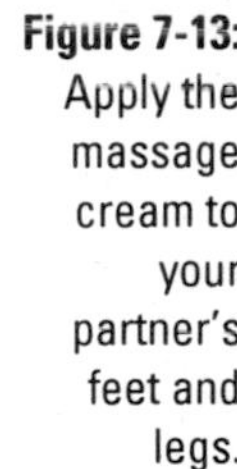

Figure 7-13: Apply the massage cream to your partner's feet and legs.

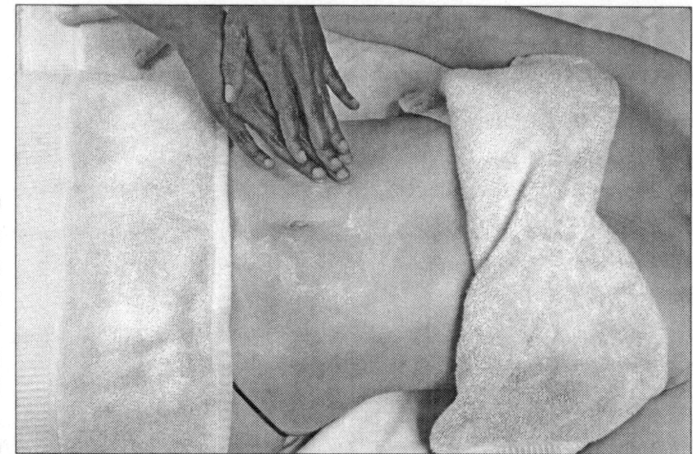

Figure 7-14: Apply the cream to your partner's torso and arms.

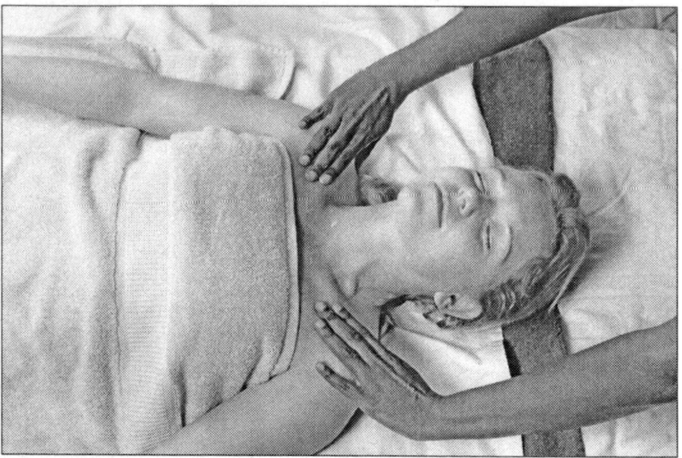

Figure 7-15: Apply the massage cream to your partner's shoulders, neck, and face.

7. **Wrap the sheet and underlying blanket around your partner's entire body and then place a pillow beneath her knees, assuring that she's comfortable.**
8. **Leave your partner wrapped for 20 minutes while you sit at the head of the table and apply light massage to her face and head as shown in Figure 7-16.**
9. **Unwrap your partner and help her sit up and stand.**

   You can leave the lotion and aromatherapy oils on to soak further into the skin.

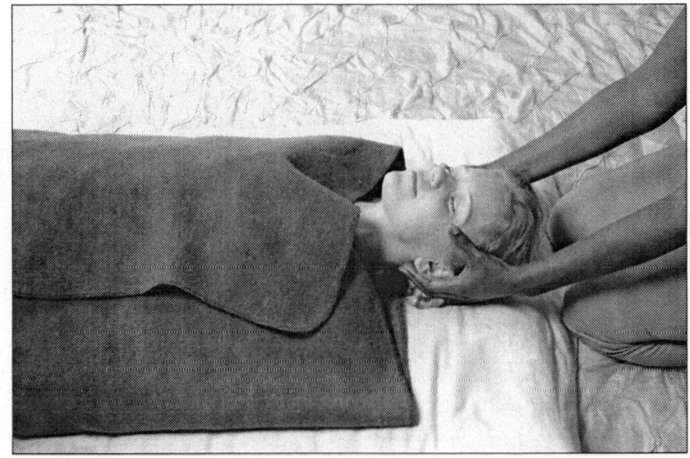

Figure 7-16: Massage your partner's face and head while she's wrapped.

Hydrotherapy

Hydrotherapy is a word that means, obviously, therapy with fire hydrants. Just kidding . . . but that description is actually quite close to the truth. Would you believe, for example, that people pay good money in spas to stand naked against a tile wall while a hydrotherapy expert sprays a blast of cold water at them from a pressure hose? It's true (it's called a *Scotch Hose treatment*).

Hydrotherapy treatments in luxury spas can also involve the use of super-expensive *hydrotherapy tubs,* which look like a cross between a bathtub and a hot tub. You don't need to be in one of these tubs to experience hydrotherapy. In fact, your own bathtub or shower at home will do just fine.

Here are a few ideas for taking advantage of your own water source to do a little hydrotherapy at home:

- **Bathe someone.** For most of us, the last time we were bathed was in early childhood by our mothers, and we've forgotten how soothing it is. Using a pitcher, pour warm water over your partner's head, shoulders, and back in the bath. Then wash her slowly and luxuriously.
- **Take a cold plunge.** Many spas have what's known as a cold plunge, which is a pool kept at a shockingly low temperature. Patrons jump in after being heated up in saunas and whirlpools. You can simulate the extremely invigorating effects of this activity by drawing a cold bath and immersing yourself for 30 seconds (or as long as you can stand it).
- **Share a bath with a friend.** First, make sure the friend wants to share the bath with you. After you determine that, slip into a tub of warm water with 10 drops of aromatherapy oil added, and see what happens next. It may not be entirely therapeutic, but it certainly will be fun.

A day of pleasure

The spa lifestyle is for everyone — unless you're the type who disdains pleasure and health, like the flagellant monks of the Middle Ages, for example, who used to wander around the streets beating themselves with sticks. If that's your idea of fun, definitely stay away from anything to do with spas.

If, on the other hand, you have what it takes to treat yourself to some healthy enjoyment in life, why not plan an entire day of spa pleasures? The sultans used to do it, and so did Cleopatra with rose petals a foot thick on the floor of her love chamber. But how about you?

You can recreate a day of luxury just like the ones people experience at spas. Trade each treatment with a lucky partner and spend the day together. Then go out and celebrate your indulgence with a healthy meal at a restaurant. The whole exchange (not including dinner) takes about 5 hours. Just follow these simple steps:

1. First, start with a body scrub to cleanse the skin and prepare you to absorb the healthy effects of the oils and other ingredients to follow.
2. Take turns soaking in a bath (or soak together if you're so inclined), with a dozen drops of your favorite aromatherapy oil or a few ounces of healing herbs added.
3. Exchange long luxurious massages, following along with the step-by-step instructions in Chapters 11 and 12.
4. Give each other a spa facial to prepare yourselves for reentry into the world.

Mud, seaweed, and other messy things

Other kinds of spa treatments work, too, but I don't go into them here, because if you tried them at home you may mess up your furniture or carpet. These treatments involve the use of such products as mud, seaweed, and clay — and they can be really messy! If you do experiment with these products (many of which are available at cosmetics counters and in beauty supply stores), try to confine your activities to the bathroom, where you're less likely to stain things.

Part III
The Art of Giving Massage

The 5th Wave
By Rich Tennant
©RICHTENNANT
My fault! My fault! Too much oil!
Dora Van
MASSAGE THERAPIST

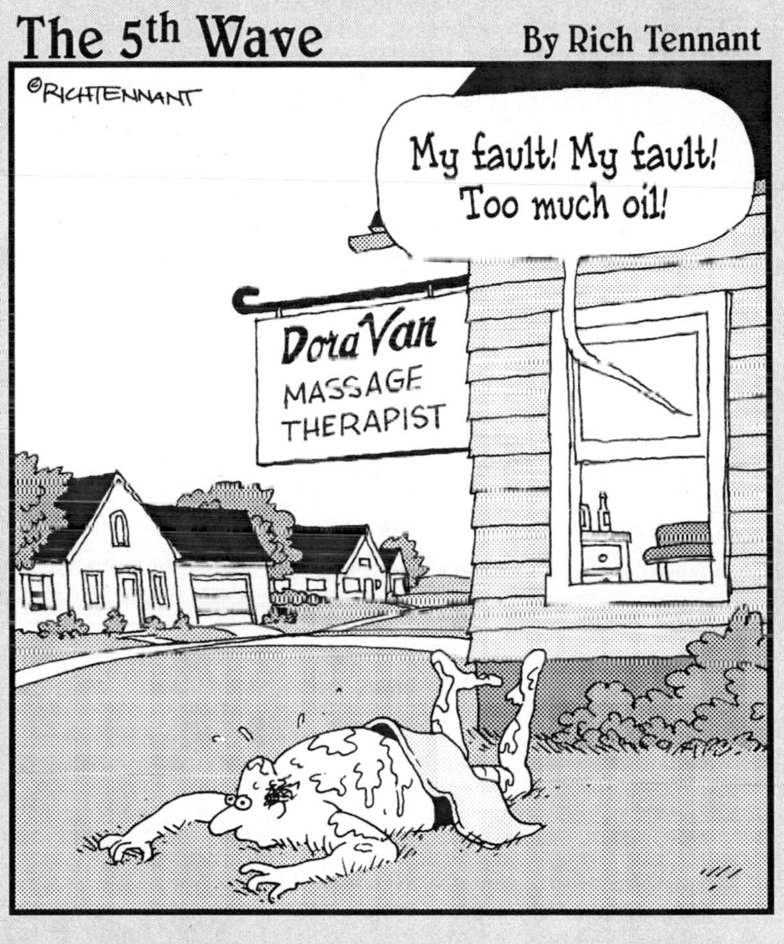

In this part . . .

You're no doubt familiar with the famous expression "It's better to give than to receive." And if you're like most people, every time you've heard someone utter that wonderful phrase, filled as it is with such a beautiful philanthropic message, you've thought to yourself, "Yeah, right. I'll take receiving any day."

But you have to admit, a certain gratification comes from giving that quite often actually feels more meaningful and fulfilling than receiving does. And the secret to achieving that kind of fulfillment is that you have to give with your whole heart. It won't work if you're just going through the motions.

This idea is especially true for massage. Massage is about cultivating the right attitude — the giver's attitude — not just applying mechanical maneuvers, which any massage text can teach you. Sure, you can rub some warmed almond oil on your partner's back for 20 minutes while watching the clock with one eye and the football game on TV with the other, but that's not what massage is all about.

But don't worry: In this part of the book, you discover how to actually give a massage, too! Just follow the simple instructions, and in no time, you'll be reproducing the very same techniques you see being performed by the highly trained models in the photographs. No problem.

Of course, you also need to know a few safety precautions and techniques for creating the most suitable environment for a great massage, and you find that information in this part as well. I also offer some advice for those considering massaging for a living (which has become a very viable career in recent years).

Chapter 8

Setting the Stage for a Great Massage

In This Chapter

- Making sure that everything smells, looks, and sounds right
- Deciding where to set up
- Creating the "massage mood"
- Trading places

Say your husband or wife or roommate sees you reading this book for hours on end and eventually says something to you like, "Hey, how about giving *me* a massage? Right now!"

Your immediate response should be

A. "Sure, lie down on the linoleum here, and we'll get started."

B. "No way, I'm too nervous about ever actually doing this stuff."

C. "I haven't finished the book yet."

D. "Okay, but first give me a few minutes to set the stage."

Yes, oh intelligent massage student, you've once again chosen correctly. The answer is D. Your partner definitely appreciates it if you take a little time to set up a special environment before you begin the actual massage. And if you're in a less-than-ideal environment, don't worry. You can materialize a magical massage mood just about anywhere if you use some of the ideas in this chapter to create your own inner chamber — a special, relaxing environment where a massage can have its best effect.

Scents, Sights, and Sounds: Engaging the Senses

One of the big secrets to giving a good massage has very little to do with the massage itself. It has to do, rather, with where the massage is happening. And I'm not talking about exotic locales like Bali or Atlantic City; I'm referring to more accessible locations, like your bedroom or the couch in your den.

So how do you turn these everyday places into someplace special? You can do it easily by involving all the senses.

Massage, of course, relies heavily upon the senses for its effects. Your sense of touch, especially, is being bombarded the entire time you're giving or receiving a massage. But it would be a mistake to neglect the other senses; they can add greatly to your massage experience, too.

The sense of taste doesn't usually play a big part in massage, unless of course you like to use edible massage oils like strawberry, almond, and mint that are . . . whoops, I think we're straying a little beyond the scope of this chapter. Check out Chapter 16 for more information on sensual massage, including the use of all kinds of flavored oils.

Anyway, for now the following sections concentrate on the three remaining senses that come into play during a massage experience, also known as the three *S*s of your inner chamber: scents, sights, and sounds.

Scents

Professional massage therapists often coach their clients through some deep-breathing techniques as part of the massage. And, as you may suspect, all that breathing includes quite a bit of smelling, too. That's part of the reason why massage pros have so much concern about the way their workrooms smell. In addition, they also know how powerful the sense of smell can be for healing and relaxation.

The following sections discuss three options for incorporating scent into the massage experience.

Just sniffing a whiff of corn muffins like the ones your Aunt Betty used to bake when you visited her on weekends as a kid is enough to send you reeling back through the years. Why is that so? Aromas trigger a mighty emotional response because the molecules that enter your nose don't mess around.

They do not pass *Go;* they do not collect $200. Instead, they take a direct route straight into the *limbic system,* which is the seat of your emotions and memories. This fact is a key to the power of *aromatherapy* — and by this I don't mean just aromatherapy oils but also other aromas used during massage, such as incense and even flowers.

Aromatherapy

If you use advanced grammatical techniques to break down the word *aromatherapy,* you discover that it means "therapy with aromas." Aha! So, does that mean therapy with just any aroma, such as the aroma of sautéed onions, for example, or the aroma of diesel fuel at dawn?

Hardly. Aromatherapy is the use of highly concentrated *essential oils* from certain plants to stimulate the brain. This stimulation causes a positive effect on the nervous and glandular systems and thus the entire body. During a massage, you can use aromatherapy in several ways. In Chapter 9 you find out how to mix up an aromatherapy massage oil, but here are three other aromatherapy products that can help you scent your massage space:

- **Diffusers:** As the name suggests, a diffuser diffuses aroma into the air. Several inexpensive models ($10 to $15) are available that use a miniature fan. Simply place a few drops of your favorite oil on a cotton pad, turn on the fan, and the scent of essential oils fills the room.
- **Candles:** Many commercially available candles have essential oils worked right into the wax, and burning one during a massage is a great way to combine effects in two of the three *S*s, sight and scent. Until recently, you had to visit a specialty shop to purchase aromatherapy candles, but now they're even available at your local grocery store or drugstore.
- **Bulb rings:** These little doodads were popular in the 1970s when they were used to cover up even more exotic aromas floating around the room at parties. Now they're making a comeback as aromatherapy aids. Basically, they're floppy little rings that you place over a light bulb. When you sprinkle several drops of essential oil into the ring and turn on the bulb, presto! — instant aromatherapy.

If aromatherapy is something you're keenly interested in, I recommend *Aromatherapy For Dummies* by Kathi Keville (Wiley), a book that promises to answer that age-old question, "How can I smell better and feel better at the same time?"

Incense

The musky, natural scents that burning incense creates can turn your inner chamber into a mystical and exotic environment, even if in reality it's just your guest bedroom. The problem is, many people overdo it with incense, fumigating the room with enough mystical and exotic smoke to choke themselves, their partner, and any unsuspecting insects living in the walls. This is not a relaxing setting.

When it comes to incense, a little goes a long way. Use it with moderation, and you can create just the right mood. If you're using one of those long thick sticks of incense, snap it off two-thirds of the way down and burn just the last bit. Also, you can crack a window open, weather permitting, to circulate a little fresh air with the smoke.

Flowers

Nothing beats the scent of fresh flowers in your massage area. You don't need a big vase and a big budget to make it happen, either. All that's necessary is a small bowl, a cup, or a mug from the kitchen cabinet that you fill with water and a single flower. Roses or gardenias work especially well. Snip the flower off the stem and float it on the water. This fills the air with scent for hours or even days.

If you want to get really romantic, spread some fresh petals on the bed or other massage surface to set the mood. Cleopatra had her love chamber filled with rose petals before Antony made his big entrance.

Sights

Focusing on the sights of a massage space may seem funny to you because, after all, the person receiving the massage probably has her eyes closed most of the time anyway. But during those few minutes when she first enters, and whenever she opens her eyes, she soaks in her surroundings. You can use a few simple items to add to the relaxing ambience (some of which also stimulate the sensed of smell; see the preceding section):

- **Candles:** Candles cast an enchanting glow over any massage experience.
- **Flowers:** Even a small bunch of silk flowers placed with care near the massage area shows this is someplace special.

- **Lighting:** You can do some simple things with lighting to make your space massage-friendly:
  - **Turn the lights down low.** This move helps the person on the receiving end concentrate more on the massage, perhaps because she doesn't feel like you are scrutinizing her body under a microscope.
  - **Throw a silk scarf over a lampshade to create instant mood lighting during a massage.**

- **Color:** Drape the area with soft, colorful fabrics.

Sounds

Carefully selected sounds serve two main purposes during a massage:

- They add to the mood.
- They mask distracting sounds like traffic noises and TVs.

You can make sound a part of your massage in a number of really interesting ways, and you may find that some massage pros carry an entire arsenal of sound makers to add to their clients' experience. Some of my favorites include

- **Meditation bowls:** These look like simple brass or ceramic bowls, but when you glide a finger or wooden instrument along the rim, they sing out beautifully with rich, vibrant tones.
- ***Ting shaks:*** A Tibetan invention, you strike these heavy brass bells together to form a clear, long-lasting tone that sets a meditative mood for a massage.
- **Wind chimes:** A classic in the relaxing-sounds category, literally thousands of types are available. If you can't be near an open window to hear the chimes, place them indoors near an oscillating fan to simulate blowing breezes.

Water

You know those cute little burbling pots filled with rocks and miniature waterfalls? You can find them in a lot of gift shops these days, and they definitely add a lot to the ambience of a massage. If you're the industrious type, you can build a little indoor fountain for yourself. All it takes is a container, some rocks, and a small submersible water pump.

Of course, being outside near a source of natural flowing water is a great choice, too, but then you have to consider other details, such as temperature, rain, insects, and privacy.

One thing to remember: The sound of running water seems to have a powerful effect on the bladder. Make extra sure your partner visits the bathroom before receiving a massage with a waterfall nearby.

Music

Music, of course, is the most popular type of sound used to complement massage. In most big spas, for example, they pump music directly into the massage rooms from a central sound system, putting the guests in the right mood to relax and unwind.

An entire industry has sprung up to provide music appropriate for massage. If you want to experience some of the most popular massage music, try putting one of the following CDs on the next time you exchange a massage:

- George Winston, *December*
- Mark Kelso, *For God Alone*
- Anything by Stephen Halpern
- Anything by George Skaroulis
- Brian Eno, *Music for Airports*
- Ray Lynch, *Music to Disappear Into*
- Enya, especially *Orinoco Flow*
- Yanni, especially *In My Time*
- Any relaxing classical music, such as Pachelbel's "Canon"

Don't get the wrong idea here, though. Massage music doesn't necessarily have to be flutes or harps or Yanni 'til you yawn. You can be creative in your choices, and sometimes the best massages are given to the most unlikely accompaniment, like the reggae classic "Jamming" by Bob Marley.

Working with the Location You've Got

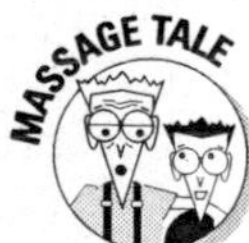

Once, in a typically cramped New York City apartment, I had to give a massage on the only available large flat surface, which turned out to be a wooden dining room table. We laid a few blankets and pillows down on it, and I scurried from side to side dodging walls and other furniture, but in the end my client reported feeling quite comfortable and loved his massage. I don't recommend this setup, but you definitely don't need a fancy expensive massage table or a special peaceful room in your house in order to give a good massage.

You can comfortably give massages in any room, including living rooms, bedrooms, family rooms, and as the story above points out, even the dining room. There are a few issues you want to keep in mind, though, when deciding where to give a massage:

- **Privacy:** Be sure to respect the level of privacy the person receiving the massage desires. If possible, choose a room where you can close the doors to keep other people out. On the other hand, some people actually prefer to be less private, and they are more comfortable in an area with some activity.
- **Warmth:** Avoid areas with a draft or air conditioning vent directly overhead.
- **Intentions:** To avoid possibly sending the wrong message, you may want to avoid giving massage in a bedroom if the person receiving is not your romantic partner.
- **Space:** You need some space to maneuver around in — perhaps more than you realize. Before you begin, make sure you have enough room on all sides to move without disturbing your partner.

Escaping the Real World

When someone's receiving a massage, she wants to pretend that she's on a secluded tropical isle with no one else around for miles. She's a Polynesian princess, the center of attention, and the person giving the massage is focused on her and her alone. Exotic birds are floating overhead, and one lone white sail puffs out on the aquamarine horizon . . . then, suddenly, she hears a voice: "Bart just threw up on my homework!"

Yes, your partner will find it difficult to achieve her ultimate romantic illusion if, in real life, she's receiving her massage on the couch in your den, with *The Simpsons* turned up full blast on the TV.

Do your partner a favor — indulge her in her illusions. Although it's not always possible to take a trip to Fiji to give your massage, you can avoid some of the more obvious distractions quite easily:

- Turn off the TV.
- Put up a little "Do Not Disturb" sign.

- Try to schedule the massage for a time when there are few interruptions.
- Turn off the ringer on the phone and turn down the volume on the answering machine.

Developing the "Massage Mood"

What I've included in this chapter so far are the external aspects of the inner chamber. But, of course, when it comes to inner chambers, the inside is what counts, and this section is about the way you and your partner feel on the inside. Even if you find yourself in a less-than-ideal situation to give massage, with distractions abounding, no music to listen to, and not a candle in sight, you can still create the most important aspect of that inner chamber, the "massage mood."

When you first lay your hands upon someone else to give them a massage, what's going through your mind? Chances are, you're a little nervous, a little uncertain of how the other person is going to receive you. And that's all right. It means you care. But how about how *she's* feeling? You, as the giver, are in charge of creating the optimal mood for her experience.

In order to create an appropriate mood for the other person, what you have to do first is get into that mood yourself. By imagining yourself in one of the following four personas as you begin a massage — saint, doctor, mother, or buddy — you can quickly adopt the mood that goes with it. Then you can give your partner something that comes from deep inside, creating the true inner chamber:

- **Saint:** Part of giving a good massage is having some simple compassion for the person you're touching. After all, you're in the same boat, both of you anchored to a fragile body in an uncertain world. You can reach out to others when you massage them, crossing the barriers of separation, sending the message that you understand how they feel. To use the golden rule, touch others as you would have them touch you.
- **Doctor:** If you're just a beginner, you shouldn't be out there trying to fix your Aunt Jeanne's sciatica with your massage techniques. However, you create a better mood by thinking in terms of helping the person feel better, not just rubbing oil on. As you begin a massage, imagine your hands filled with healing energy, communicating the intention to soothe and make whole.
- **Mother:** Who ever cared about you more than good ol' Mom? She had a level of acceptance for your quirks and shortcomings that was just plain astounding. You can aim that same kind of unconditional love toward

your massage partner (at least for that one hour), making him feel perfect just the way he is.

- **Buddy:** Don't let all this serious stuff about saints and doctors scare you away from giving a massage. Another, more lighthearted giver's personality is that of the buddy. You can just hang out together and have some fun while you're exchanging massage. Go ahead, put a little reggae on the CD player. Tell a few jokes to break the ice. Relax and have an easy conversation during the massage. Sometimes this is the best choice when your partner is apprehensive about receiving the massage.

Finding Someone to Swap Massages with after the Mood Is Set

Finding a professional massage therapist with whom you can trade money for massage is not difficult. Money seems to be a great motivational tool when it comes to getting people to massage you. Finding an amateur, however, can be very tricky. By definition, you are not going to pay the amateur, and therefore you must offer some other form of incentive to get him to give the massage. Most frequently this incentive comes in the form of a reciprocal massage. But what if that's not enough to motivate your partner?

Say you've got this really neat environment set up, with lavender-scented candles flickering, and you've meditated for half an hour, eventually entering a state of transcendent Zen sainthood, ready to give the best massage of your life. Then you slowly open your eyes and discover that you're alone in the room with nobody to massage. You must find somebody to trade with.

Your mate is not the only person with whom you can form a massage-trade relationship. Other potential partners include

- Somebody who practices massage professionally. It may surprise you how many pros don't receive massage nearly as often as they'd like — your offer to trade, although you're less experienced, is likely to be met with considerable enthusiasm.
- Members of your church.
- Members of your family.
- Friends of the family.
- Members of a sports team you're on.

Finding a way to be comfortable trading massages may be challenging at first. It's an admittedly intimate form of sharing, and not everyone takes to it right away. One good alternative to jumping straight into a full body massage is to try offering a back massage. Or try some massage with your partner's clothes still on. You find plenty of nonthreatening options in the chapters to come.

Fighting "TFS"

I'm trying not to be sexist here, but statistical evidence suggests that one gender in particular has motivational problems when it comes to *giving* massage. Yes, I'm talking about males, 95 percent of whom, when asked by their loving partners to give a massage, develop an instantaneous and very debilitating case of temporary fatigue syndrome (TFS). Even the thought of moving just a pinkie finger suddenly makes them feel very tired. As soon as the request for massage is withdrawn, however, they bounce back incredibly fast and can often be observed playing touch football just moments later.

Here are some ways to motivate a partner who is the unfortunate victim of TFS:

- Suggest to him that his love life might suffer dire consequences unless he gives you a massage.
- Suggest to him that his love life could be greatly enhanced were he to be so kind as to give you a full-hour massage.
- In exchange for the massage, offer to let him go shopping at his favorite store (camping store, hardware store, computer store, beer store, and so on) and don't bug him about spending time there.
- If he agrees to massage you at least three times, let him pick the destination for your next vacation (yes, even if it's bass fishing on Lake Okeechobee).

Chapter 9

Stocking Your Massage Tool Chest

In This Chapter

- Preparing a comfortable setting
- Working with massage oils
- Strengthening your body to give better massages
- Finding out the rules for massage

This chapter is all about stocking your massage tool chest with oils and sheets and towels and so on, but first I just wanted to say that this stuff is not what's most important. What really matters are your *self* and your *good intentions*. The rest is just icing on the cake.

That said, many people believe that the tastiest part of a cake is usually the icing, so getting the "massage icing" just right is important so that you can enjoy the entire dessert that is a great session of massage therapy. Therefore, this chapter focuses on some simple yet essential topics that make your massage experience that much more delicious.

First, you discover where the best places are to perform a massage, making yourself comfortable in whichever environment you happen to find yourself, even on the floor. Next, I give you a little advice about sheets and towels and oils and such because the wrong oil can spoil an otherwise perfect massage. I help you build up a few muscles you didn't even know you had, your "massage muscles," so you can keep going when your partner begins raving about how wonderful your hands feel. Finally, I offer a few basic "rules" to help you give the best massage you can possibly give.

Setting Up

I assume here that you've created a suitable *inner chamber* for your massage experience as I discuss in Chapter 8 and that now you're chomping at the bit, all ready to get your hands on somebody for gosh sake. Whoa, there! You can practice massage moves in Chapter 10. Here, you find out how to set up and organize your supplies before you begin.

Table (or floor) for one?

You may notice that the massage in this book is being given on the floor. You always have a floor available someplace to work on, right? But you probably don't have a massage table like the ones the pros use. For those of you not familiar with them, massage tables are oblong, padded tables. Most of them have legs of adjustable height, and some of them are even portable like the one in Figure 9-1. These tables are great tools, and if you get serious about massage at some point, you may want to consider investing in one. New ones cost a few hundred dollars.

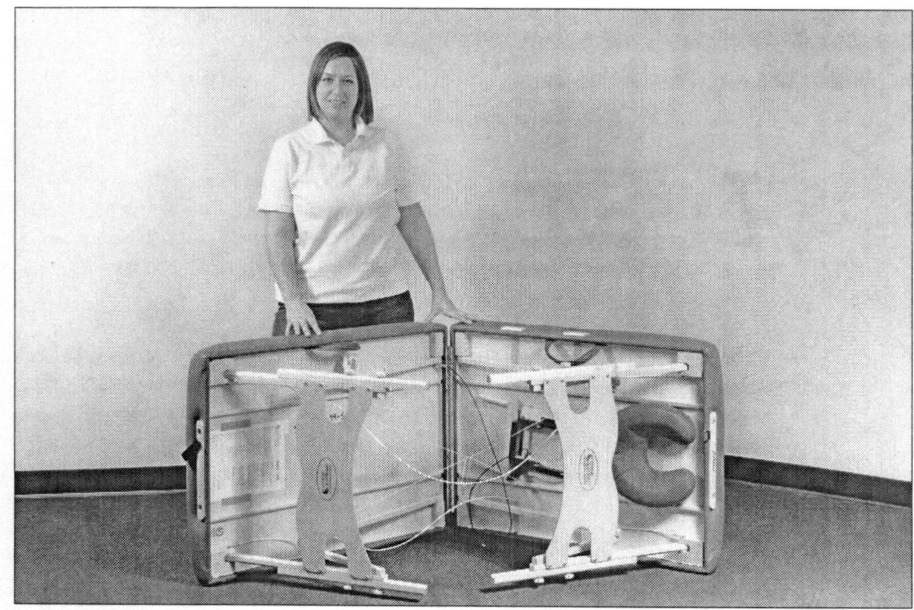

Figure 9-1: Massage tables look like oblong, upholstered card tables.

Massage tables are nice, but the floor can be quite a comfortable place to get a massage, especially if you add a few pillows, a sofa cushion or two, plus a sheet and towels, as you can see in Figure 9-2.

Many massages have been given on beds, but in those cases the massage often leads to other activities — like sleeping! That's right, it's very tempting for the giver to just roll over and lounge around instead of working like he should. When you do give a massage on a bed, have your partner lay on towels near the foot or along one edge of the bed so that you don't have to be up on the bed yourself the whole time you're giving the massage.

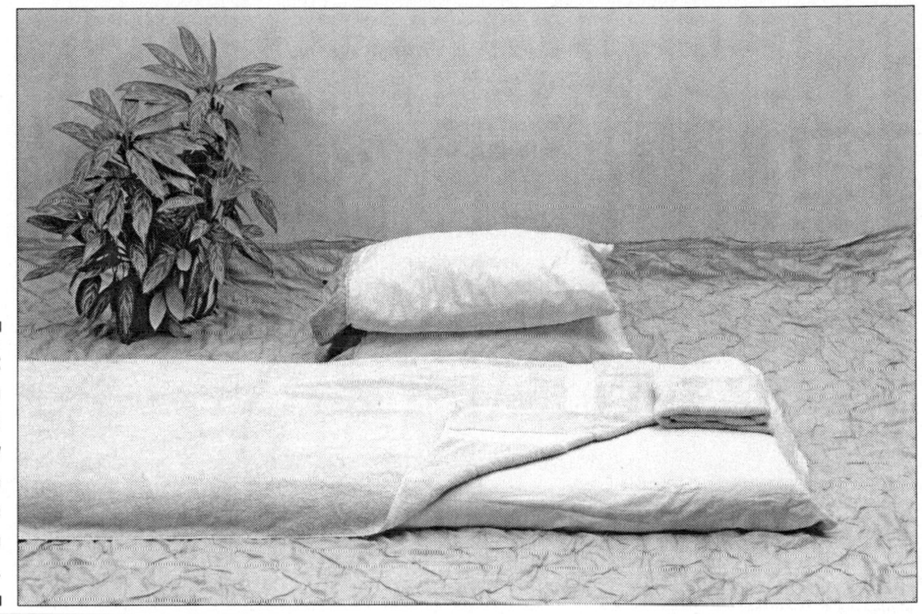

Figure 9-2: You can create a perfectly comfortable massage space on the floor.

Sheets, towels, and so on

You want to have one sheet to cover the surface you are working on and one sheet or towel to cover those areas of your partner you aren't currently massaging. Bath sheets are nice to use over the body because they're thick and fluffy and provide an extra feeling of security and warmth, especially if you warm them up in a dryer for a few minutes prior to beginning the massage. This extra step is a nice touch when the weather is cold, and your partner will greatly appreciate it.

Don't use your best sheets and towels to do a massage on because the oils and creams can leave stains and a musty oil smell behind. Also, the color white seems to show off oil stains the most. Many spas and massage studios use darker colored linens, like brown, green, or blue, for this reason.

Other things you may want to have around include heating pads, blankets, bottle warmers, and other such comfort-creating devices. Nothing's worse than getting a massage and not being able to concentrate on how good it feels because you're shivering the whole time.

You can further increase your partner's comfort by supporting his knees and ankles with some extra pillows used as *bolsters,* as shown in Figures 9-3a and 9-3b. Massage pros use special bolsters made out of foam covered with fabric and shaped into contours that fit the body, but don't you worry about that. You can just say, "Bolsters? I don't need no stinkin' bolsters," and then grab the closest pillow instead. If you use one of your nice pillows, cover it with a towel to keep it from getting stained by oil.

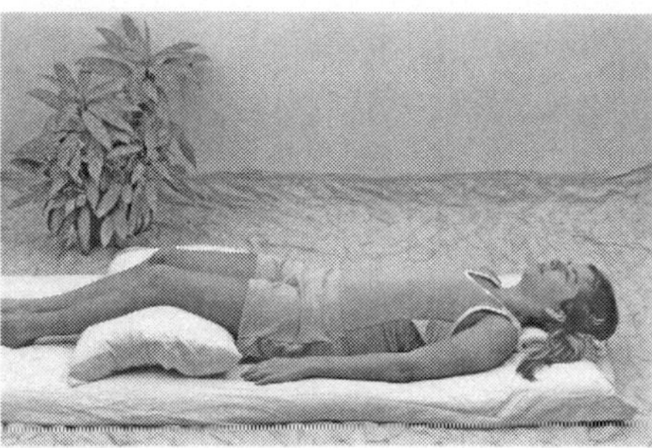

a

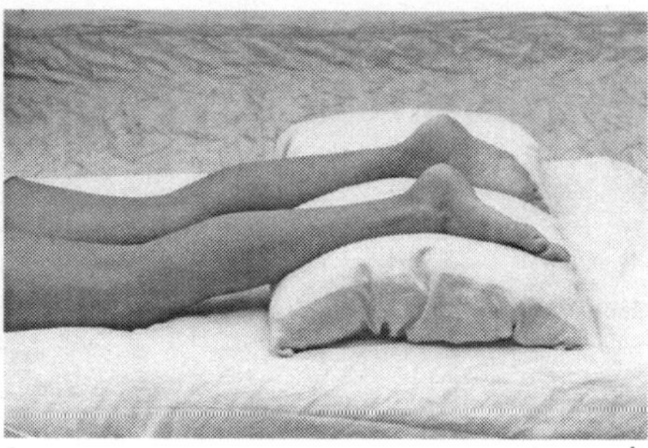

b

Figures 9-3: Pillows come in handy to support your partner when faceup or facedown.

Oil's Well That Ends Well: Massaging with Oil

Massage can be an oily endeavor. In fact, in some countries, such as India, oil plays a major part in the whole procedure, and about halfway through a massage people in Delhi end up glistening with a layer of lubricant. The Indian system prescribes large amounts of oil — usually sesame oil — on purpose for its reported health benefits. This method is okay (as long as you have lots of towels around to sop up the extra oil afterward), but the common wisdom in most other countries is that you should use just enough lubricant to, well, lubricate.

Choosing your oil

Walk into any bath and body shop or health food store and you see at least a dozen choices in massage oils. Which is the best one, you ask? Is it the special formula designed by the spiritual healer Edgar Cayce who "received" the recipe while in a trance? Or is it the "mango tango" scented blend that your favorite boutique down the street recently released?

Several oils available straight from the shelf in your local grocery store are usable, if not ideal, for massage. Almond oil is used in spas around the world, and you can use sesame oil and olive oil, too. But the special oils formulated just for massage really are better. They have more nutrients for the skin, and they create just the right amount of lubrication. In my opinion, spending the extra money for a high-quality massage oil is worth it.

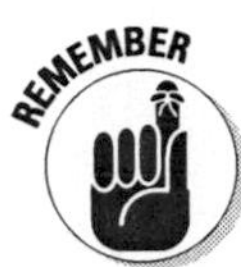

A few things you want to look for when choosing an oil:

- **Ingredients:** Check the ingredients. A common addition to several oil blends, for example, is lanolin, which comes from an animal source and turns some people off.
- **Scent:** Make sure the scent isn't overpowering or synthetic.
- **Viscosity:** Everyone has his or her own preference as far as the right viscosity goes. Thin oils, such as mineral oil, feel a little watery and spread unevenly; I don't recommend them. Some thick oils like coconut can leave a greasy feeling. Test a little on your palm before buying to find an oil somewhere in the middle of this spectrum that works for you.

Knowing how to use the oil you've chosen

Follow the steps below to properly use oil during a massage:

1. **First, choose the oil (see the preceding section).**
2. **Second, make sure the oil isn't cold.**

   If you apply cold oil to your partner's skin, it may cause an undesirable reaction, like him hitting you. Warm the oil first by placing the bottle in hot running water for a few minutes or using a baby bottle warmer until the oil is warm to the touch. Don't microwave the oil, which can potentially overheat it, causing an equally adverse reaction from your partner.
3. **Cup one palm and pour a small amount of oil into it.**

   Ideally, you want to keep the back of your cupped palm in contact with your partner so that you maintain a constant connection, as so artfully shown in Figure 9-4. The amount of oil depends on the size of the area you're massaging, the amount of body hair in the area (the hairier the skin, the more oil you need), and the maneuvers you plan to use. You may have to experiment a few times to get the amount right.
4. **Rub your palms together for a few seconds to further warm the oil and then glide your hands over the skin, spreading a smooth layer of oil over the whole surface you're massaging.**

   The correct amount of oil leaves the skin lubricated but without puddles of oil or greasy spots.

Getting creamed

Skin creams and lotions are a good alternative to oil, and in fact many professional massage therapists wouldn't be caught using anything else. Creams and lotions absorb more quickly into the skin than oil, so you don't slide around so much. Good ones leave a lubricating layer that makes it easy to work.

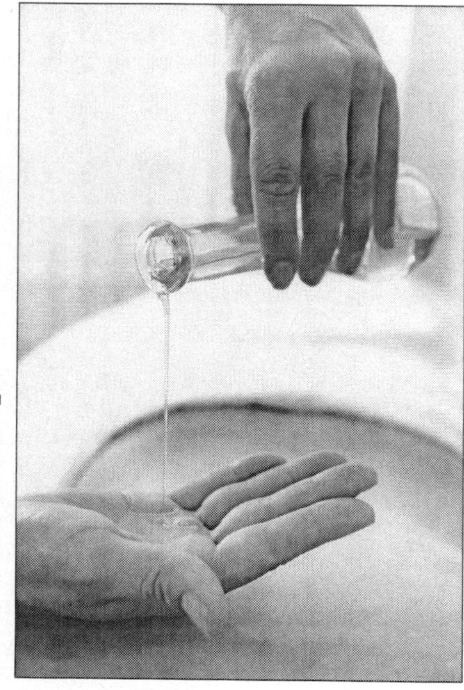

Figure 9-4: Keep contact with your partner while pouring the oil into your palm.

Considering bottle placement

An age-old feud exists among massage therapists over where to place the oil bottle during the massage. I know that this may seem silly to you, but you can rest assured that the debate is taken very seriously by otherwise intelligent adults. There are basically two camps:

- Those that propose placing the bottle next to the person, where it's handy but liable to get knocked over.
- Those that propose keeping the bottle out of harm's way, where it's harder to reach but less likely to get kicked or spilled.

Some people go as far as to keep their oil bottles in a specially made holster strung around their waist like a six-shooter. This gives the average massage therapist a Wyatt Earp kind of look that is perhaps not ideal for inducing relaxation.

Where should you put the bottle of oil during a massage? In my professional opinion, speaking as a massage therapist who's been working in the field for over 20 years, it doesn't really matter. Whatever's most comfortable for you is best.

The type of bottle (and especially the cap) does matter, though. You can make things much easier for yourself if you choose a squeeze-top or pop-up type cap that pours a tiny bit of oil at a time. Pump tops work well, too. If you use a wide-mouth opening, chances are you may end up with oil all over the place, especially if you have your massage area dimly lit with candles.

Making your own oil blends

You can incorporate the concepts of aromatherapy into your massage by adding *essential oil* (oils that are distilled essences of plants) to the oil you're already using, which is then called the *carrier oil.* Typical carrier oils include grapeseed, sweet almond, jojoba, avocado, and sesame, which are all good as a base for the essential oils.

To make your own aromatherapy oil, blend 24 drops of essential oil with 2 ounces of carrier oil. For added aromatherapy benefits, place a few drops in a *diffuser* to fill the room you're in with the same scent you're using for the massage, as I suggest in Chapter 8.

Table 9-1 lists the essential oils I use in my spa therapy workshops and a description of their basic effects:

Table 9-1 Essential Oils

Oil	*Properties*
Cedar	Reduces fluids in body tissues; diuretic. Warming in baths.
Clary sage	Balances female hormones. Good for scalp problems.
Eucalyptus radiate	Excellent for lungs, respiratory system. Muscle tonic.
Geranium rose	Balances the skin by affecting sebum. Balances emotions, too.
Juniper	Calming and purifying.
Lavender	Antibacterial (first-aid kit in a bottle); calming; good for skin.
Lemon grass	Stimulates digestion. Antiseptic, detoxifies lymph. Uplifting.
Orange	Mood elevator.
Peppermint	Stimulates alertness. Good for headaches, colds.
Pine	Painkiller. Natural deodorant.
Rose	Excellent for the skin.
Rosemary	Hair tonic. Astringent. Good for oily skin.
Sandalwood	Grounding and relaxing. Spiritually uplifting. Aids aging skin.
Tea tree	Antiseptic; antifungal; antibacterial. Good for the skin.
Vetiver	Grounding and calming.
Ylang ylang	Aphrodisiac. Relieves tension/stress. Balances dry skin.

Building Your Massage Muscles

You may not think of your body as a massage tool in the same way that oil and towels are, but it's a tool you can't do without. Massage requires the sustained dexterous use of certain muscles in your hands, forearms, shoulders, and in fact your entire body. You may not be using these muscles for any particular purpose right now. Like any other muscles that come suddenly into use, they may be sore when you begin using them. Don't be alarmed; the soreness fades away as you get stronger.

Here's a list of a few exercises and devices that massage pros sometimes use to help build massage muscles:

- **Walking a quarter:** Balance a quarter on your thumb. By using only the one hand, try to turn it over onto the top of your index finger. If you succeed, then try to flip it over onto your middle finger, and so on. When you get good, you can walk the quarter over all four fingers and catch it with the thumb again from below.
- **Finger dancing:** First, hold your hand in front of your face, with your palm facing away from you. Keeping your thumb out of the way, hold all four fingers loosely together. This is the starting position. Next, separate your fingers down the middle, two on each side. This position is shown in Figure 9-5. Finally, bring those fingers back together again, and then take just the pinkie finger and index finger away from the center. This position is also shown in Figure 9-5. Practice until you can repeat these steps over and over in a continuous loop.
- **Fingertip pushups:** For you fitness fanatics, try doing some fingertip pushups; these not only strengthen your fingers for massage but also give you the added benefit of some powerful exercise. Be careful not to overdo it, and always check with a physician before starting a new exercise regime.
- **Grape squeezing:** In order to sensitize your fingers for delicate massage moves, you can practice squishing grapes. Simply place a grape between your thumb and your first two fingers and squeeze till you burst the skin. Practice squeezing new grapes until they're just about to burst, maintaining a constant sensitive level of pressure.
- **Lunges:** Lunges strengthen your legs and hips, making standing, bending, and squatting easier when you're giving a massage.
- **Dance:** Any kind of dance class is great to prepare you for using your whole body to do massage.
- **Yoga:** You won't believe how quickly you get tight and tired just from giving a simple massage. Doing yoga may help keep you limber.
- **Fist squeezing:** You can pick up a little stress-relief squeeze ball just about anywhere these days, even at the checkout counter in most drugstores. These items are great not only for relieving stress but also for building hand muscles, too. A special compound called *power putty* is made just for this purpose and is sold in massage stores.
- **Dumbbells:** Lightweight dumbbells (5 to 12 pounds) are great for building strength and endurance in your forearms and wrists. Simply sit with the dumbbell in one hand, support your elbow on the top of your leg, palm up, and curl and extend the forearm.

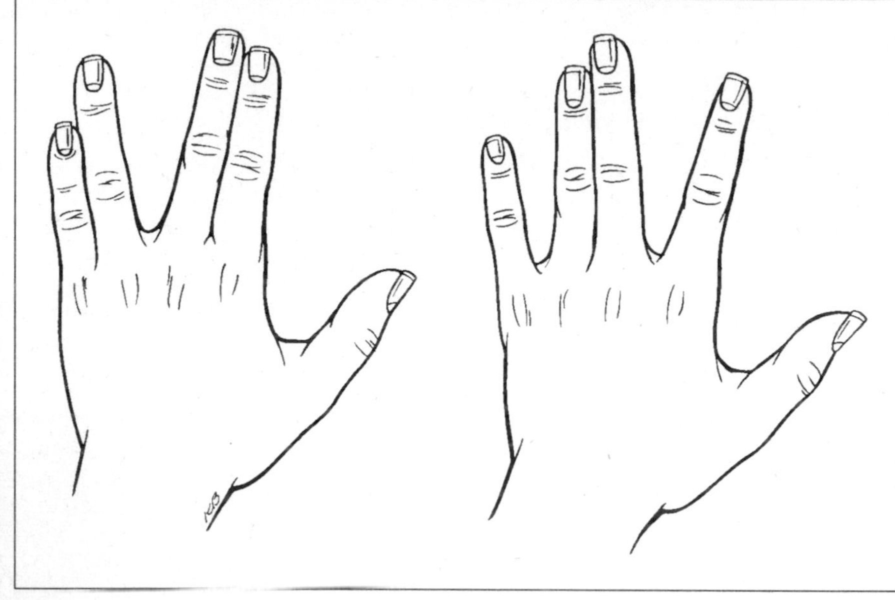

Figure 9-5: Finger dancing is great for building hand strength and coordination.

Following the Rules for Giving Massage

Just as Chapter 6 discusses the rules for receiving massages, here you find out the rules for *giving* massages. These rules are valuable tools that enhance your technique, making your massage something of purpose and focus instead of simple touch. While you're prepping your massage area, setting out your oils, and so on, be sure to focus your mind and remember the following:

- **Do no harm.** This is the number-one rule for giving a massage. Refer to Chapter 10 and make sure you're aware of the moves that you shouldn't make, the places that you shouldn't press, and the conditions you shouldn't treat.
- **Think 3-D.** Try to visualize the physical structures beneath the skin that you're affecting with your hands during the massage. Refer to Chapter 3.
- **Use your whole body.** Remember to use correct *body mechanics* (see Chapter 10) in order to save your own body from overexertion while applying just the right amount of pressure for your partner.

- **Focus on the other.** A massage is no time to be thinking about politics, sports, the weather, or your upcoming turn to receive a massage yourself. As fully as you can, focus on your partner, what he's feeling, and how you can make him feel better.
- **Go out of your mind.** After you figure out the moves, practice the technique, and focus on your partner with all your concentration, you can stop thinking. That's right. Let go of your extraneous thoughts, and even your thoughts about doing a good job.
- **Get creative.** Go ahead, go crazy; just let yourself feel whatever you're feeling and go with your intuition. Want to leave one palm on your partner's forehead and the other on his stomach completely motionless for ten minutes? That's probably exactly what he needs. As long as what you're doing is generated from caring and commitment to your partner, it's going to be the right thing.
- **Let love flow.** Certain people develop an ability to send a very distinct and palpable sensation of love into their fingers and palms. You can feel it when they touch you. Everyone else has the potential to develop that ability. Why not use massage as an opportunity to explore your own innate abilities to send a powerful message of caring to others through your touch and presence? You could spend your time in worse ways.

For the most part, these rules are things I mention throughout earlier chapters, but reviewing them right before you actually give a massage is helpful.

Good hands

What does it mean to have *good hands?* It's the one quality that millions of massage lovers around the world use to describe the essence of an excellent massage therapist. As in, "Oh, that was the best massage I ever had. You've got great hands." But because that quality is so vague, it's a little difficult to reproduce or teach to someone else. Good hands? What does that mean?

Having good hands, as it turns out, is not really about your hands. It's about *you.* It's the way you focus on your partner, the way you become sensitive to her, and the way you care. It's also about following some very simple guidelines, which I call the rules for giving massage. You can find those rules right here in this chapter.

Follow these simple principles, and you may even go beyond having good hands to having great hands one day.

But do I have to cut my nails?

Once I was hired to present a massage workshop at a huge annual convention of nail technicians (manicurists) in Detroit. I never knew so many manicurists existed before. I demonstrated some basic massage moves on the feet of one class member and then told them to exchange similar moves. Soon the room was filled with sounds of pain and discomfort.

These women had nails an inch and a half long. Sharp nails. Some of them had holes drilled in the ends of their nails, and miniature charm bracelets dangled through them. It was impossible for them to practice massage.

If you have long nails, you'll have an awfully hard time giving a good massage. One of the first things people are told when they sign up for massage school is to cut their nails, and you can often tell a massage pro by her short and neatly trimmed nails.

Does this mean you have to lop off your own dearly beloved nails in order to give a massage? Not necessarily. If your husband is the only person you're going to be massaging, and he likes it when you run your long nails down his back, don't worry about cutting them. You can improvise massage moves by using your palms and the bottoms of your fingers, keeping your nails lifted up out of the way. However, if your nails are long and your intention is to get better at massage and perform all the moves described here to their fullest, you have some serious trimming and filing to do in your near future.

Chapter 10

All the Right Moves

In This Chapter

- Doing the moves
- Finding out about contraindications

This chapter is where you find all those massage moves that you can use to turn your everyday, ordinary hands into instruments of irresistible pleasure. Your fingertips and palms will be sought after by friends, family, co-workers, and complete strangers alike. Everybody will say, "Use some of those moves on me! Me me me me me!"

Then, inflated by your newfound abilities and the quick expertise you acquire in these pages, you may find yourself thinking, like many folks do in the beginning, that these neat new massage moves you've gained actually are the massage itself. But you'd be wrong! Massage moves aren't the massage; they're just the medium.

Picking up massage is like learning to play a musical instrument: The moves in this chapter are the notes on the scale, plus some basic chords and combinations. They're great ways to warm up your fingers and make some rudimentary noises, but if you continue to play them over and over again, you're going to drive the people close to you crazy.

In massage, you have to go beyond the moves pretty quickly. You need to develop a "moveless movement," or *flow*, in which you're concentrating not on your own technique but on your partner's feelings, sensations, and reactions, just like a musician who forgets all about notes and scales, sharps and flats, and even the instrument itself. Your movements are the technique, the body you massage is the instrument, and it's the interaction between the two that makes the music. In other words, massage — not the movements required to produce the sensations — is the music, the communication, the thing that you create.

Whoa! Getting a little deep here, aren't I? Sorry about that. Don't worry — the rest of this chapter is very practical and concrete. After all, you still have to learn your scales before you can play Carnegie Hall.

You Got the Moves

So, what do you actually do when you place your hands on a body and start giving a massage? Well, the first thing many people do is panic. They stand there with their hands motionless on an arm or a leg or a back, and they think to themselves, "Oh my gosh, what do I do now?"

This situation is where the seven types of massage moves you find in this section come in handy. After practicing them, you can rest easy that you won't draw a blank when it comes time to give a massage.

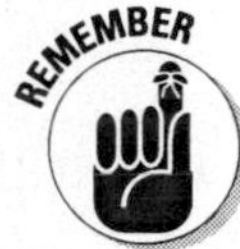

Here are some simple general guidelines that you can apply to all the upcoming maneuvers and use in every massage you give:

- **Follow the contour.** When in doubt about what particular move to make, just trace the body's outlines with your fingers for a few moments, applying pressure according to what you feel. Try to keep moving in a constant flow rather than stop and say something like, "Now, what was that next maneuver again?", which can be annoying to your partner.
- **Do no harm.** Don't press too hard or work on areas that may be too delicate, such as sprains, strains, or scar tissues soon after injuries. Of course, avoid all contraindicated areas and conditions. (The term *contraindication* is massage-therapist speak for any condition that makes massage unadvisable.) Ask for a physician's advice if you see anything that gives you concern.
- **Stay in the moment.** The easiest way to look at a massage is piece by piece. Concentrate on one movement and one area at a time. Work on just that leg first, and worry about what you're going to do on the arm later. One move at a time, one after another, creates a whole massage.

Feeling versus doing

Massage is as much (or more) about feeling as it is about doing. In fact, without really doing anything, you can still give a good massage. Through simple touch alone, you can have a profound effect on somebody else.

When I was in massage school, during the very first day in class, the instructor had us do a little experiment, which you can try for yourself: Have your partner sit barefoot in front of you. Gently grasp one of her feet in your hands and then *don't do anything.* Just feel. Feel her foot, the weight of it in your hands, the contours of it against your fingers and palms, its warmth, and the pulse of the blood. Resist any temptation to squeeze or press or knead.

After just five or ten minutes, slowly pull your hands away and ask your partner to note the feeling in both of her feet. Almost everyone notices a large difference; the touched foot feels as though it's been vigorously massaged. It's tingling and alive.

All you had to do to achieve that effect was to feel. No need to do anything at all. So, if you ever find yourself at a loss when giving a massage, remember that you can get by (and make your partner perfectly happy) by simply concentrating on what you're feeling in your hands. It really works.

Slip-sliding away: The pleasures of gliding

Usually the first move you make on any particular part of the body is gliding. Why glide first, you say? Why not just get right to the pressing and muscle-squeezing part of the massage — isn't that what feels best? Four reasons:

- Gliding is a great way to warm up the skin and underlying muscles for the massage moves to come.
- Gliding is the best move for spreading your massage oil or lotion over the skin.
- You cover a lot of territory during a glide, so it's perfect for "introducing" your hands to your partner.
- You get a feel for your partner's body and discover which areas may need the most attention during the rest of the massage.

Methods of gliding

The following list shows you the three basics types of gliding you can choose from. Depending upon the amount of pressure you use, a glide can be light and ethereal or downright intense. Usually, you want to start with lighter gliding at the beginning of a massage and then progress to the more heavy-duty stuff later, after your partner trusts your touch.

- **Long, soft, light:** You can create the lightest type of gliding by just barely brushing the fingertips or palms across the skin in a feather-light fashion (see Figure 10-1a). This type of movement is also known as a *nerve-stroke* because it calms the nerves.
- **Sliding down the banister:** This movement follows the contours of the body more closely. As you glide, you mold your hands to fit the body, just like a little kid who molds himself to fit over the banister as he slides down it into the foyer (see Figure 10-1b). This technique is the primary form of gliding, the type you use to spread oil, warm the body, and so on.
- **Squeezing toothpaste through a tube:** This intense gliding may stun your partner at first. With this method, you wrap your hands around a leg or an arm and squeeze firmly while you glide, as if you were trying to squeeze toothpaste from a giant tube (see Figure 10-1c). The most typical places for this maneuver are on the calf and the forearm.

Start out slowly, and always, always make the motions toward the heart because you actually move blood through the veins with the deepest gliding moves. Watch out for the contraindications of varicose veins and phlebitis, which I discuss in more detail later in this chapter.

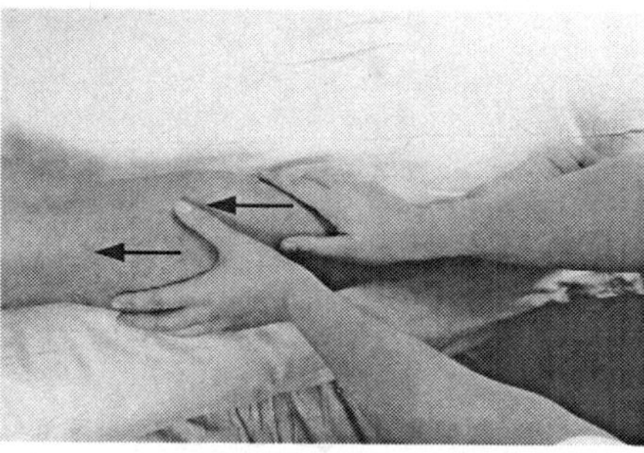
a

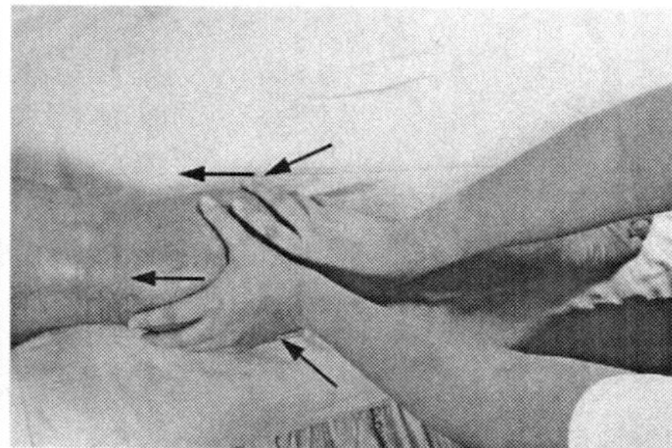
b

c

Figure 10-1: The three types of gliding.

For all types of gliding, you need to turn your hands into supersensitive, micro-adjusting instruments that constantly change to conform to each and every little hill and valley on your partner's body. Imagine yourself trying to smooth out a sheet of plastic wrap around an irregularly shaped piece of fruit, allowing no air-pockets or wrinkles.

Good places to glide

You can glide just about anywhere you can find an expanse of skin to move over. Tight little nooks and crannies, such as those between the toes, aren't good places to glide because they don't have enough open territory. However, you can still glide on smaller surfaces. Simply adjust your hands to the area you're touching. Thus, a forehead glide includes just your fingertips, and a glide to the leg includes your whole palm.

X marks the spot: Pressing

If you've ever received a back rub from someone and suddenly felt him press exactly the right spot, you know the sensation is swift and unmistakable. Immediately, you say something like, "Yes, that's the spot!"

So, what is "the spot" anyway? Massage pros have all kinds of fancy names for it, like *trigger points, muscle spasms,* or *adhesions.* Whatever you call them, these points of tension or pain are what you're trying to get rid of in massage, and pressing on them skillfully can help achieve that.

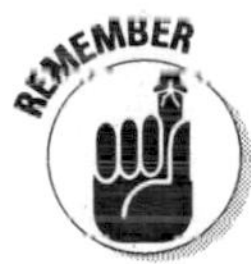

The spots I'm talking about in this section aren't *shiatsu points* or *acupressure points,* which are spots along energy pathways in the body. You get to know a few shiatsu points in Chapter 11; the spots in this section are occasionally found in the same areas as shiatsu/acupressure points, but they're a different animal altogether.

I envision these spots as tenacious little criminals who invade the body and take some of your muscles hostage. They're tough and resourceful, and they thrive best when you don't know exactly where to find them. Massage helps you locate where your tension spots are hiding so you can ferret them out.

Pressing out spots correctly

When the spots don't leave your muscles alone, you have to go in with some heavy firepower. That's where pressing comes in. Here are a few steps you can follow to find spots and press them into submission:

1. **While you're warming the tissues up during your preliminary gliding strokes, feel for areas that are unusually tight, hard, or sensitive.**

2. **After you're done gliding over a certain area, come back to these targeted spots one at a time and zero in on them by using just your fingertips or thumbs.**

   You know those little rubberized buttons that you push to change the light to green at intersections? They give a little at first, but then you get the feeling that you have to push harder. You can't quite tell whether you're holding it down or not, so you hold it in firmly for a few seconds, much longer than you'd hold, say, the on/off switch on a desk lamp. Well, that's the same kind of pressing you can use in your massage — good, firm, sustained pressure is what makes pressing work.

   The best way to apply pressing is with either with your fingertips or your thumbs, as you can see in Figure 10-2. When you do this move, be careful to keep your thumbs or fingers lined up straight all the way to your shoulders (as shown in Figure 10-13 later in the chapter) so you don't put too much stress on your joints.

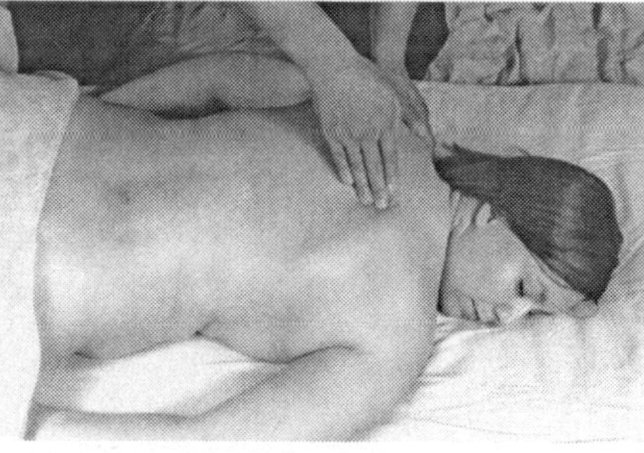
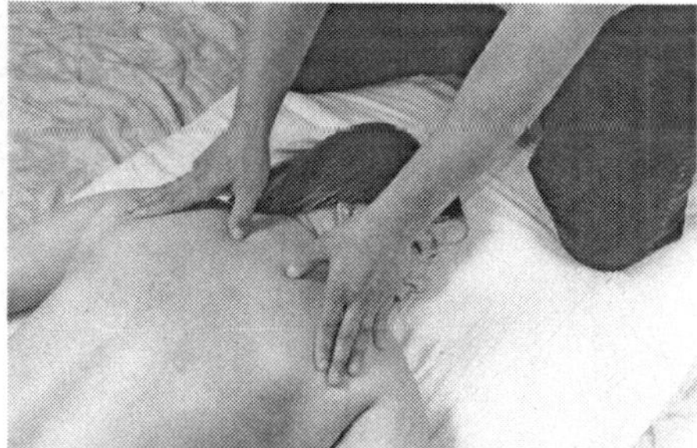

Figure 10-2: Finger pressing (a) and thumb pressing (b).

3. **Keep feeling around until you can tell you're directly on top of the spot.**

   Pinpointing the spot's position can mean an itty-bitty micro-difference in the location of your fingers or thumb. If you're in the exact spot, you usually feel like you can easily slip off of it on either side.

4. **Keep adjusting.**

   As you feel your partner's body respond, you can adjust your pressure accordingly, lightening it as the tension dissipates.

Good places to press

Finding the right spots to press may sometimes feel a little tricky to you. After all, the body has about a million different points on it. How do you tell where's a good place to apply pressure and where's not a good place? Two answers:

- You have to practice feeling for these points (this process is the art of *palpation*, which you find out about in Chapter 3).
- Certain points are common to most people. After you practice on several willing massage partners, you build your skill in locating spots. Some of the most common tension hotspots can be found on top of the shoulders as you get closer to the neck and on the back near the shoulder blades.

Let's do the twist: Kneading

By definition, to *knead* something means you have to grasp it between your fingers or palms to press, rub, or squeeze it, which makes kneading a valuable massage tool. After you master the art of kneading, you may be in great demand because kneading, in my opinion, produces the most pleasurable sensations of all the maneuvers. It gets in deep to flush out tension while at the same time stimulating a large surface area on the skin.

Methods of kneading

Your kneading technique can make or break you as a massage giver, so I recommend practicing quite a bit on this one. If you practice building your massage muscles as I suggest in Chapter 9, you can be a better kneader because this particular maneuver requires a lot of strength in the hands.

In order to knead effectively, you must banish fear! The biggest mistake novice kneaders make is kneading too timidly. As a massage teacher, I've spent hundreds of hours hunched over students guiding their hands into bigger movements. "Get more flesh between those fingers!" I cajole them. "Twist your arms around some more. Use your whole body to make the movement."

This advice is good for you, too. A wimpy knead is much worse than no knead at all. Here are some ways to make your kneading big, bold, and beloved by all who encounter it:

- **Use your whole body.** Chubby Checker would have been disappointed if he'd looked out on the dance floor to find dozens of people just standing there and sort of half-heartedly bending a little at the waist. When he said twist, he meant *twist*, as in twist-tie, twist-off tops, and wow-look-at-that-twister-about-to-destroy-the-barn! The number-one rule for kneading is to use your whole body to create a twisting movement around the area you're working on. Figure 10-3 shows how your hands can move around a thigh in a circular wringing motion, using your whole body to make it happen.

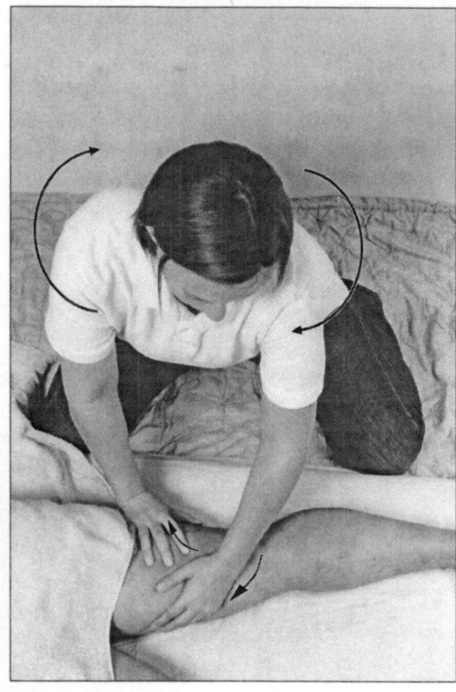

Figure 10-3: Notice how your entire body moves around the area you're kneading.

- **Act like a baker making bread.** The word *kneading* often conjurs images of a baker with his hands wrist-deep in pliable flour, constantly squeezing, rolling, and pushing the dough. In fact, those are the three components of a successful knead. After you have twisting down, add these steps to complete the picture:
  - **Squeezing:** During your twist, the hand that's farthest away (the right hand as shown in Figure 10-4a) is *squeezing* in as much flesh as possible between the fingers and palms.
  - **Rolling:** The far hand *rolls* the squeezed flesh back toward you while the near hand begins its journey away from you, pushing more flesh into the fold, as shown in Figure 10-4b.
  - **Pushing:** Finally, you're in the position shown in Figure 10-4c, and your far hand starts *pushing* while your near hand takes over the squeezing and rolling.
- **Utilize skin rolling:** *Skin rolling* is reserved for areas that normally don't respond too well to bigger twisting, squeezing, and rolling maneuvers. It's a little tricky to do, but most people love the way it feels. First, pinch a roll of flesh between your thumb and the first two fingers. Then, keeping your thumb locked in position, glide your whole hand over the skin while "walking" your first two fingers forward so that they push a constant roll of skin back against your thumb as shown in Figure 10-4d.

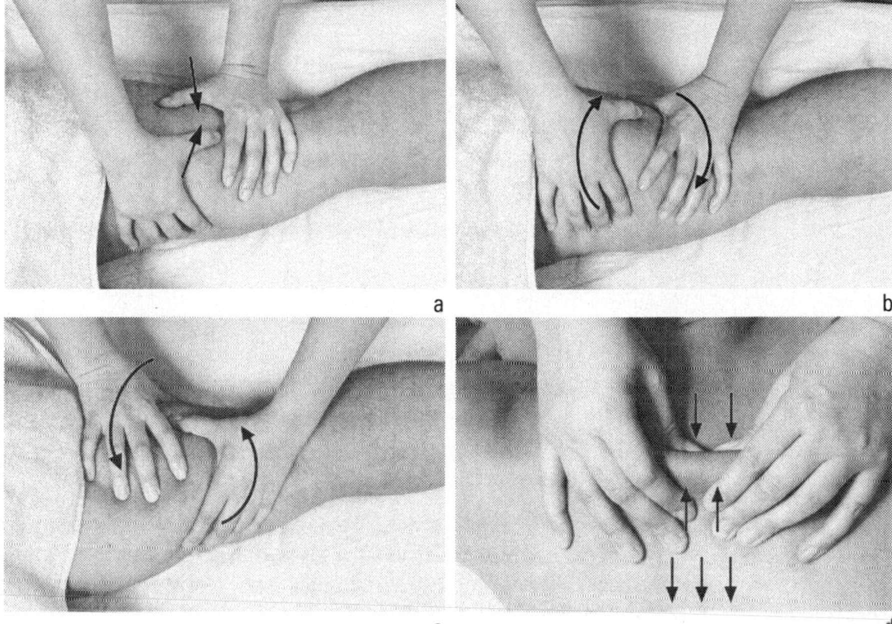

Figure 10-4: Squeezing (a), rolling (b), pushing (c), and skin rolling (d).

Good places to knead

Because kneading requires you to grasp, areas of the body that you can't grasp, you can't knead. That's why kneading skinny people is trickier than kneading fleshy people and kneading a knee is tougher than kneading a thigh. That doesn't mean you need to knead a whole handful of flesh to get the job done, though. You can perform skin rolling even on areas with almost no fat, like a supermodel's upper back. For regular baker-making-bread kneading, the most popular places are the shoulders, thighs, calves, and back. You can also knead the arms, but your movements have to be a little smaller.

Wax on, wax off: Rubbing

The secret to successful *rubbing,* or *friction* (as massage pros call it), is to make the pressure from your fingers or palms strong enough to stay stationary on the surface of the skin while moving the layers below. In other words, your fingers don't glide while they rub, although they can definitely move around quite a bit. Take, for example, the maneuvers you receive on your head when you get a shampoo at a salon. A good shampoo person employs friction techniques, holding his fingers steady on a certain part of your scalp while manipulating your head beneath it. If he simply glides his fingers across your scalp, the sensation is disturbingly inadequate.

Another analogy for rubbing is waxing your car. You take a buffing pad in one hand and rub the wax on. Then with a rag in the other hand, you rub the wax off. Your fingers are never in contact with the car itself, but the car receives the effects, not the buffing pad or rags. So it is with massage. Your fingers are in contact with the skin, but you're affecting the layers below.

Rubbing techniques

Here are a few rubbing techniques that work well for various parts of the body:

- **Miser's rub:** Especially good for the fingers and toes, the miser's rub may remind you of someone rubbing a gold coin between his fingers, as shown in Figure 10-5a.
- **Circular:** Making sure your fingers are planted securely, move the skin over the tissues below it in small circles as you see in Figure 10-5b. You can move your hand gradually along the skin's surface, creating a series of circles over an entire area.
- **Cross-fiber:** In any given area of the body, the muscle fibers run predominantly in one direction or another. On the inside of your upper arm, for instance, the biceps muscle runs from your shoulder to your elbow, up and down. If you rub in a cross-wise direction over these fibers, from the inside of your arm to the outside, you're making the *cross-fiber* movement shown in Figure 10-5c. This action is especially good for people who exercise a lot or are in the later stages of recovering from an injury because it promotes the repair of scar tissues.

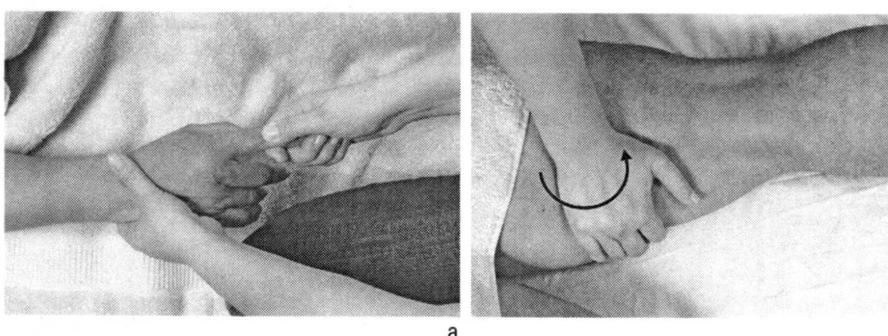

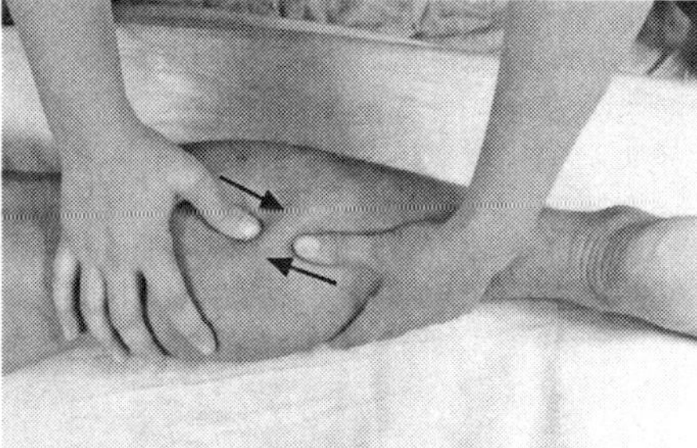

Figure 10-5: The miser's rub (a), circular rub (b), and cross-fiber rub (c).

Good places to rub

You can rub most everywhere, but you have to be careful in sensitive areas because rubbing can be a little annoying if you do it, say, on areas with very little flesh.

Shake, rattle, and roll: Shaking

Shaking is like loosening fruit from a tree. Imagine that you're standing on the ground in front of an apple tree, and one big perfect juicy apple is still left just barely clinging to a high branch. Grasping a lower limb, you shake with the intention of loosening that apple at a distance from you. Loosening distant areas is the essence of shaking in massage, too.

Of course, you don't want to literally loosen muscles from bone so that they fall off, but you do want to help ease the muscles' tight grip of chronic tension, especially in the joints. Shaking is great for this goal, but it's a fine art. The following sections describe three different versions you can practice.

Vibration

No other massage move feels quite as dramatic as vibration. It's a move with pizzazz, but it isn't always easy to pick up; it takes concentration and a willingness to look spastic. The following steps and Figure 10-6 walk you through the process.

1. **Placing just your fingertips on the area to be vibrated (try the back, which is easiest to start with), stiffen all of your joints from your fingers all the way up to your shoulders.**

   Be careful not to vibrate a fingertip directly on top of the spine, because you may cause some discomfort or bruising.

2. **Try making your entire arm tremble as one unit, as if you were extremely cold and shivering uncontrollably.**
3. **Pressing firmly, concentrate all of that trembling down into your fingertips.**
4. **Simultaneously, drag your fingertips slowly down over your partner's back, remembering to imagine your movements loosening muscles all along the way.**

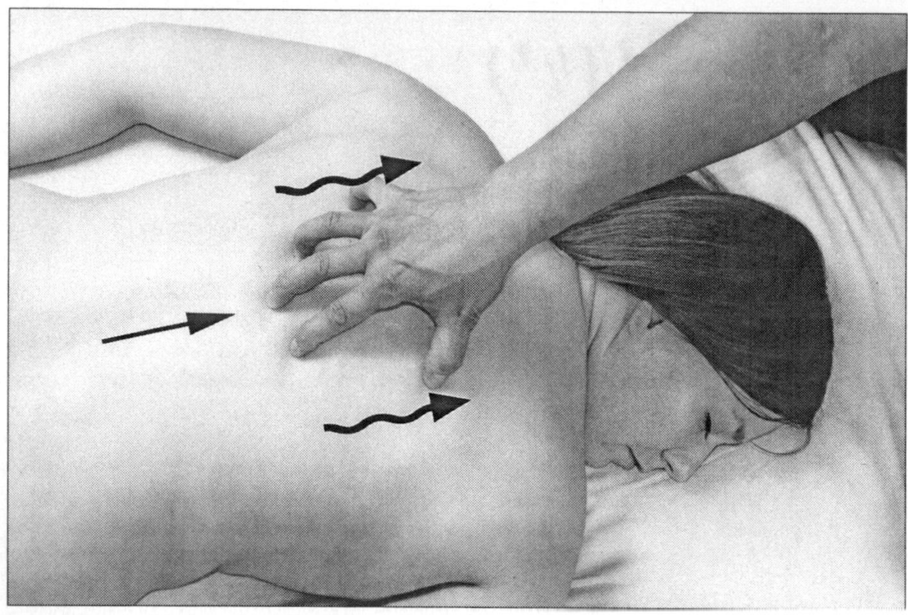

Figure 10-6: Vibration creates a dramatic massage effect.

Shaking

In this move, you grasp one part of your partner's body (usually an ankle or wrist) and then recreate the same kind of rigid trembling you do for vibration. It can be a slower trembling, though, even languid, but the intent is still to loosen deep muscles. See Figure 10-7.

Rocking and rolling

A doctor named Milton Trager developed a kind of massage (appropriately called *Trager*) that includes rocking and rolling the entire body from side to side, as shown in Figure 10-8. One of the results of a really good Trager massage is a deep release of tension from areas that you wouldn't be able to get to with your fingers, like deep inside joints. You can recreate some of the effects of this type of massage by doing some very gentle rocking and rolling of your own. You find out more about how to apply rocking and rolling to specific areas in Chapters 11 and 12.

Good places to do shaking moves

Larger areas such as the back and thighs respond well to vibration, and you can rock the whole body, especially when your partner is lying facedown. The limbs also respond exceptionally well to shaking.

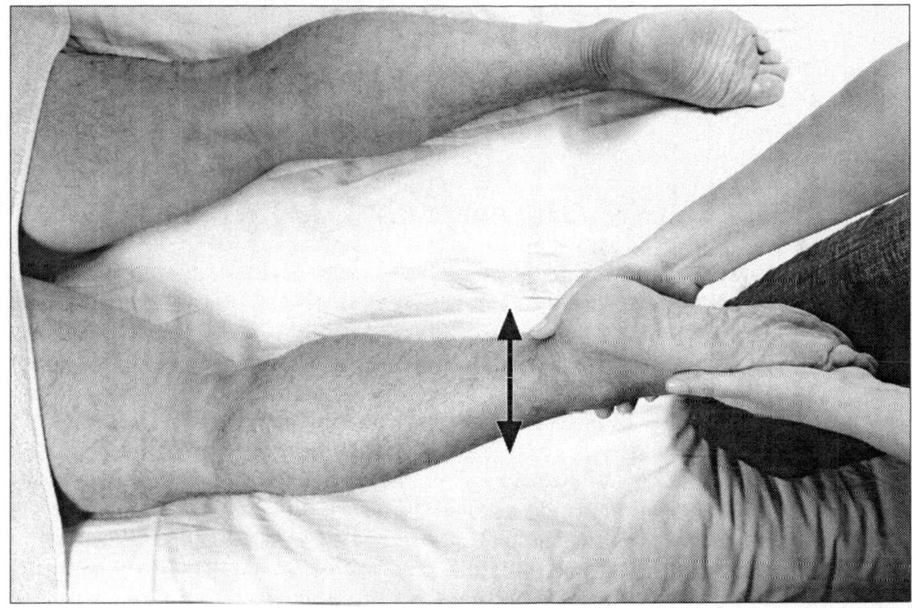

Figure 10-7: Shaking is similar to vibration, but you grasp rather than press.

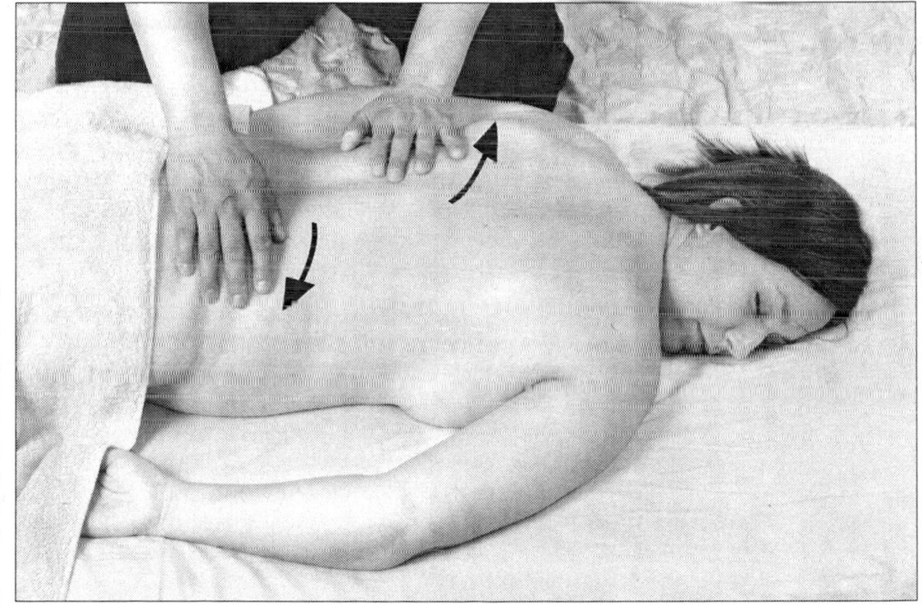

Figure 10-8: Rocking and rolling affects the surrounding muscles and distant joints as well.

If you shake the head, you're coming dangerously close to a chiropractic maneuver, which is a definite no-no. If you were to inadvertently make some chiropractic adjustments without knowing what you're doing, you may potentially hurt somebody.

Get into the rhythm: Tapping

Tapping (the famous karate-chop family of massage maneuvers) is the type of movement that you see actors performing when they think they're doing some really authentic massage on-screen. It also seems to be the preferred move for overweight Russian men giving massages in bathhouses.

This family of moves is based on one major concept: Getting pounded on feels surprisingly good. This is true as long as you tap judiciously, with the right amount of pressure. To achieve seasoned tapping prowess, practice with the following three basic hand-shapes for tapping. You do them all with *soft hands* (hands that feel and respond to what they feel without jabbing or prodding) because, after all, your intention isn't to attack ninja-style but to increase circulation and soothe sore muscles.

- **Fingertip tapping:** This method is the lightest tap and is excellent for faces and the top of your head. A lot of cosmetologists use this move to bring extra circulation to the cheeks, creating that rosy glow look. Check out an example in Figure 10-9a.
- **Karate hacking:** Make sure to keep your hands limp, and don't treat your partner's body like a board you're trying to break. Don't hack directly on bony areas, of course (think about what happens when you whack the bony part of your ankle even lightly). Keep your wrists loose and let the edges of your flopping fingers do a lot of the hacking for you, as Figure 10-9b illustrates.
- **Loose fist pounding:** You have to be extra careful when using your fists for tapping, but they definitely come in handy if your partner is one of those NFL linebacker types who doesn't seem to respond to normal massage manipulations. Don't tighten your fists completely when pounding, and resist the temptation to do a Rocky-Balboa-side-of-beef-in-the-freezer move. Figure 10-9c gives you an example of proper pounding.

The secret to all good tapping is the rhythm. If you're not a natural born drummer, try slowing your tapping down until you reach a rhythm that you can sustain easily. Consistency, not speed, is what counts.

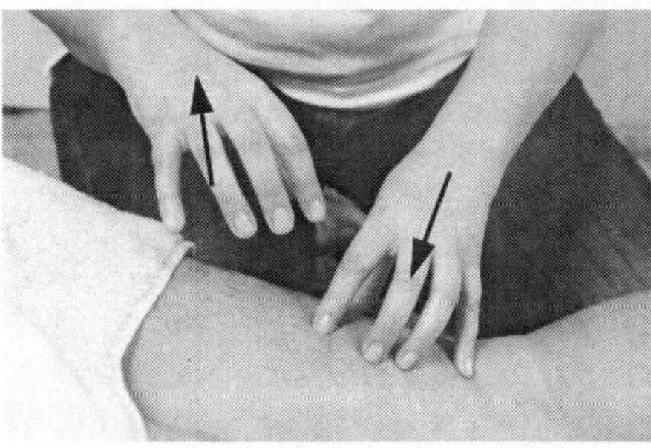
a

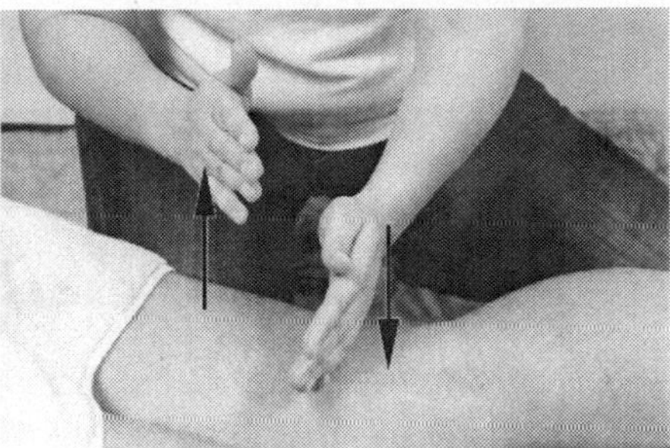
b

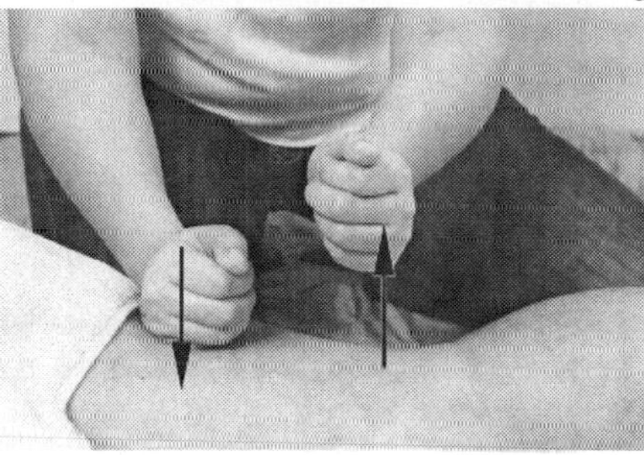
c

Figure 10-9: Fingertip tapping (a), karate hacking (b), and loose fist pounding (c).

Good places to tap

Tapping feels good just about anywhere, but if you tap someone too hard on the top of his head, he's likely to think you have something against him. The usual rule is the more flesh in an area, the more force you can tap with, progressing up the scale from fingertips to hacking hands to loose fists. Bony areas like the knees need light tapping with just the fingertips. Also, go feather-light on the kidney area on either side of the spine in the lower back. Certain spots you may not think of, like the bottom of the feet for example, are great places to hack. And of course the ever popular back, buttocks, and thighs are great places to practice getting into the rhythm.

Keep it loose: Stretching

Stretching is really good for you, and a lot of people don't stretch as much as they should in order to stay limber and youthful. You can help solve this problem by incorporating a few stretching moves right into your massage.

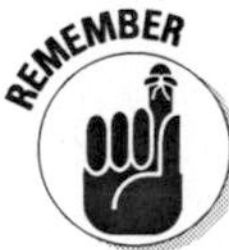

Stretching feels really good as long as you follow three easy guidelines:

- Ease your partner into it.
- Easy does it while you're doing it.
- Ease your partner out of it.

Remember that each joint has a *range of motion,* a limit as to how far it can stretch in any and all possible directions. Don't try stretching any part of the body past its normal range of motion because if you do, it hurts. A lot. Stop long before you think you reach the maximum stretch. Always ask your partner for feedback about how the stretch feels. Some people are super limber, and you can twist them like pretzels, but others can take very little stretching before it becomes uncomfortable.

Be especially careful when stretching your partner's neck, moving it slowly and in only one plane at a time: left to right, up and down, or ear to shoulder. And don't *hyperextend* the neck, or any joint for that matter. (See "Being Aware of Contraindications for Massage" later in this chapter for more on certain dangerous moves to avoid.)

Basic types of stretches

You can apply three basic types of stretches during a massage:

- **Passive stretching:** *Passive stretching* doesn't mean you should have a ho-hum attitude about the stretch. As Figure 10-10 shows, it means your partner just lies there passively and doesn't assist you at all while you stretch her.

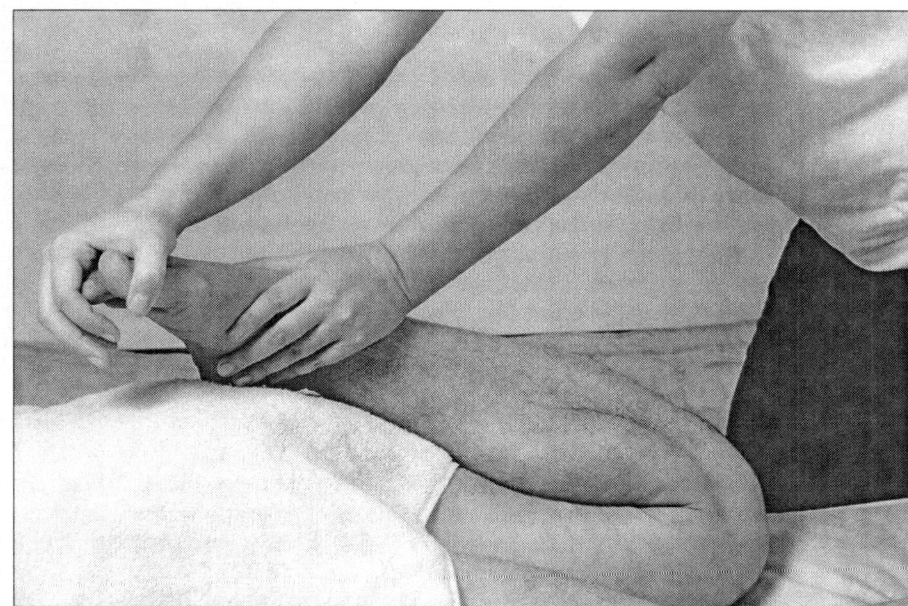

Figure 10-10: In a passive stretch, the person just lies there.

- **Active assisted stretching:** This type of stretching, shown in Figure 10-11, requires your partner to move through the stretch while you help her stretch a little farther. It's not recommended for lazy partners who just want to lie back and have you do all the work during the massage.
- **Active resisted stretching:** This stretch is the deepest of the three. In this one, your partner resists the movement of the stretch that you're giving him. When he stops resisting, you're able to stretch him even farther. This one's good for strengthening muscles and can be considered a kind of mini-workout.

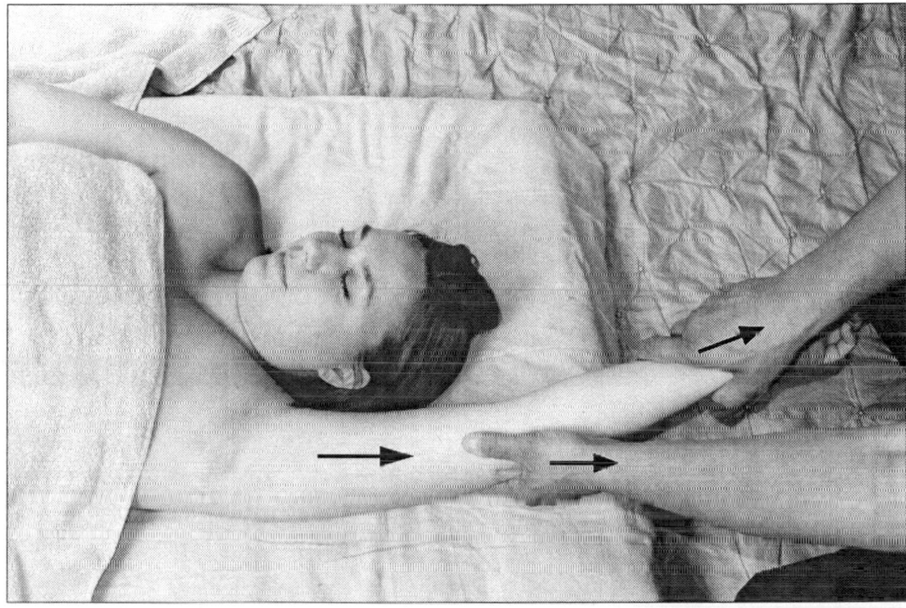

Figure 10-11: In active assisted stretching, you help your partner stretch a little further.

Good places to stretch

The multitude of joints in the body means you can do a large variety of joint manipulations and stretches in many areas such as the toes, ankles, knees, hips, shoulders, elbows, wrists, and hands. You find out about a few all-time favorite stretches in Chapters 11 and 12.

A ticklish situation

Some people flat-out refuse to even consider the possibility of getting a massage because they're afraid they'd giggle so hard they'd fall right off the massage table. These folks consider themselves "ticklish," but what is a ticklish person, anyway? Most people are sensitive to getting poked in the ribs or stroked lightly on the bottom of the feet, but some people claim any kind of touch at all elicits the tickle response.

When someone complains of being overly ticklish, you can follow these steps to help them get over it:

1. **First, explain that surface tension in the muscles causes excessive ticklishness.**
2. **Explain that you're going to get underneath this layer by applying firm pressure that affects tissues below.**
3. **Gradually apply pressure with as broad a surface as possible — for example, use your entire palm rather than your fingers.**
4. **After you sink down to a depth that isn't ticklish anymore, make your movements slow and steady, gently rocking back and forth and pulsing up and down; avoid kneading, pressing, and vibration.**
5. **Move slowly from one area to another, staying away from the areas your partner reports as most seriously ticklish.**
6. **If your partner shows any signs of discomfort, discontinue movement and simply apply steady firm pressure.**

The Massage Dance: Using Proper Body Mechanics

You may ask yourself, "What am I supposed to be doing with the rest of my body while my hands are massaging someone?" Quiz time! Here are some possibilities (and eyes on your own paper):

A. It doesn't matter, as long as you remain in a generally upright position and don't fall asleep.

B. Something constructive, such as learning a foreign language with audiocassettes, because otherwise you're just wasting your time.

C. Absolutely nothing; stay as stiff and still as possible so you don't distract the person you're massaging.

D. Make every move a whole body move by engaging your entire self in what you're doing, turning the massage into a dance.

The answer, of course, is D. In fact, using your entire body properly while giving a massage is so important that massage pros have given this practice a name — *body mechanics*.

It may seem like a lot of extra effort at first, but in the long run massage is easier if you use proper body mechanics and engage your entire body while giving a massage instead of relying on the strength of your arms and shoulders alone. Actually, using your arms and shoulders alone is guaranteed to burn you out really quickly. You may end up quitting after ten minutes, offering muscle-fatigue as an excuse to your disappointed partner.

Here are a few guidelines to help you fine-tune your body mechanics:

- **Position yourself properly:** Whether you're kneeling next to your partner on the floor, leaning over her on the edge of the bed, or actually using a professional massage table, maintaining proper positioning is important. First, get into a comfortable position. Many people like sitting on their own heels when doing massage on the floor. You can also kneel when working on a bed. Whatever position you're in, remember to keep changing it periodically so you don't get sore or your limbs don't fall asleep (nothing worse than a sleeping massage giver).
- **Root yourself:** Your movements should feel like they're coming from the place where your body is rooted to the earth. Don't get off balance and lose your center of power. You need to ground yourself enough so that you're steady when you're giving a massage.
- **Move from below:** Whether you're kneeling down on the floor to give a massage or standing next to a massage table, generate your movements from your legs and hips, not just from your upper body. Figure 10-12 illustrates proper form in both a kneeling position (a) and standing (b). Keep your knees soft.
- **Maintain straight lines:** Apply pressure in a straight line from your shoulders down to your fingertips. Bending your joints and then applying pressure puts extra unwanted pressure on your thumbs, wrists, and elbows. Figure 10-13 shows you what I'm talking about; a is the wrong method, and b is the better option.
- **Be kind to your thumbs and wrists:** Thumbs take the biggest beating when you're giving a massage, and wrists come in a close second. Be extra careful not to rely only on these delicate instruments to do your heavy-duty massage work. Give them a break every once in a while by using your knuckles and forearms.
- **Lean a lot:** Instead of straining your muscles to get the job done, use your body weight. Simply lean on the person you're massaging by placing your center of gravity several inches away from her and then falling forward and supporting yourself on her body. This movement may take a little practice because your civilized instincts tell you not to use other people's bodies as counter tops. Go ahead and try it, though. It saves you a lot of work.

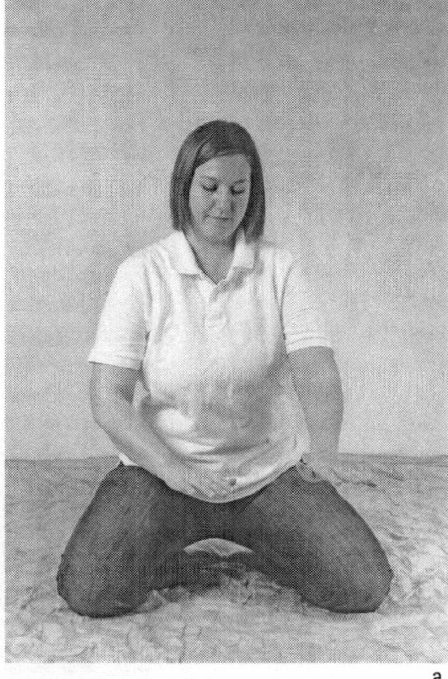
a

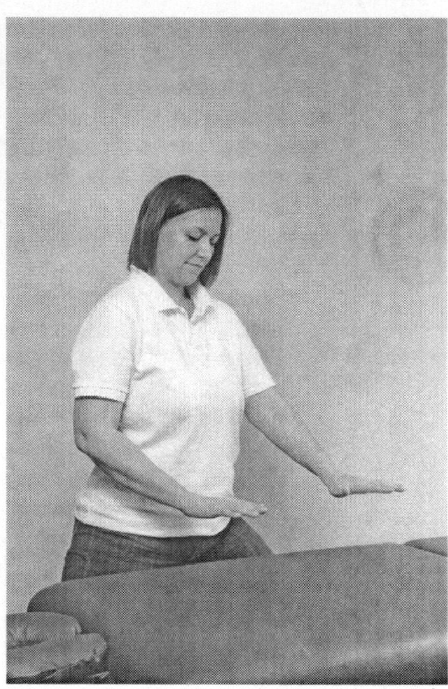
b

Figure 10-12: Move from your hips (and legs, if you're standing) while giving a massage.

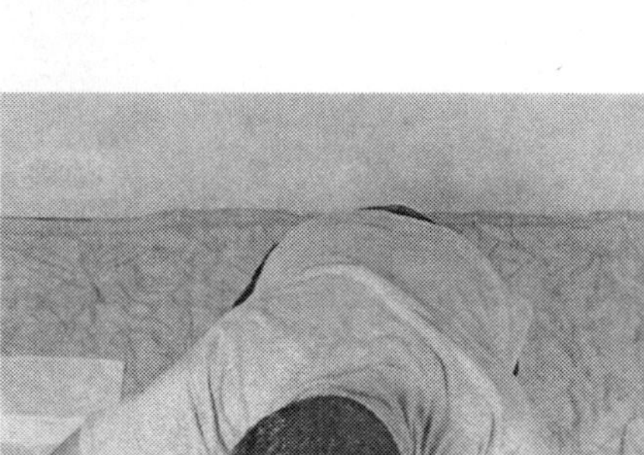
a

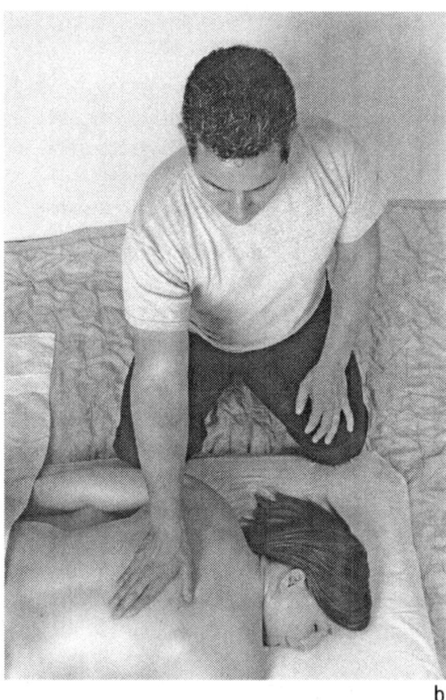
b

Figure 10-13: The wrong way (a) and the right way (b) to apply pressure.

Being Aware of Contraindications and Other Massage Risks

As innocuous as massage may seem, sometimes you should refrain from giving one because it may adversely affect a health condition of the recipient. As I mention earlier in the chapter, these contraindications are warning signs telling you to stay away.

The list of contraindications for massage may be longer than you expect, and it includes some conditions that at first glance don't seem like massage would affect them at all. Take a look:

- **Fever or infectious diseases:** When you have a fever or infectious disease, your body is trying to isolate and expel an invader of some kind. Massage increases overall circulation and can therefore work against your body's natural defenses. And to make matters worse, you expose yourself to your partener's virus as well.
- **Inflammation:** Massage can further irritate an area of inflammation. Inflamed conditions include anything that ends in *-itis*, such as *phlebitis* (inflammation of a vein), *dermatitis* (inflammation of the skin), *arthritis* (inflammation of the joints), and so on. In the case of localized problems, you can still massage around them, however, avoiding the inflammation itself.
- **High blood pressure:** High blood pressure means excessive pressure against blood vessel walls. Massage affects the blood vessels, and so people with high blood pressure or a heart condition should receive light, sedating massages and check with their physicians to see whether they can receive more vigorous massage.
- **Hernia:** Hernias are protrusions of part of an organ (such as the intestines) through a muscular wall. Surgery is a better strategy for getting these organs back into their normal areas.
- **Osteoporosis:** Elderly people with a severe stoop to the shoulders often have this condition, in which bones become porous, brittle, and fragile. Massage may be too intense for this condition.
- **Varicose veins:** Massaging directly over varicose veins can worsen the problem. However, applying a very light massage next to the veins in question, always in a direction toward the heart, can be beneficial.
- **Broken bones:** Stay away from any area with mending bones. A little light massage to the surrounding areas, though, can improve circulation and be quite helpful.

- **Skin problems:** Avoid anything that looks like it shouldn't be there, such as rashes, wounds, bruises, burns, boils, and blisters. These problems are usually local, however, so you can still massage in other areas.
- **Cancer:** Massage increases lymphatic circulation, and cancer can spread through the lymphatic system, so massage may potentially spread the disease. Simple, caring touch is fine, but massage strokes that stimulate circulation are usually not recommended. Always check with a doctor first.
- **Other conditions and diseases:** Diabetes, asthma, and other serious conditions each have their own precautions, so get a doctor's okay before administering massage to a sufferer.
- **HIV infection:** HIV isn't contraindicated itself — it can't be transmitted during massage if there's no exchange of bodily fluids (blood, semen, vaginal fluids, or mother's milk). However, some of the infections that people suffering from the later stages of AIDS experience are contraindicated, and you should avoid those infections. Loving, soothing contact is extremely important for people at any stage of infection, but in the case of any visible rashes, sores, lesions, or swelling, massage is best left to a professional. If you have any cuts, scrapes, or scratches on your hands, wearing thin surgical gloves while massaging an HIV-infected person with any signs of open lesions is an especially good idea.
- **Pregnancy:** Most women love to receive massage during pregnancy, and it's perfectly fine to give them one, but you do need to observe a few precautions. See the nearby sidebar about pregnancy and massage.

This list may make you think your massage partner practically has to get a medical checkup and a doctor's okay before getting a massage, and in many cases, that's exactly what it means. Always err on the side of caution when you're considering giving a massage to a person with any health concerns. Check it out with his or her physician first.

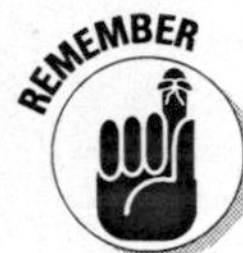

The first and foremost rule here is "Do no harm." If you're not sure about a particular condition, don't give the massage.

The following sections bring you up to speed on other potential massage risks.

Pregnancy: A contraindication?

Some people believe that pregnant women shouldn't receive massage. Most of these people, needless to say, aren't pregnant women, whose backs and legs are often quite sore and who love massage. Chapter 17 delves more fully into this topic, but for now I want to put your mind at ease and say that it's perfectly okay to massage a pregnant woman as long as you observe a few simple precautions:

- Always make sure her legs and head are supported with pillows.
- Never put her in a face-down position to massage her. In her last trimester, she should lie only on her side.
- Use only light gliding strokes directly on the abdomen. Don't press directly onto or knead in this area.
- Always give soothing, relaxing massage moves, never heavy or deep.
- Avoid the ankles and heels because, according to the theory of reflexology, the heels contain special points that may stimulate labor. Going into labor during a massage isn't recommended. Chapter 14 has more info and a diagram showing the location of these reflexology points.

Avoiding bad moves

Ever watch an infant pet a cat? They often have the best of intentions, but they just can't seem to get it right. Wham! goes the beefy little hand on top of the cat's head, and the poor feline scurries away before the infant does any serious damage. Similarly, some moves you shouldn't make during a massage, no matter how good your intentions are. They all cause discomfort, and some of them may even cause harm:

- **Neck pulling:** Don't grasp the head firmly and pull upward, attempting to lengthen the neck.
- **Neck twisting:** Only a very gentle and slow turning of the neck to one side or the other is appropriate during massage. No sudden movements!
- **Neck pulling and twisting together:** Never ever, for any reason, pull and twist the neck at the same time. This movement can be very dangerous (for obvious reasons).

- **Bone cracking:** Never ever try to do a chiropractic-type adjustment if you haven't been trained as a, you know, chiropractor.
- **Bone pushing:** Don't press directly on bones, especially the spine. Instead, glide lightly over these areas.
- **Hyperextension:** Basic stretches are okay, and I explain several in Chapter 15. However, don't try to *hyperextend* any joint past its normal range of motion unless you receive some serious schooling in massage. Hyperextension is hard to do accidentally with the knee or elbow, which resists such maneuvers, but you can easily hyperextend the neck, for example, so use caution.

Taking the highway away from the danger zones: Endangerment sites

Endangerment sites are super-sensitive areas on the body that contain important pieces of your anatomy, like nerves and blood supply, in exposed and vulnerable positions. Highly trained massage therapists can sometimes work in these areas, but if you're not a professional massage ace yourself, stay away from the following spots:

- **Front of the neck/throat:** You've heard of the expression "Go for the jugular," right? Well, this area is where you find it. Unless you're trying to choke someone, avoid this area that also contains the carotid artery and major nerves.
- **Side of the neck:** It's not quite as sensitive as the front of the neck, but you should still treat it delicately.
- **The ear notch:** Just behind your jawbone and beneath your ear you find a little notch that contains a sensitive facial nerve. Don't jam a finger into this notch unless you're trying to extort money or favors from the person receiving the massage.
- **The eyeball:** Unless you're trying to do a Three Stooges massage (popular among college males), don't poke your fingers directly into the person's eyes.
- **The axilla:** *Axilla* is a fancy term for the armpit, which, as you know, is a sensitive area filled with nerves, arteries, and lymph glands. Not to mention, most people are very ticklish there.
- **The upper inner arm:** Just down from the armpit, along the inside of the upper arm, is a sensitive, nerve-filled area along the length of the arm bone. Pressing here too firmly gives you that yucky-nervy feeling.
- **The ulnar notch of the elbow:** Otherwise known as the funny bone, this spot contains the ulnar nerve which, if you touch it too hard, causes normally discreet people to curse in several languages.

- **The abdomen:** Houdini was killed by an unsuspected punch to this area, which is filled with many squishy important bits known as organs. Be especially gentle around the upper abdomen along the ribs, where you find the liver, gall bladder, and spleen.
- **The lower back:** Just to both sides of the spine, and below the ribs, is where you find the kidneys. Don't press too hard here or pound on them.
- **The femoral triangle:** Not to be confused with the Bermuda triangle, this area is often referred to as the groin. It's the inner part of the line in front where your leg meets your body. If you press hard here, you can actually cut off circulation to the leg.
- **Popliteal area:** Popularly known as the back of the knee, you should always treat this spot gingerly. It's very sensitive to pressure.

Please don't do that!

The ultimate contraindication is a request from the person receiving the massage that you stop doing what you're doing. Immediately. Quit it. No more!

When a person says, "Please don't do that," don't do that. This guideline is especially true for well-meaning beginners, who have a tendency to press ever forward with their newfound massage skills in spite of the complaints issuing from the poor soul beneath their fingers.

The following isn't proper massage etiquette:

> Massage partner: "It really hurts!"
>
> You: "Oh no, it doesn't. That's just your tension melting away. Visualize your muscles as butter . . . ."

In massage, more than any other business, the customer is always right. But sometimes the person receiving the massage either doesn't know or won't tell you he's uncomfortable. How do you know what to do then? That's where body language clues, such as the following, come in:

- Curling the toes
- Arching the back
- Inability to speak in a normal tone
- Facial grimaces and contortions
- Excessive sweating, especially in a cool room

So, what should you do when your partner starts showing signs of discomfort? The answer is simple — talk about it. Simple, straightforward communication clears up most situations immediately. Some people just won't be able to believe that you honestly want them to tell you how they feel. Go ahead, surprise them.

The one word never to say when you're giving a massage

You can get away with almost any kind of amateur commentary while giving a massage to friends and family because after all, they understand that you're an amateur. Thus, when you say, "Geez, am I pressing too hard there?" they're likely to respond with some positive criticism. However, there is one particular word that neither amateurs nor professionals should ever utter while giving a massage. Hearing it strikes fear into the poor vulnerable person lying there receiving. And that word is . . .

"Oops."

Like a surgeon saying "oops" in the middle of an operation or a pilot saying "oops" while making the approach for landing, your saying "oops" in the middle of a massage, although hopefully not life-threatening, simply doesn't inspire confidence. It may lead some people to imagine horrible scenarios — injured muscles, crushed arteries, or indelible marks left on the skin.

The person receiving doesn't know what kind of massage move you're attempting to perform at any given moment. So, if you don't get the move exactly right each time, don't worry; she's not going to know the difference. Not unless you say "oops," that is.

Chapter 11

Putting the Moves Together: Massaging the Back of the Body

In This Chapter

- Getting into position and preparing mentally
- Starting off slow and easy
- Taking care of the back
- Working on the back of the legs

Okay, here it is, the moment you've all been waiting for. Time to massage! And you can only talk about it for so long without realizing that massage is not really about talking, it's about feeling. And as Bob Marley once sang, "He who feels it, knows it."

But first, let me fill you in just for a second regarding what, exactly, a massage actually is. "But I already know what a massage is," you may protest. "It's when you rub somebody, right?" Well, yeah, but how long do you rub them for? Where exactly do you massage them and in what sequence? How do you know when to stop? What's the shortest amount of time you can massage your girlfriend and still have her think that you gave her a "real" massage?

I'll try to answer all these questions here. First of all, what most people refer to as a massage is also referred to as a *full body massage*. *Full body* doesn't mean that you massage the Adam's apple, the belly button, the inside of the nasal passages, and every other possible inner and outer surface area of the body, however. What it generally means, and what people have come to expect when they get a massage, is that it lasts a minimum of about an hour (though an hour-and-a-half or two-hour massage is super awesome; just ask anyone who's gotten one), it covers the legs, feet, arms, hands, back, head, neck, shoulders and sometimes the abdomen, and it progresses in some kind of logical sequence. You can definitely get creative with your massage, but if you're jumping all over the body like a rabbit on an energy drink, you may just end up disorienting or annoying your partner.

So, in this chapter and Chapter 12, you sail away toward a full hour of massage bliss that covers the full body as I've just described. This chapter shows you how to massage the back of the body, and Chapter 12 shows you how to massage the front of the body. Of course, I, as your long-distance massage teacher, will be extra proud if you take what you find in these chapters and make it your own by customizing moves, adding moves of your own, swapping one move for another, and so on. These two chapters are not meant to constrict you — far from it. If you stay safe, as counseled in these chapters, you can simply use the suggestions here as signposts along the road to massage heaven. If you're ever lost, come back to the step-by-step instructions and follow along until you go off on a riff of your own once more. Also, you can use this sequence as a launching-off point that you can practice, get used to, and then improvise and improve upon.

Starting Off Right: Five Preliminary Steps

So, as you get started with the actual massage, make sure you cover these five preliminary steps:

- Cleanliness first
- Draping
- Take your positions
- Invocation
- Use the force, Luke

Cleanliness first

You're all set up, the mood is right, the lights are low, and now, before you do anything else, you must follow one critical procedure before starting the massage — wash your hands!

Washing cleanses away dirt and grime, and it also protects you and your partner from nasty bacteria. Just like your mother always told you, it's a good habit to get into.

Draping

The word *draping,* when uttered by massage therapists, refers to the various ways in which the body is covered for modesty during the massage. If you are massaging your significant other, draping may not be an issue, but a large number of people really do want to be modestly covered at all times during a massage. That's where sheets and towels come in. You can have your partner get completely undressed and covered with a bed sheet or bath sheet (basically a large bath towel) before the massage starts and then just uncover the area you're working on at any given time. You can see an example of a modest draping technique when massaging the legs in a face-up position in Figure 11-1. First, tuck the towel between the legs (a), tuck it upwards slightly (b), and finally pull one edge out on the outer edge of the leg (c).

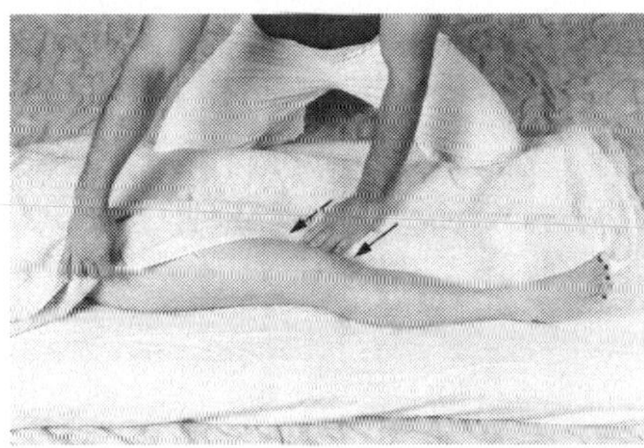

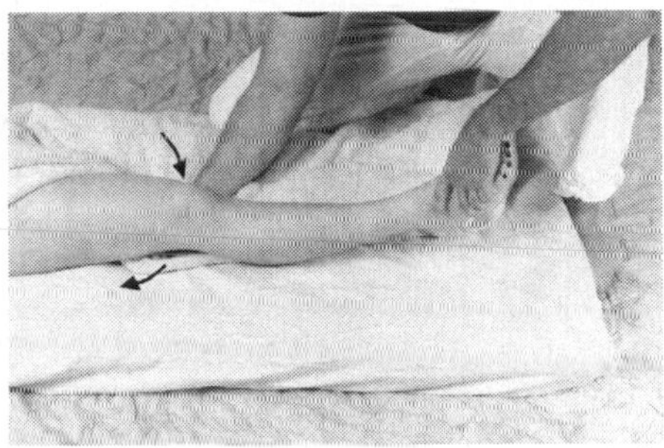

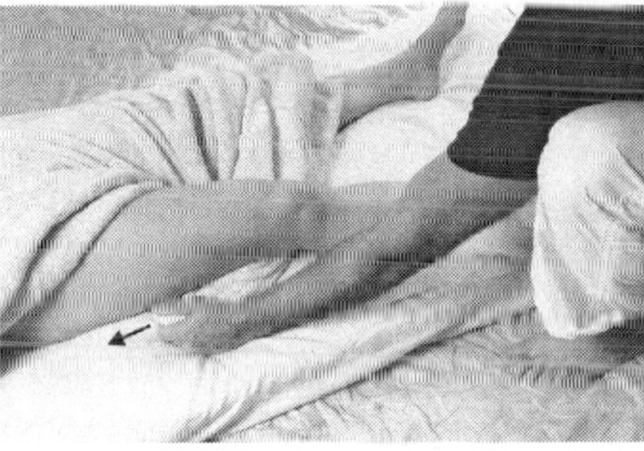

Figure 11-1: Make sure your partner feels comfortable and modestly covered.

When it comes to draping, you basically want to cover up what a bathing suit would cover up, which can be a little tricky with a towel while administering all kinds of nifty massage moves. When your massage partner is a female, it may be appropriate to use what we therapists call a *breast drape,* shown in Figure 11-2. First place a smaller towel, usually a hand towel, over the larger drape (a), and then hold it in place over the breasts while pulling the larger towel down beneath it (b).

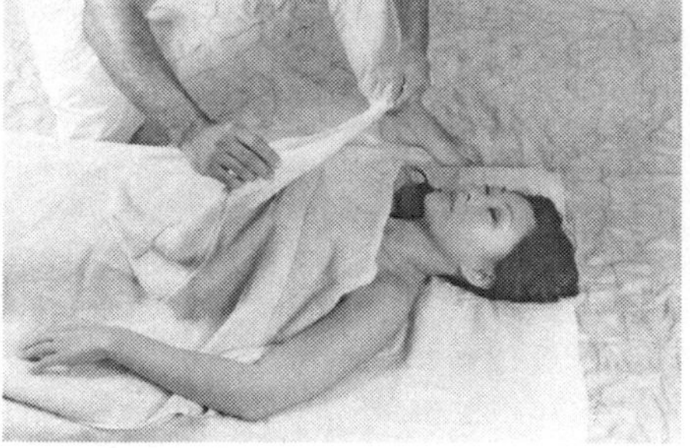
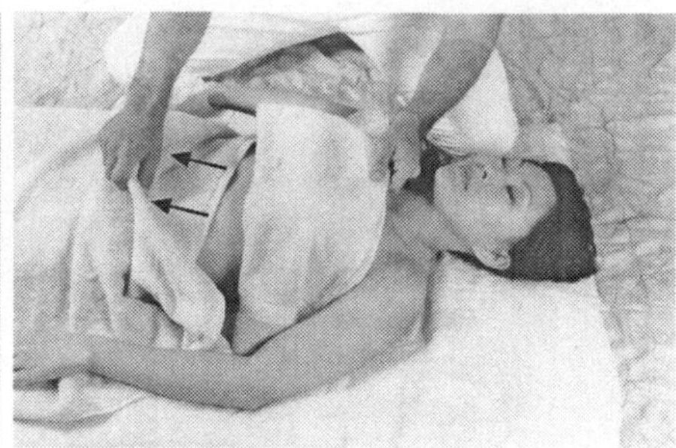

Figure 11-2: The breast drape technique.

Take your positions

To begin the massage, you and your partner both have to be in the right positions. In the routine shown in this chapter, you start with your partner lying on her stomach, and you sit alongside her back.

Some people are sticklers about this whole positioning issue, but I don't believe in starting every massage in the same position every time. In fact, starting over and over again in the same position can lead to a boring massage. Instead, begin each massage where your intuition, your partner's suggestion, and your observations lead you. The sequence of the massage shown in this chapter is not the only acceptable way.

Invocation

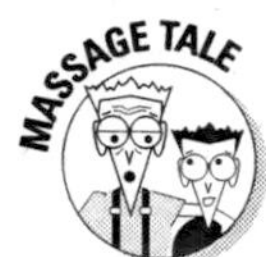

In Chapter 4, I describe a massage I received from Wesley, who's a native Hawaiian massage therapist and healer on the Big Island. What I didn't describe was the prayer Wesley used to begin the massage, sitting humbly on the floor beside me, melodiously intoning some words in Hawaiian: *"Kou makou makua iloko okalani."* This invocation was meant to make both Wesley and me at one with the source of life. He learned it from his teacher, Auntie Margaret, and she in turn was taught it by her elders.

Although you may feel a little funny at first, it may be appropriate for you to say a couple of words of invocation as you're about to start your massage. They don't have to be in Hawaiian; something simple is fine, such as, "I summon the spirit of health and relaxation to be with us during this massage." Just say them from your heart, and you get your message across.

Use the force, Luke

Remember, you're not just dealing with a pile of flesh and bones here. Your partner is more than a series of points to be pushed and muscles to be kneaded. She has a magical inner spark, too. According to many massage philosophies, especially those from the East like shiatsu, the body is filled with invisible pathways that are pulsing with this inner energy, variously known as *chi*, *ki*, *prana*, *universal-life-force-energy*, and *the-force-Luke-remember-the-force*.

You can give a better massage if you simply stop for a moment at the beginning of the massage and focus on that force that exists within you and your partner. Remember the scene from Star Wars when Luke is zeroing in on the Death Star using nothing but his intuition? The voice of his mentor is there in his head urging him to "use the force." Tune into your own inner guidance as you begin the massage, and you may surprise yourself with how well you do.

Performing the First Touch

The first touch is the crucial moment when all of your preparation and practice is put to the test. Ninety-five percent of what your partner needs to know about your massage is completely obvious in the first few seconds, with the very first touch. At this juncture, you go forward into the realm of being and doing rather than thinking, and a new thing is created: the massage.

Reaching both hands down, place them gently and consciously on your partner's back, as if you were touching a sleeping child and trying not to wake her. Put one hand up on the top of the spine near the head, and the other down by the base of the spine. Then just touch for a moment, with no need to move. You can actually summon the force and say your invocation (see the preceding section) at this time, too. (See Figure 11-3.)

Hold this position for half a minute, with your hands on your partner's spine, simply communicating your presence and loving intentions. Then you can begin.

Note: You may notice that I haven't included any stretches in this chapter or Chapter 12. That's because I explain stretches when I discuss sports massage in Chapter 15. This fact doesn't mean you can't use them during your full body massage, too, though. In fact, I highly recommend stretches. After you master some of the stretches, sprinkle them liberally throughout your massage for optimum effect.

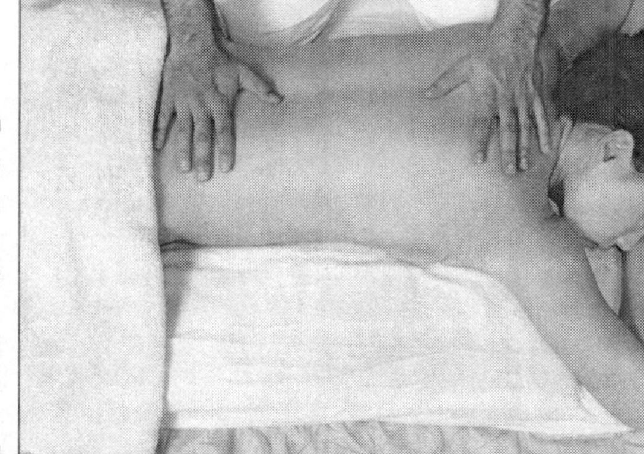

Figure 11-3: After you summon the forces within, reach out and touch someone.

Working the Back

The back is a great place to begin a massage because many people equate massage with a "back rub." Although it looks large and solid, the back is actually prone to lots of little aches and pains, and much of the tension and everyday complaints people have can be found there. Thus the famous phrase, "Oh, my aching back." And finally, the back is the least vulnerable area to touch someone, psychologically speaking, so people are more likely to relax and "let you in" when you begin there.

Check out Chapter 10 for details on the various massage techniques I mention here. Follow (or at least consider) the general steps in the following sections to fully massage the back:

Beginning the back massage

Work with these steps to get your back massage going.

1. **Without moving your hands from the position they're in, simply begin to rock your partner gently from side to side by using the tailbone as a kind of handle for the heel of your hand.**

   When you get good at it, you can extend your rocking maneuvers further up the back and down onto the buttocks and even the legs. The idea is to get a wave-like motion going through your partner's body so that she starts to melt into the floor.

   When you want to get someone out of the mood they were just in and into the mood of getting a massage, nothing beats rocking.

2. **Try a little skin rolling.**

   People either love skin rolling, or they really don't like it at all, so you have to experiment a little and ask your partner how it feels. Start by repositioning yourself up by your partner's head and getting a grasp on the skin at the base of the neck between your thumb and your first two fingers. Walk this roll down the back, keeping it between your fingers the whole time, as in Figure 11-4. This takes some practice, so start with a partner who doesn't mind playing guinea pig.

3. **Use your fingertips to "hook" into the muscles alongside both sides of the spine near the tailbone; start vibrating your hand while dragging it with medium pressure back up toward your partner's head, as shown in Figure 11-5.**

   Repeat this three times.

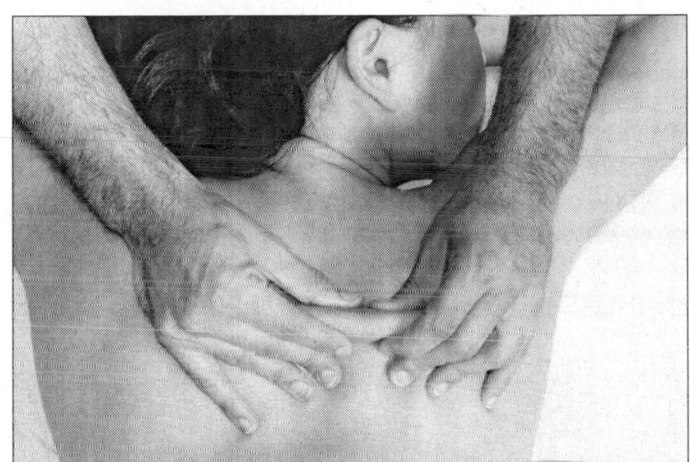

Figure 11-4: Skin rolling.

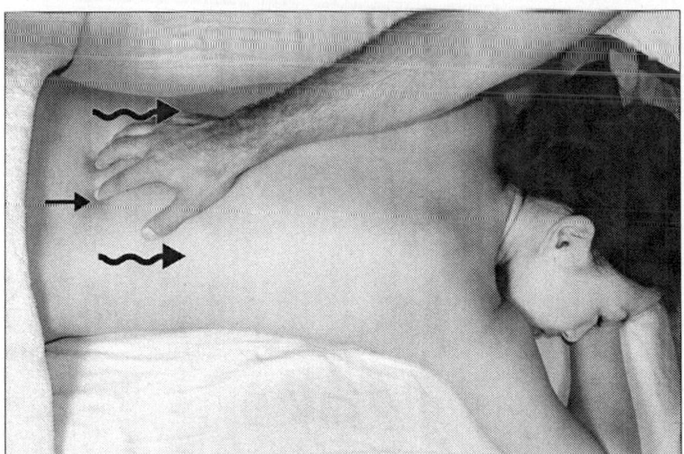

Figure 11-5: Vibrating up the back.

4. **Glide down with both hands on the muscles on either side of the spine, with your fingers pointed in toward the middle; when you reach the base of the spine, swivel your fingers toward the outside and glide back up as shown in Figure 11-6.**

   Repeat this gliding four or five times, using light pressure at first and then slightly firmer pressure.

   This long gliding movement spreads oil and further warms up the entire area. See the section on oil in Chapter 9 for the proper oil-spreading technique.

5. **When you reach the base of the spine on the fourth or fifth glide, stop and apply circular rubbing all over the *sacrum,* or tailbone, as shown in Figure 11-7.**

   You may notice that when your partner is lying down, this bone is tilted in such a way that it presents a relatively flat surface, so you can lean your weight forward from your partner's head and apply pressure to it.

6. **Start with your thumbs at the top of your partner's back (one thumb on either side of the spine) and *very slowly* push your thumbs down along the ridge of the muscles one inch on either side of the spine with medium to firm pressure, as Figure 11-8 illustrates.**

   This move should take 30 seconds or more. When you get to a tight spot, slow down and let your thumbs sink into it even more slowly, making a mental note to revisit this area later.

   After you reach the base of the spine, glide your way back to the top.

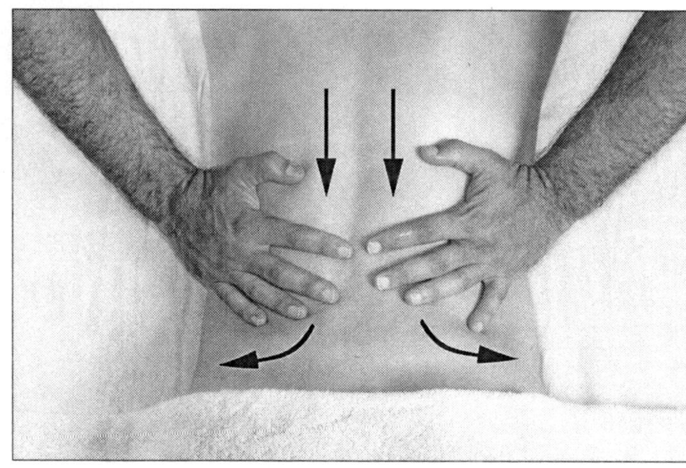

Figure 11-6: Gliding along the spine.

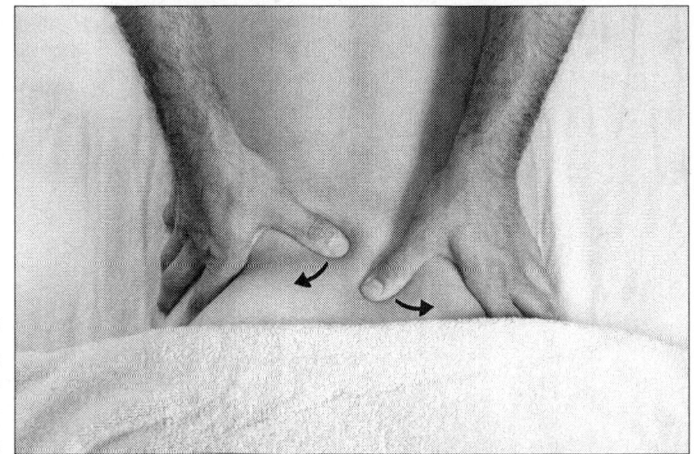

Figure 11-7: Circular rubbing.

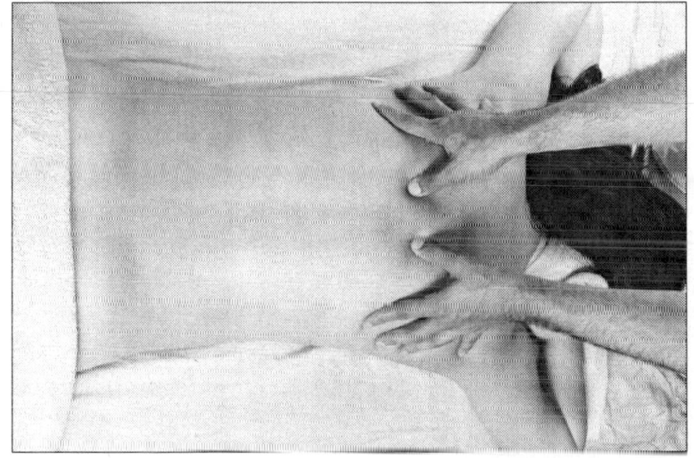

Figure 11-8: Gliding/ pressing along both sides of the spine.

7. **With your thumbs atop the shoulders and your fingers up on your partner's back, knead the tops of the shoulders, also called the *trapezius muscles*, as shown in Figure 11-9.**

   While you're doing this kneading, you can feel for tight spots and then stop for a moment to apply pressure with your thumbs directly on those areas.

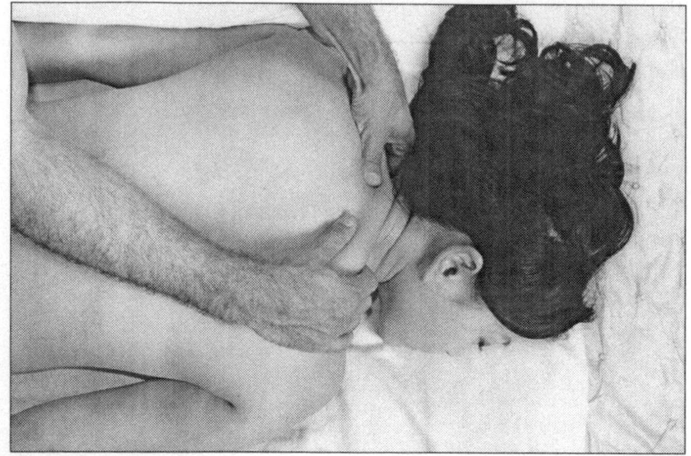

Figure 11-9: Kneading the trapezius.

Continuing the back massage

This section helps you finish off a great back massage. Just remember these steps:

1. **Switch your position to your partner's side facing toward her head and then, using medium pressure, glide your hands up the back, separating them at your partner's shoulders and gliding back down with lighter pressure.**

   Do this move two or three times, being careful not to press too hard directly over the spine.

2. **Reaching across your partner's back, drape your fingers over her side and then pull back slowly all the way to the spine, actually lifting her body up a tiny bit and then letting it back down again as you engage in a nifty reverse glide, as shown in Figure 11-10.**

3. **With small kneading movements that use mostly just the fingers, reach down and pull up the muscles along the back of the neck, alternating one hand after the other as Figure 11-11 demonstrates.**

   You can be firm, but be careful not to pinch your partner. Also, make sure not to pull her hair when you're doing this maneuver. You should also avoid reaching around too far with your fingertips because you may end up on the front of the throat, which can hurt or even cause damage.

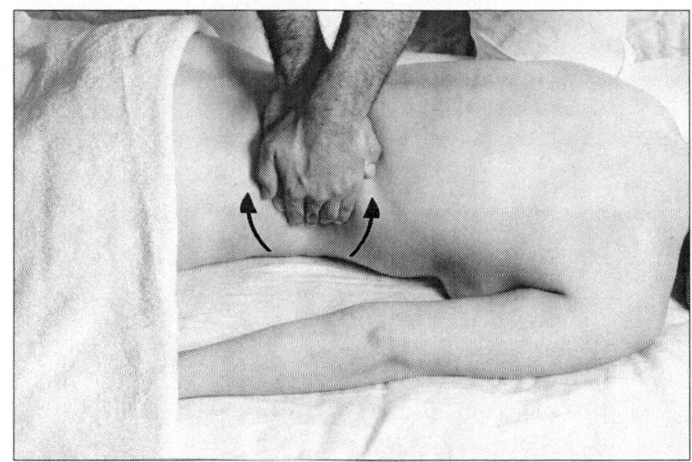

Figure 11-10: Reverse gliding.

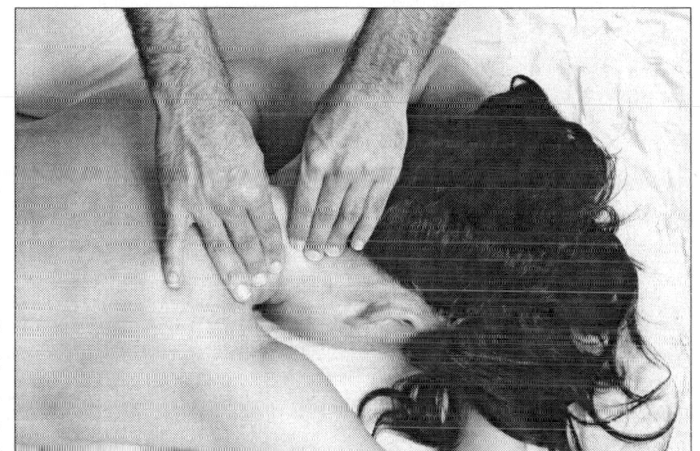

Figure 11-11: Neck kneading.

4. **Start at the base of the spine and place your thumbs in the little groove that's formed between the spine itself and the band of muscles that run up alongside the far side of the spine, pressing out toward the opposite side of the back and moving your thumbs in a little reverse *J* motion over the muscle as shown in Figure 11-12.**

Never press directly on the spine itself while you're doing this move. Instead, keep your thumbs pressing away from the spine at all times.

The main difference between a good massage and a mediocre one is that a good massage is always custom-made for each person every time. So customize this maneuver and apply it exactly where your partner needs it this time, seeking out and concentrating on the tight spots you find during your gliding in Step 6 in the preceding section.

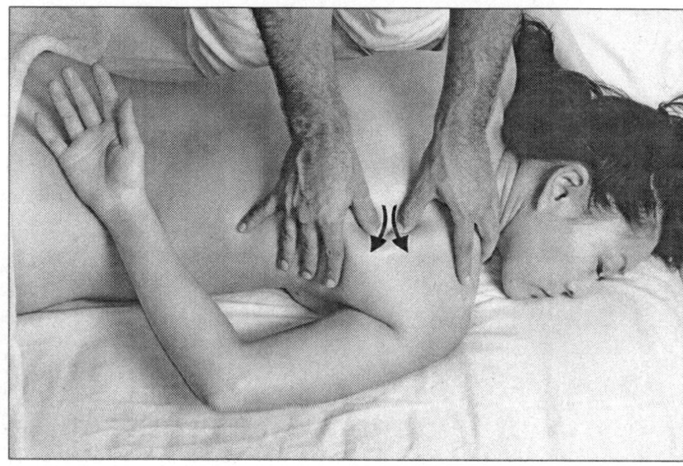

Figure 11-12: *J* motion pressing alongside spine.

5. **Release tension by running your fingers along the lifted inner edge of the shoulder blade, pressing in and down while you do so as Figure 11-13 shows.**

   If you lift your partner's hand onto her lower back, the shoulder blade automatically lifts up and you can easily see it. Sometimes you can feel the shoulder blade lifting even further from the back as you relax the muscles. For some people, this movement can be uncomfortable, so go slowly putting the arm into position.

6. **Use your thumbs to zero in on the spot that lies about midway out from the spine at the level of the armpit, as shown in Figure 11-14.**

   It's right at the base of the inner edge of the shoulder blade and is usually tight on almost everyone. If you can find this spot and do a thumb press with firm pressure for ten seconds or longer, you may feel the entire shoulder fall away from the back in relaxation.

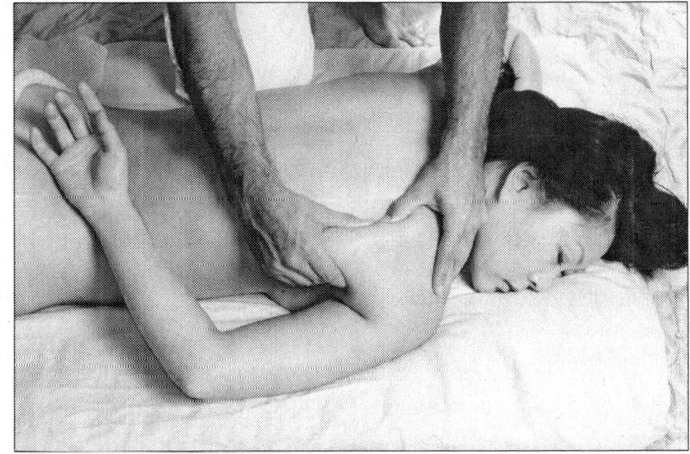

Figure 11-13: Lifting the shoulder blade.

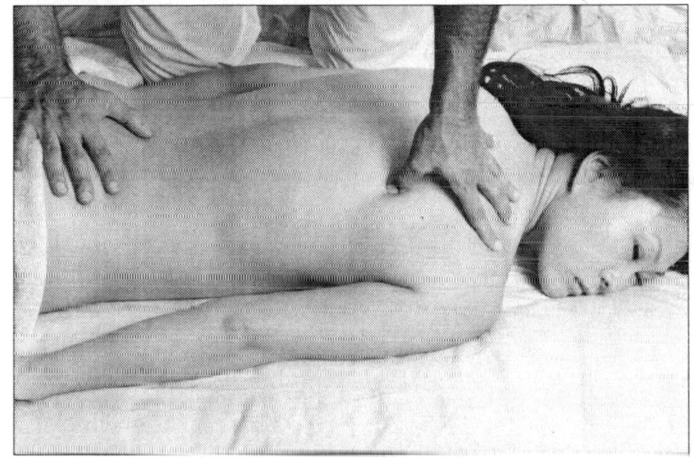

Figure 11-14: Pinpointing pressure.

7. **Tap all across the upper and lower back, being careful to avoid the spine, as shown in Figure 11-15.**

   This method is a typical way to finish massaging the back (and every body part, for that matter). It feels good, but I find it sometimes disrupts the calming, soothing effect of the massage. Only use tapping if your partner wants it, or if he's about to jump off the table to engage in some activity, in which case some serious karate chops and loose fist pounding are called for. Otherwise, stick to some soft fingertip tapping at this point or leave it out altogether.

Knots, and what to do with them

As you get used to gliding over people's bodies with your hands, you may quickly realize that no two bodies are the same and that, in fact, the same body can even feel different on different days. Eventually, you'll know how to distinguish a *knot* (a tense lump of muscle tissue) from an area of normal muscle tone. Then you can apply the techniques you find in this book to start relaxing those tight places.

You could easily spend an entire hour just dealing with your partner's knots, so you have to decide when enough is enough and move onto the next area. This decision is a tough call because your partner's knots and sore spots are the areas that need the most attention. In general, during a full body massage, spend no more than five minutes on any particular tight spot. If you want to focus on it more later, schedule a special session just for that purpose.

When working on a tight spot, don't just dig in like you're excavating for copper in a rocky mine. Instead, use gentle but insistent pressure, precisely locating the tight spot and touching it as if your fingers were saying, "Whoa, there big fella, everything's gonna be okay now. All ya gotta do is let go. Soften up. Relax. Melt. There ya go. . . ."

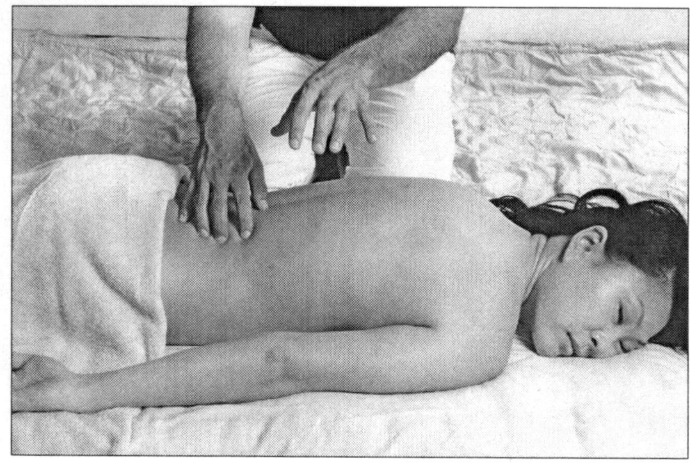

Figure 11-15: Tapping to complete the back massage.

8. **Make your departure from the back by using gliding connective strokes (see the later sidebar "Creating wholeness" for more).**

   Remember to make your departure from the back a gradual one, lest you shock your partner and cause sudden back-massage withdrawal symptoms.

Moving to the Back of the Legs and Buttocks

The buttocks contain the largest muscle in the human body, and they do a large percentage of the work. Without them, you couldn't walk, sit, or dance the Bump. Buttocks really deserve a lot of respect, but they're often disparaged and have unfortunately become the butt of many off-color jokes. Don't let this flippant attitude about buttocks keep you from spending some serious time there during your massage. And don't forget about the backs of the legs, including the hamstrings (which can get very tight on many people and merit a good deal of massage) and the calves (which are prone to cramps).

To give the buttocks and back of the legs the attention they deserve, follow these steps (and flip to Chapter 10 for more on the specific massage moves):

1. **After you glide your way down from your partner's back and reposition yourself by your partner's legs, apply some oil to the entire back surface of one leg with firm gliding strokes, circling your outer hand around the buttock and gliding more lightly back down as in Figure 11-16.**

   Your partner can relax more if you can get her to let go of her lower leg and allow you to take the full weight of her limb in your hands. Take a look at Chapter 6 for a reminder on how to do this.

2. **Lift your partner's foot, supporting it with both of your hands while applying circular rubbing all around the anklebone with your thumbs and fingertips of both hands, as shown in Figure 11-17.**

3. **Before you put your partner's foot back down, do some gentle shaking movements, using the foot as a handle to move the leg as Figure 11-18 illustrates.**

   This tactic can help relax the muscles of the entire limb, right up into the joints, in this case the knee and hip. Practice until just using a gentle shaking at the foot can produce a rhythmical movement throughout the body up to the head.

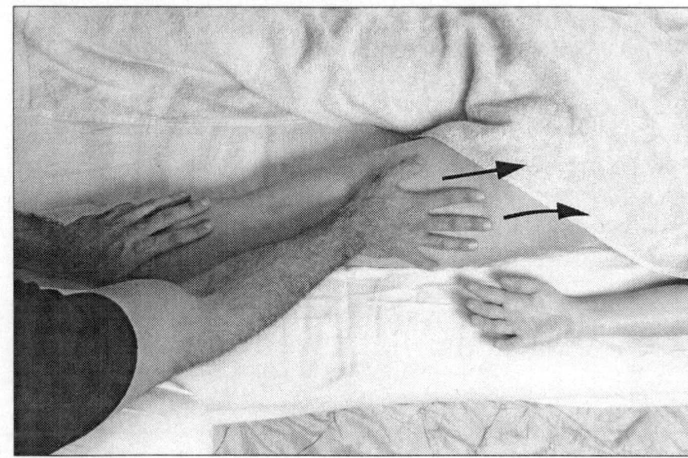

Figure 11-16: Gliding over the backs of the legs.

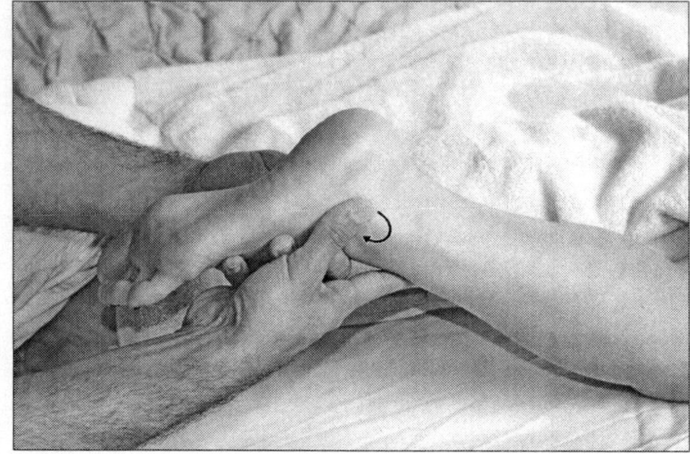

Figure 11-17: Ankle rubbing.

4. **Run your thumbs or the tips of your fingers up the middle of the calf, separating the two sides, as shown in Figure 11-19.**

   The largest muscle in the calf is actually separated into two "bellies." You can also make a straight line up on either side of the middle.

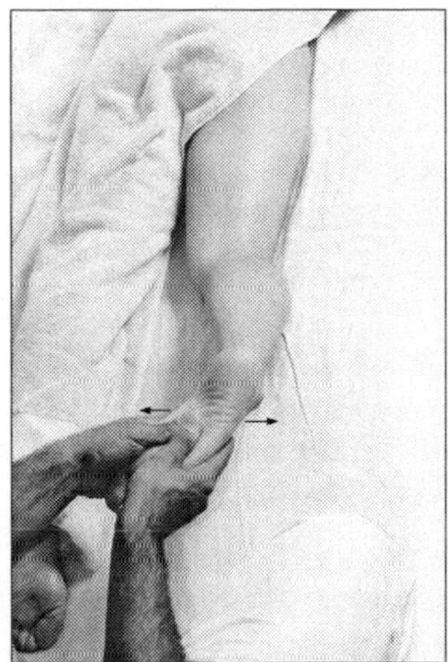

Figure 11-18: Foot shaking.

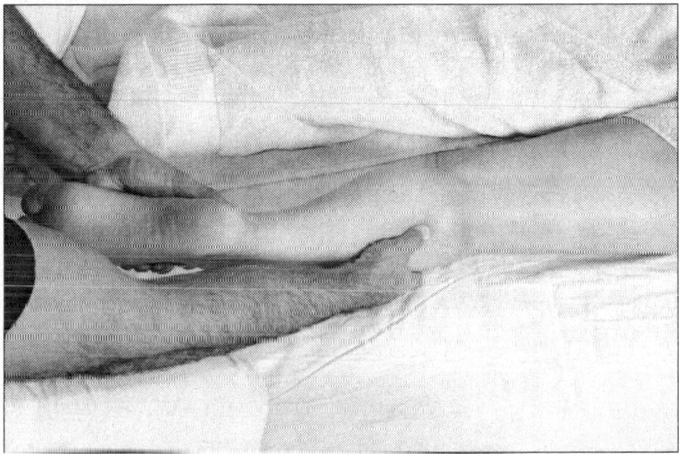

Figure 11-19: Thumb gliding on calves.

Creating wholeness

You can create a better experience for your partner if you never really "finish" one part of the body. Because, if you finish, that means the clock is ticking, and the massage is slowly dripping away. You'll provide a better experience if you create the illusion of timelessness by connecting all the pieces of the massage together into one whole.

So, just because you've already massaged the back, that doesn't mean you shouldn't allow your hands to move there again. In fact, you should add some *connective strokes* (meaning the stroke starts on one part of the body and ends on another, such as the leg and back for example) throughout the massage so that it feels as though you never completely finish with any particular part of the body. You can even connect the front of the body to the back by reaching beneath your partner during certain moves.

5. **While you knead the calf muscle with a back and forth motion, move your hands up and down so that you cover the entire muscle as Figure 11-20 demonstrates.**

   Stop about two-thirds of the way down from the knee because the calf tapers down to the Achilles tendon there and becomes too thin to knead. At that point, you can continue by squeezing the tendon between your thumb and fingers down to the ankle.

6. **Grasping the leg just above the ankle with both hands, use the webbing between your thumbs and forefingers to create a tight seal; squeeze in and glide up the leg at the same time, as shown in Figure 11-21, moving slowly and stopping when you reach the back of the knee.**

   With this maneuver, you can actually help move stagnant blood out of the limb, improving circulation. If you do it correctly, this move may incite your partner to say something like, "Whoa, that's intense!" Take this as a sign that you're doing things right, but also make sure that you're not squeezing too hard — there's a fine line between intense and painful.

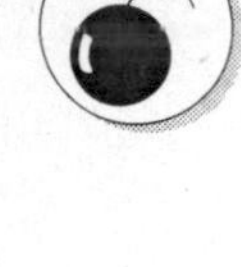

   Apply only very slight pressure over the back of the knee, which is an area with blood vessels and nerves close to the surface. And be careful to avoid any varicose veins because massaging against the blood flow over them could have a negative effect on the one-way little valves in the veins.

7. **Making your hands into fists, apply pressure with the knuckles into the back of the upper legs, called the *hamstrings*, as shown in Figure 11-22.**

   Knuckling is a form of gliding that is especially appropriate to this area because each knuckle slides between the long bands of muscles here.

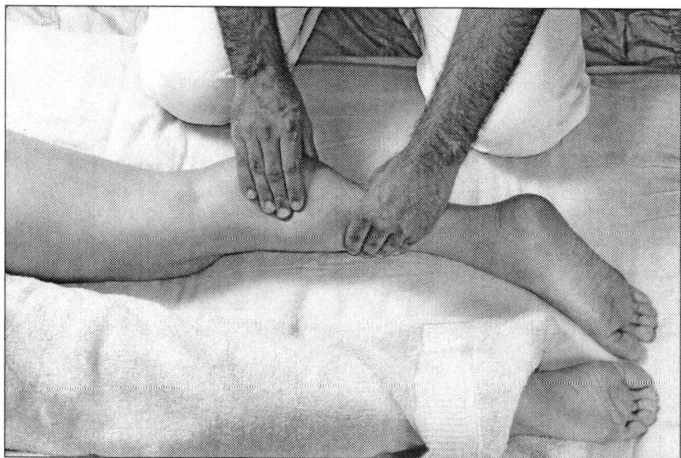

Figure 11-20: Calf kneading.

8. **Knead from the top of the leg down to the knee, moving up and down three to four times as in Figure 11-23.**

   This move feels like an ice cream sundae for the leg muscles. To make it most effective, try keeping as much of your hand in contact with the skin as possible as you squeeze, roll, and push.

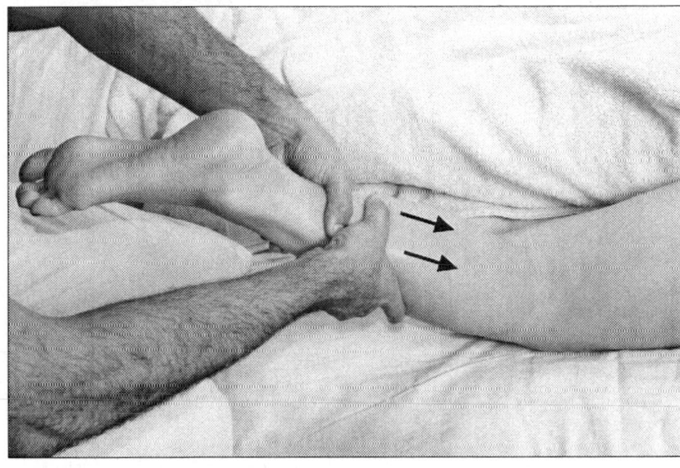

Figure 11-21: Calf squeezing.

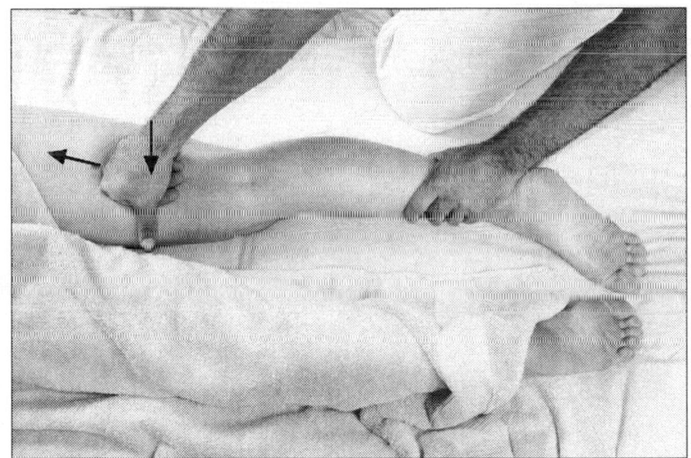

Figure 11-22: Knuckle gliding on hamstrings.

9. **To find just the right spot on a buttock to press, palpate the outer upper edge of the tailbone (sacrum) and then go straight down toward the leg halfway across the buttock and press directly in here with your thumbs as in Figure 11-24.**

Depending upon how big any particular buttock is, you have a variety of choices of where to press, but this move should get you right in the middle. Use your fingers, fist, or elbow at an angle perpendicular to the surface. Hold this move for five to ten seconds.

This move is particularly beneficial for sciatica pain which can run from the buttock all the way down the leg but is usually felt in the upper leg.

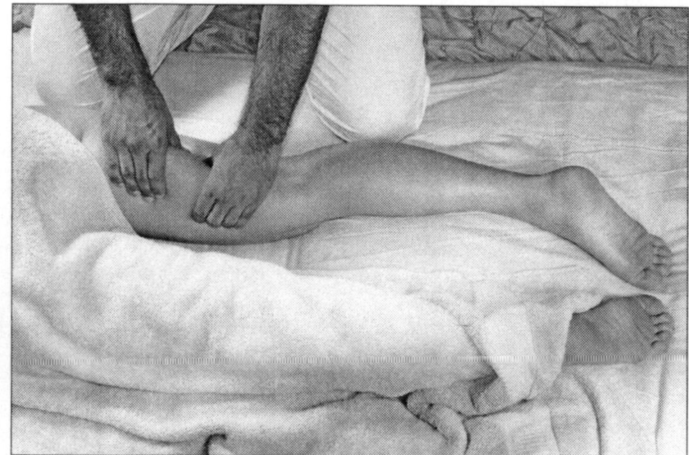

Figure 11-23: Hamstring kneading.

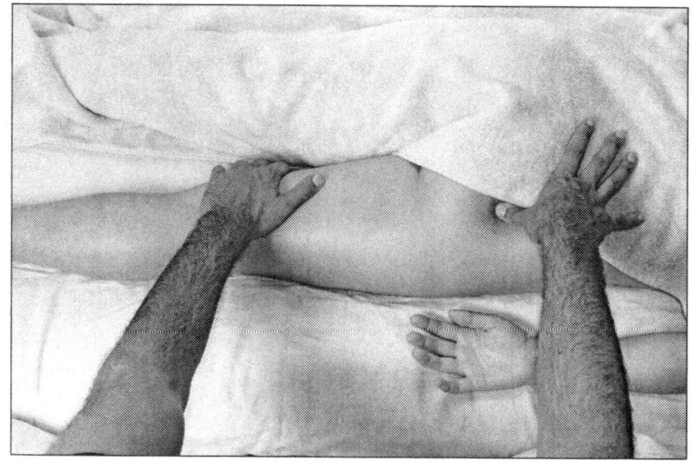

Figure 11-24: Pressure point on buttocks.

10. **Knead the thick muscles of the buttocks as shown in Figure 11-25, particularly on the upper, outside portion, which often tends to be the sorest.**

    You have to watch where your fingers are going while you squeeze, roll, and push here, though! It's kind of a tight area to work in.

11. **Use loose fists and firm pressure to provide some tapping here (as Figure 11-26 illustrates); move the tapping down the leg, opening your fists so that you're doing karate-chop moves.**

    Because the buttocks include the largest muscles in the body, they can withstand some heavy percussion movements; however, be sure not to pound with your fists on the tailbone, which is much more delicate. And remember to lighten up over the back of the knee!

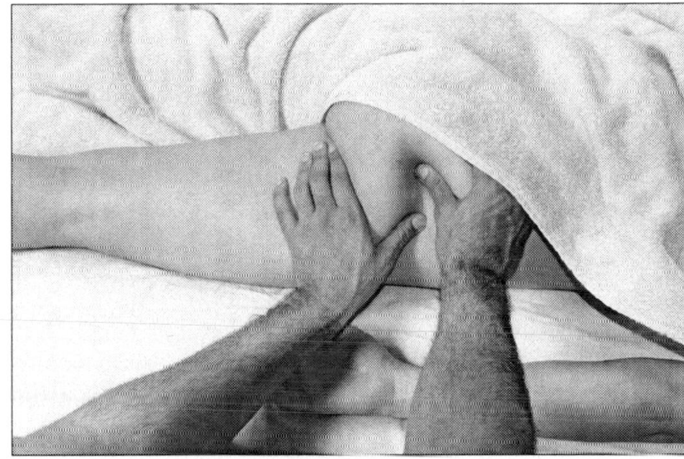

Figure 11-25: Kneading buttocks.

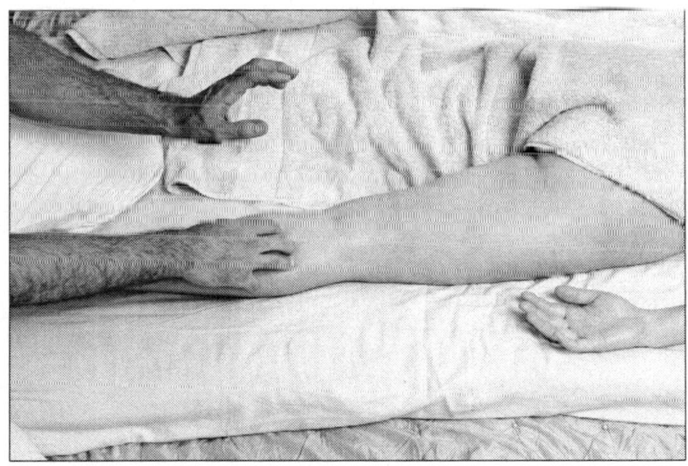

Figure 11-26: Tapping down legs.

12. **Apply light fingertip brushing up the back of the leg and onto the back and then back down again (see Figure 11-27).**

    After pummeling, pressing, squeezing, and kneading your way across your partner's back, fingertip brushing is a really good way to remind your partner how nice you are. You can extend the move from the feet all the way to the head.

After you finish the first leg, switch to the other leg and repeat. Remember, because you already connected the back with the first leg, you want to do some connecting strokes when you begin the second leg as well. So, make your initial gliding on the second leg go up and over the buttocks and onto the lower back.

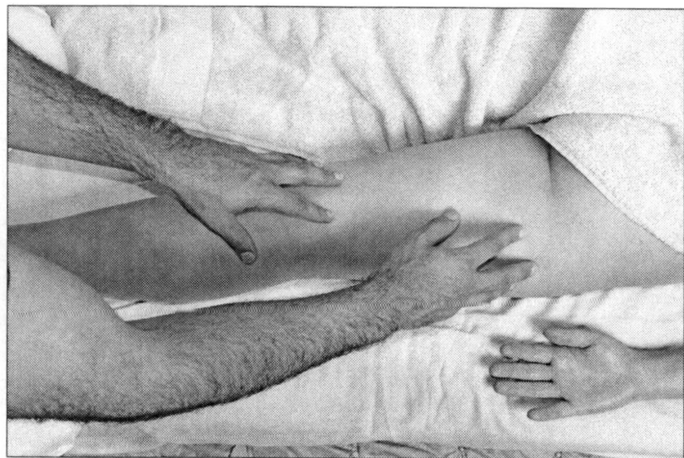

Figure 11-27: Fingertip brushing.

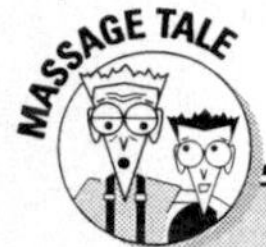

Turning over

In my opinion, not enough is said about the art of turning over during massages. Often, this turn is the only physical effort a massage recipient has to make for over an hour. And, as it comes right in the middle of the experience, it has the potential to be disruptive and a little jarring. For these reasons, most massage pros are quite gentle with their clients when it comes time for them to turn. In a soft, soothing voice, they say something like, "All right, Mr. Smith, I'm going to ask you to gently roll over onto your back now. Take your time."

You have to watch your wording carefully because there are those who take what you say too literally. I have one client who is a world-class athlete, and once when I asked him to "flip over," he literally flipped, springing a foot off the table and twisting over in midair to come crashing back down on the table, splintering one of its wooden legs.

When it comes time for your own partner to turn over, follow the example of the pros:

- Be gentle.
- Speak softly.
- Give them as much time as they need.
- Assist them if necessary, offering support.
- Use the phrases *roll over* or *turn gently* instead of *flip.*

Chapter 12

Putting the Moves Together: Massaging the Front of the Body

In This Chapter

- Starting with the face and scalp
- Working on the upper body: Neck, shoulders, arms, and hands
- Moving down to the front of the torso, legs, and feet
- Ending the massage well

Here you are, smack in the middle of giving a full-blown massage. Do you know how much good karma that's building up in your favor? Those people who give full body massages all the way through to the end are held in extremely high regard by those people who receive the massage. Just wait, you'll soon see (if you haven't already) the look of swooning gratitude on your partner's face. It's really worth the effort!

For a moment here, I'd just like to be your own private little cheerleading section, shouting out some support from the sidelines. You're doing great! Keep up the good work! Don't stop now!

You're halfway through the whole massage, but some of the most interesting and intricate stuff is about to come. This chapter is all about the front of the body and how to massage its various parts. ***Note:*** You can start a massage on either the front or back of the body, so Chapters 11 and 12 are reversible at your discretion, especially if your partner is feeling a little sore in a particular area and wants you to concentrate there first. Whichever side you start with, make sure to do some nice opening and closing moves like those at the beginning of Chapter 11 and the end of this chapter in order to make your massage a nice package that fits together perfectly, whichever way you choose to start.

Providing Relaxation to the Face and Scalp

After your partner is on her back, you are presented with entirely different terrain to massage. The front of the body is a little more perplexing. You have to deal with more intricate surfaces, as well as more private, vulnerable, and delicate areas. Therefore, you need to be more of a diplomat while massaging the front of someone's body. Most people allow just about anyone to give them a backrub, but when it comes time for you to touch the front of their bodies, they have to trust you.

The face, for example, is quite a private area. Although it's exposed to the world for all to see, it's not there for all to touch. You have to be sensitive as you begin to massage your partner's face. Avoid large gestures and quick movements. All of your maneuvers here, including those you make before you even touch your partner, should be smooth, deliberate, and slow.

You probably don't need any extra oil for the face. The oil leftover on your hands from massaging the back is sufficient.

Follow these steps for massaging the face and scalp (and head to Chapter 10 for more on the specific massage moves mentioned):

1. **Place your hands gently on the side of your partner's head, thumbs resting on the forehead and glide your thumbs out from the middle toward the sides, starting low by the brow and making three to four lines progressively higher; as shown in Figure 12-1, begin making circles with your thumbs all across the forehead.**

   This position is a perfect place to start massaging the forehead with some thumb gliding and firm circular rubbing.

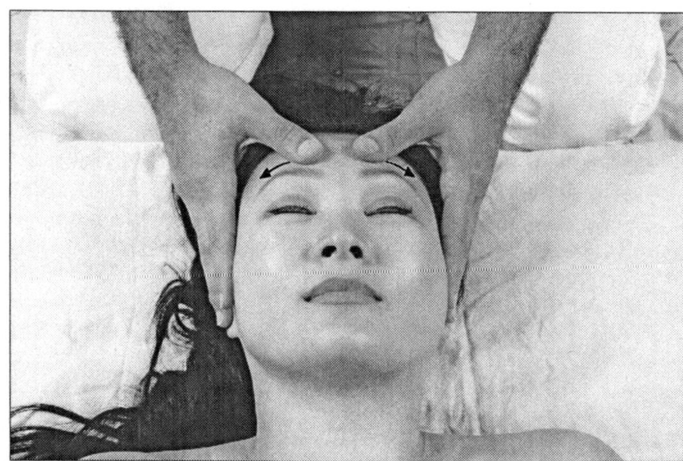

Figure 12-1: Thumb lines on the forehead.

2. **Leaving your hands in about the same position, begin using the fingertips to circle into the side of the head around the spot where sideburns would start if your partner had some, as Figure 12-2 illustrates.**

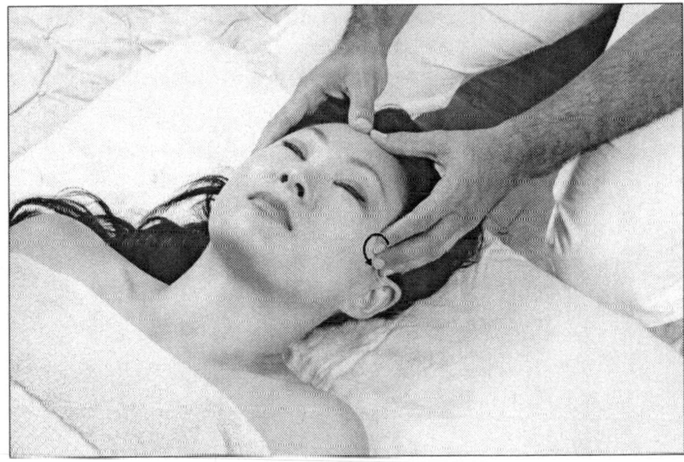

Figure 12-2: Fingertip circles on the temples.

3. **Using your thumbs (or the tips of your first two fingers), trace around the edges of the bones that surround the eye — across the brow, down along the nose, and around the top of the cheek bones, as shown in Figure 12-3.**

   You may try a little mini-kneading along the same path with your thumbs and fingertips.

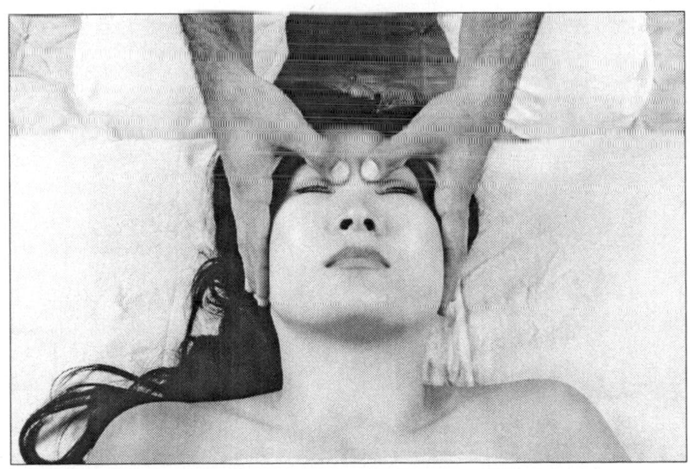

Figure 12-3: Tracing thumbs around the eyes.

Make sure your partner isn't wearing contact lenses before applying any pressure, even if it's very light, near the eyes or directly on the eyelids.

4. **Glide your fingertips lightly across the top and down along the sides of the nose, being careful not to block your partner's breathing passages.**

   The base of the nose, near the outside edge of the nostrils, is a good place to apply light to moderate pressure and small circular rubbing as in Figure 12-4, which helps open sinuses in the area.

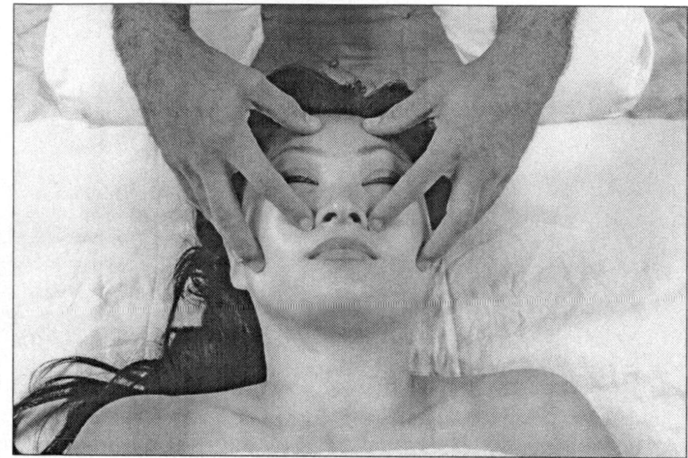

Figure 12-4: Circular rubbing to the base of the nose.

5. **Use your thumbs in an opening gesture to fan out across the cheeks from just under the inside corner of the eye down toward the jawbone (see Figure 12-5).**

   The pressure you apply should be light to medium.

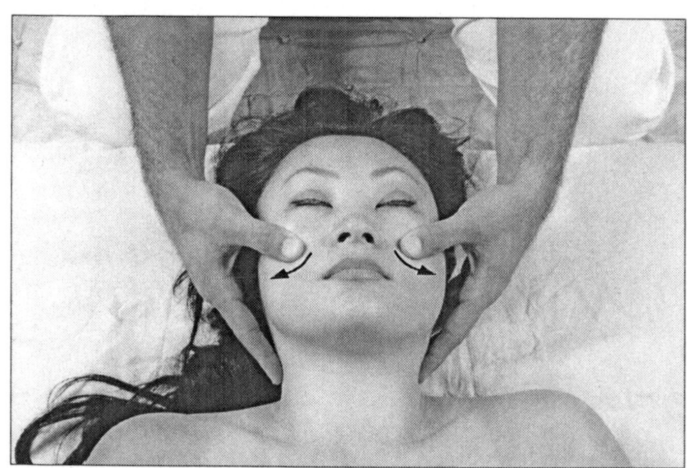

Figure 12-5: Thumbs fanning across the cheeks.

6. **Apply circular rubbing all around the chewing muscles with your fingertips as Figure 12-6 demonstrates.**

   You find the chewing muscles slightly in front of and below the ear at the corner of the jawbone. In order to locate them, ask your partner to clench her teeth, which makes these muscles bulge slightly out to the side.

   Locate the highest point on this muscle, directly in the center, and use some pinpoint pressure directly inward for five to ten seconds while suggesting to your partner, "Relax your jaw, let your mouth open slightly, and just breathe."

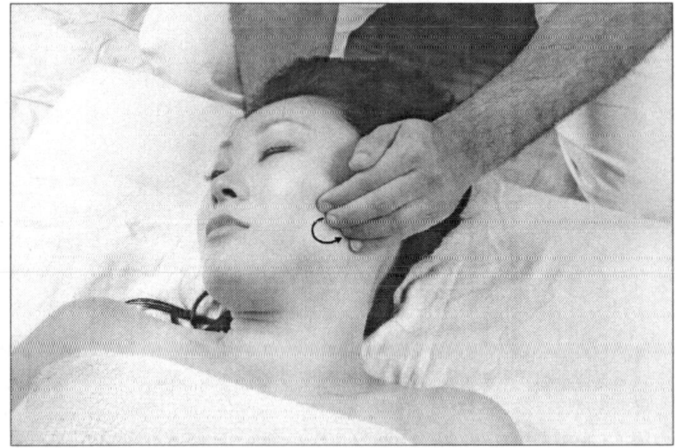

Figure 12-6: Circular rubbing to the jaw.

7. **Use some pinch-and-roll kneading to walk your fingers and thumbs from the jaw muscles out onto the chin, as shown in Figure 12-7.**

   Glide back softly and repeat twice more.

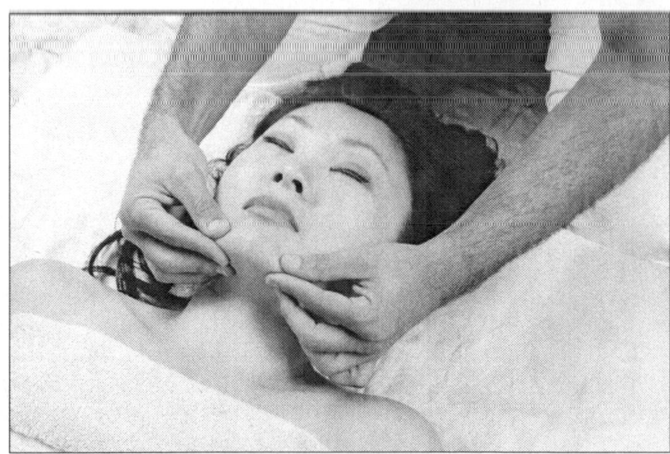

Figure 12-7: Finger kneading along the jaw.

8. **Massage the ears, using your fingers and thumbs to pinch and roll the ear from the lobe up around the edges to the top, as shown in Figure 12-8.**

   Repeat this twice and then tug gently for a second on the top, back, and bottom of the ear. Most people love to have their ears massaged.

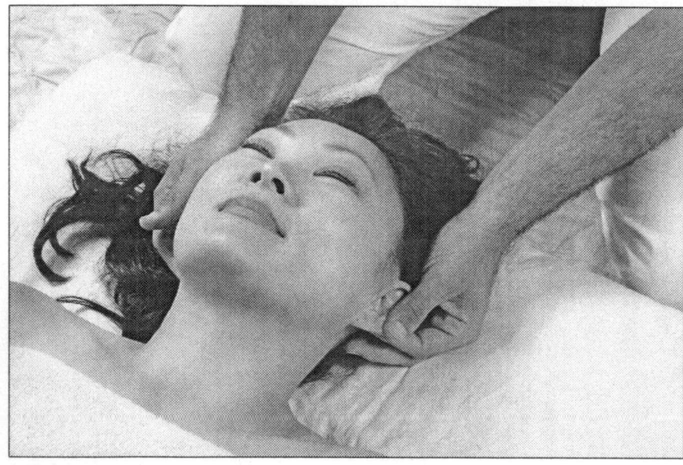

Figure 12-8: Ear massage.

9. **Massage the scalp using medium to deep circular rubbing with the fingertips as indicated in Figure 12-9.**

   Keep lifting your fingers up slightly, moving them a half-inch or so and then placing them firmly on the scalp again. During the rubbing, keep your fingers glued to the scalp and move the muscles below it over the cranium. Be careful not to pull your partner's hair while doing this move.

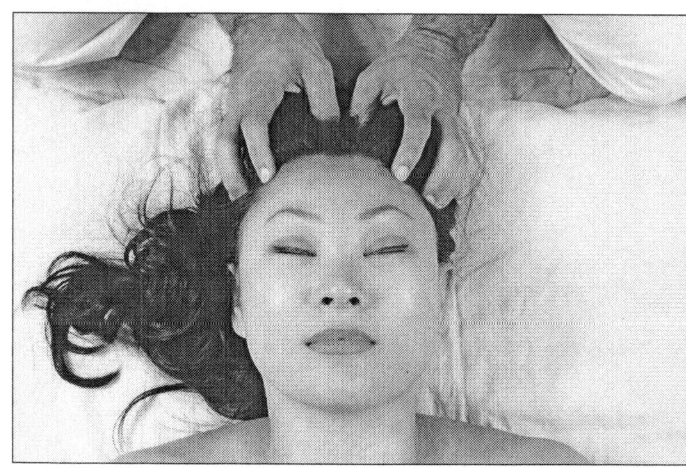

Figure 12-9: Circular fingertip rubbing on the scalp.

Favorite places

Everyone has his or her own particular favorites when it comes to getting a massage. Some swoon over an ear massage, while others go into ecstasy as soon as you lay a finger on their back. Oftentimes, you can find these favorite places somewhere on the head, neck, or face, although other areas like the hands and feet are popular, too.

Encourage your partner to communicate with you about any areas that feel particularly therapeutic or pleasurable. Then, during her next massage, spend more time focusing on the area she likes the most. She'll enjoy the sensation and appreciate you for remembering.

Relieving the Neck and Shoulders

Most people refer to just about anything that bothers them as "a pain in the neck," perhaps because the neck is particularly vulnerable to feeling pain. Filled with delicate nerves, vertebrae, and vessels, your neck can give you pain if you simply turn your head too quickly. Massage is a great way to soothe some of the minor complaints that people experience in this area, many of which are a reaction to stress.

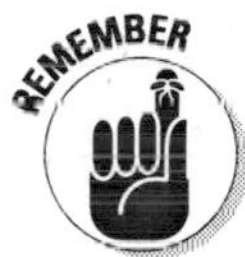

Be especially sensitive when massaging here, tuning in to your partner's muscles and letting what you find guide your movements. Sometimes simply by adding your awareness to the equation you can help your partner get rid of that pain in the neck she's been complaining about.

Here's a good sequence to follow for a relaxing neck and shoulder massage; Chapter 10 gives you the lowdown on the basic massage moves:

1. **Start with the shoulder swoop.**

   The *shoulder swoop* move may be a little tricky at first, but after you master it you have a great tool under your massage belt:

   A. Pour a small amount of oil into one palm and rub your hands together; place them on your partner's upper chest, with your fingers pointing inward, as shown in Figure 12-10a.

   B. Slide your hands outward, pivoting your palms on top of the shoulder so that your fingers end up beneath your partner's upper back as Figure 12-10b illustrates.

   C. Glide your hands in and up the back of your partner's neck to the base of her head while lifting slightly as shown in Figure 12-10c.

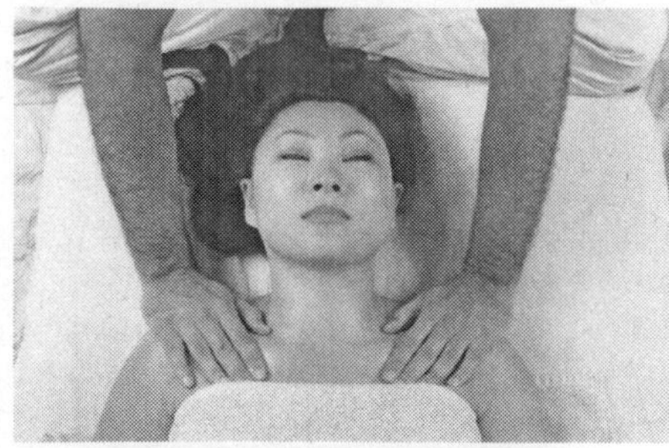

a

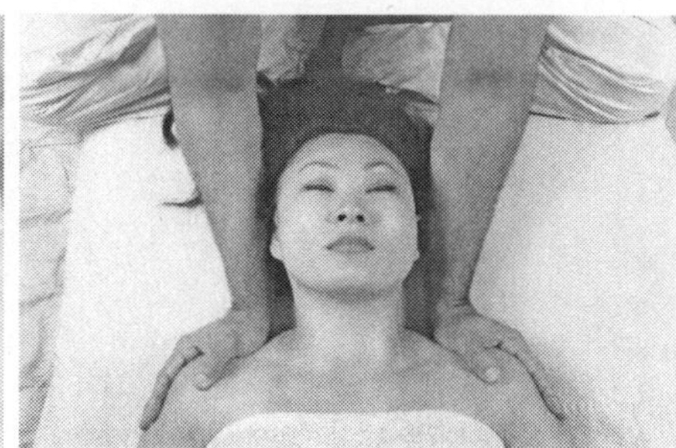

b

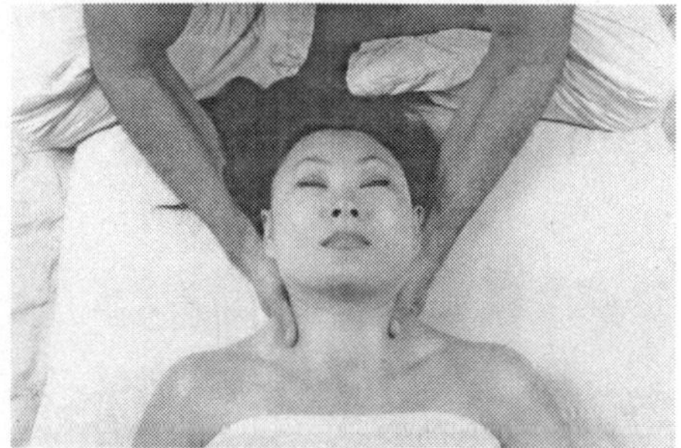

c

Figure 12-10: Shoulder swoop.

2. **Slip your fingers beneath your partner's neck, cradling her head in your hands and lift very gently just until you can turn her head to one side, supporting it in your bottom hand; rock her head back and forth slightly until she no longer tries to hold onto her own neck muscles.**

   You can then use the other hand to apply circular rubbing to the muscles in the back of the neck, as shown in Figure 12-11. Move your circles up and down, and when you find a tense spot, apply some pinpoint pressure.

   By using both hands for different purposes (one massaging, the other cradling the head), you have extra-effectiveness with this move.

   Be careful not to let your fingers stray to the front of the neck, which is a delicate area that may be harmed by vigorous massage.

3. **Still supporting your partner's head in one hand, use the other to knead up and down the back of the neck (see Figure 12-12).**

   Practice switching the position of your hands during this maneuver until you can create a fluid sensation for your partner — left, right, left, right. This feels darn good.

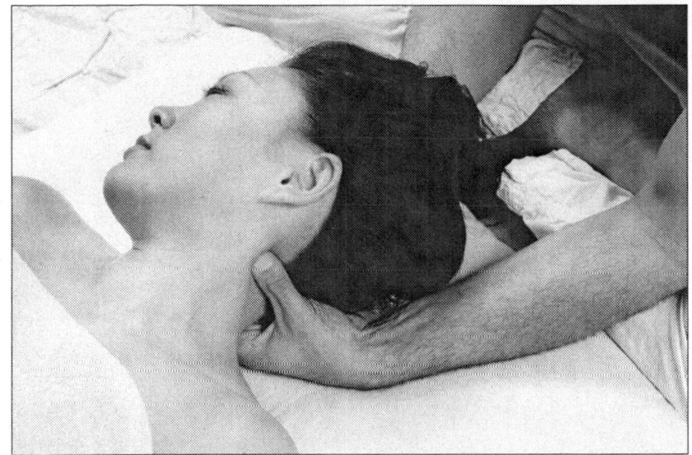

Figure 12-11: Circular rubbing to the back of the neck.

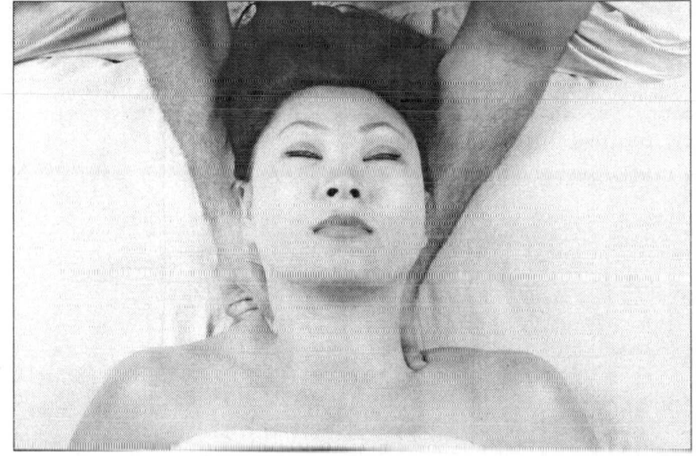

Figure 12-12: Alternate-hand neck kneading.

4. **Supporting your partner's head with both hands, lift up and forward, bringing her chin toward her chest as shown in Figure 12-13; hold this position for about five seconds, being careful not to twist your partner's neck, and then slowly lower her head back down.**

I believe this is the only stretch you should try with the neck until you receive further training.

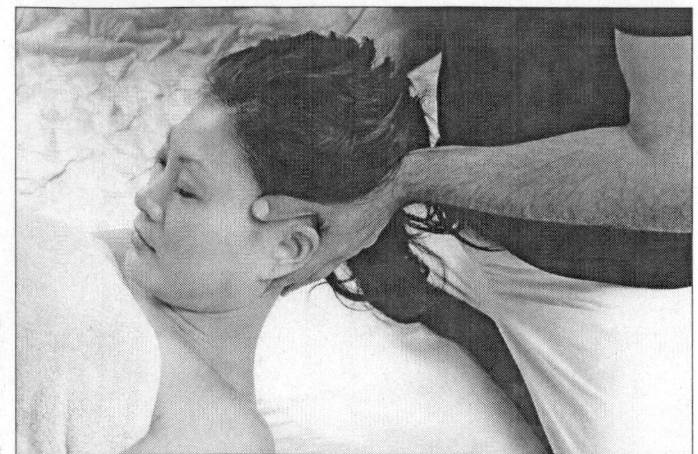

Figure 12-13: Neck stretch.

5. **Pushing down with your palms, glide across the tops of your partner's shoulders, also known as the *trapezius muscles.***

   The tops of these muscles often hold a lot of tension. As a more intense alternative to this move, you may try using your knuckles to glide in this area, too (see Figure 12-14).

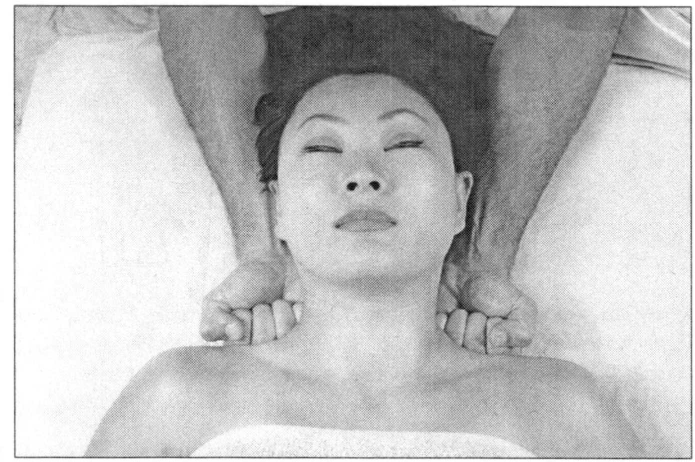

Figure 12-14: Gliding atop the shoulders.

6. **Take the muscles on top of your partner's shoulders between your thumbs and fingers, kneading with a good amount of pressure, as Figure 12-15 indicates.**

   As your fingertips reach down beneath your partner's back, curl them up so you're applying pressure in that area at the same time.

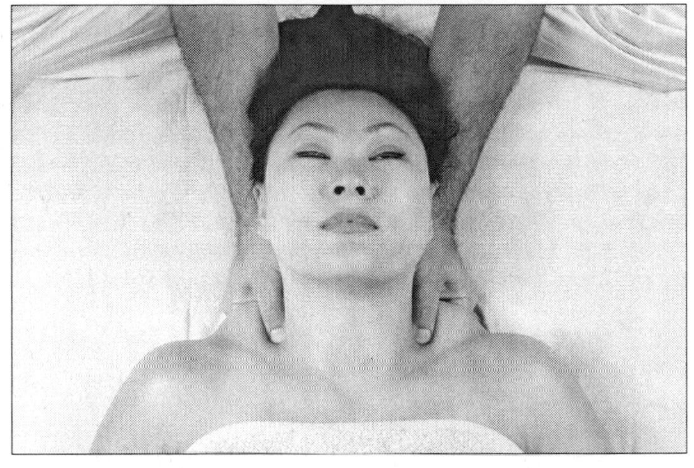

Figure 12-15: Kneading the tops of the shoulders.

7. **Use some pinpoint pressure with your thumbs to zero in on the tight spots you find, as shown in Figure 12-16.**

   Remember to keep a straight line from your elbows and shoulders to your thumb so you don't stress your joints.

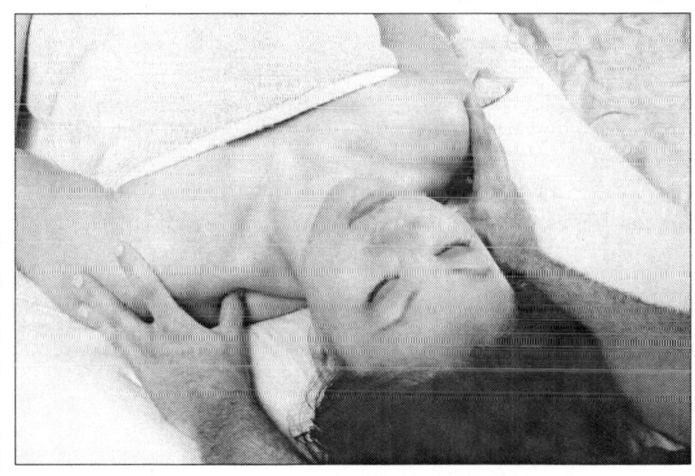

Figure 12-16: Pinpoint pressure to the neck and shoulders.

To create a smooth transition, finish the neck and shoulder area with another shoulder swoop. Then move down onto your partner's left shoulder and arm with a long flowing glide, which leaves you in position to begin massaging the hand (see the following section).

Soothing the Arms and Hands

Arms and hands are some of the most active parts of most people's bodies. Think about it: Even couch potatoes use their arms and hands to reach for the potato chips and to open cans of beer. In fact, just about everybody is so used to doing things with their arms and hands that, at first, you may find it challenging to get your partner to let go in this area (see Chapter 6 for help in getting your partner to let go). However, this tendency doesn't mean that you can't perform some spectacularly beneficial and pleasurable massage moves here.

The secret of good arm and hand massage is to make your moves smaller and to focus on the little details. Every pinkie finger counts!

A typical reaction you may get when you begin massaging in this area is, "I didn't know my arms were so sore until you started doing that!" Good massage techniques can put vitality back into this active, expressive part of your partner's anatomy.

Follow these steps to see if you can get such a reaction, looking at Chapter 10 for guidance on the specific massage moves:

1. **Position yourself at your partner's side and begin with some gliding moves.**

   Your initial gliding in this area spreads the oil, of course, but it also does much more. At this time, you help your partner let go and loosen up by offering some support to the limb at the wrist and elbow while you're gliding. This technique means you're actually picking the arm up and supporting it with one hand while gliding with the other (see Figure 12-17). Practice switching hands with this lift-support-glide maneuver until you get fluid with it.

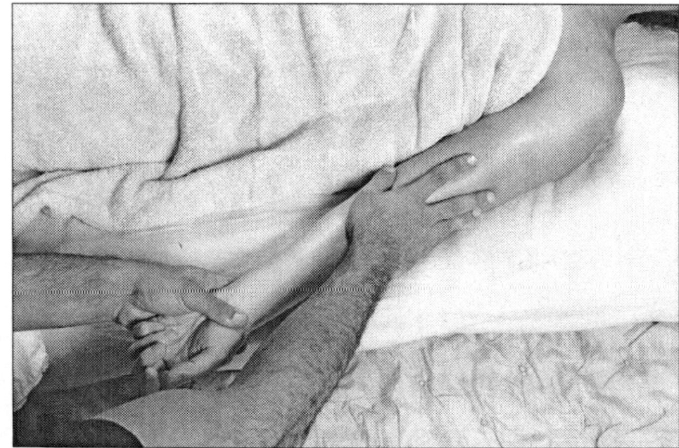

Figure 12-17: Arm gliding while supporting the wrist.

2. **Begin kneading the palm.**

   You've already picked up your partner's hand, so you're in the perfect position for this move, shown in Figure 12-18. You can flip your partner's hand up and down to work at different angles, spreading open and squeezing between the bones of the palm.

3. **Do some knuckle rolling on the palms.**

   You have to build up a little dexterity in your fingers in order to get this knuckle-rolling technique down. One at a time, curl your fingers closed into a fist and then open them back up again over your partner's palm, as shown in Figure 12-19.

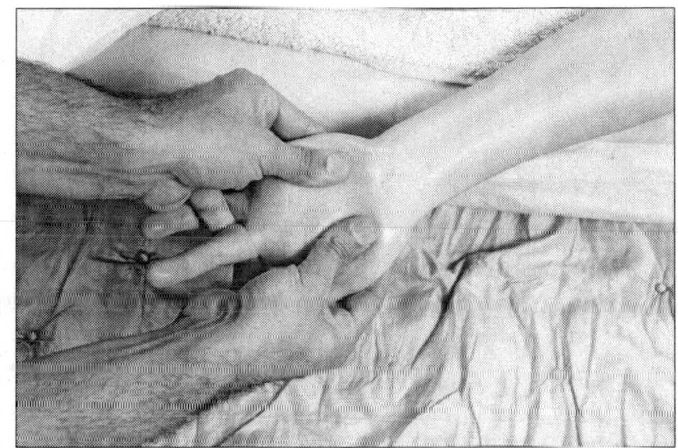

Figure 12-18: Palm kneading.

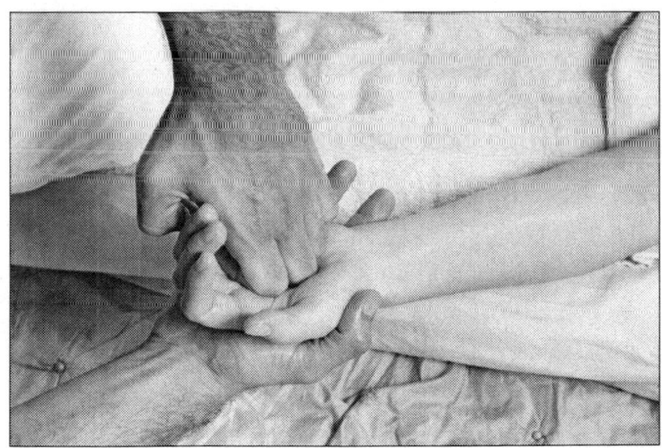

Figure 12-19: Knuckling the palms.

4. **Squeeze each finger as you pull slightly at the same time, moving up from the base of the finger to the tip as Figure 12-20 demonstrates.**

   Make sure to rub the sides of the fingers as well as the tops and bottoms.

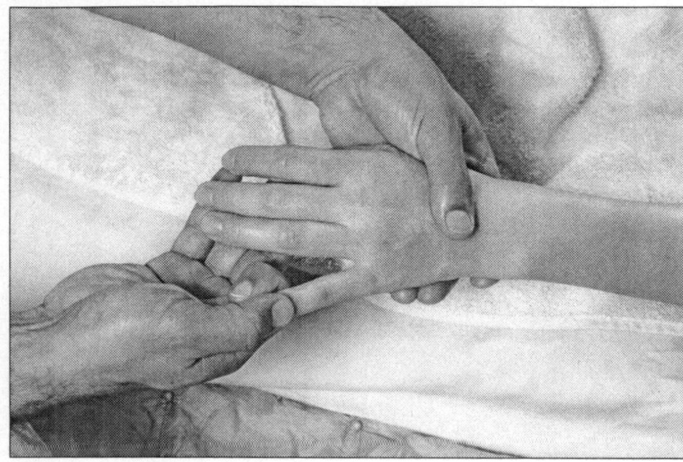

Figure 12-20: Finger squeezing.

5. **Massage the webbing between the thumb and index finger.**

   The pressure point in the webbing between one's thumb and index finger is especially good for helping to relieve headache pain. The best way to massage it is with direct pressure from your thumb, as shown in Figure 12-21. Hold this pressure point, pushing in toward the bones of the hand, for approximately five seconds.

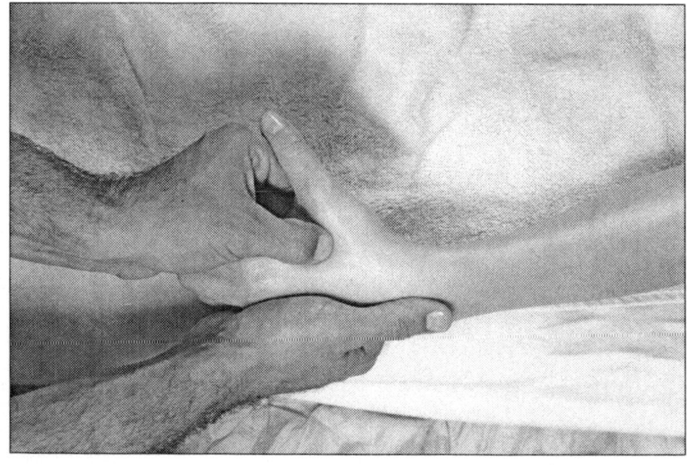

Figure 12-21: Hand pressure point.

6. **While holding your partner's hand palm-down, apply circular rubbing over the top of the wrists as in Figure 12-22.**

   This little move feels surprisingly good.

7. **Use your thumbs to trace lines straight up the forearms from the wrists to the elbows, as shown in Figure 12-23.**

   The forearms are jam-packed with muscles all crying out for attention, and this deep gliding is meant to sink down between the bands of muscle in this area.

   You can find special massage moves for the forearm that are effective on tennis elbow in Chapter 16.

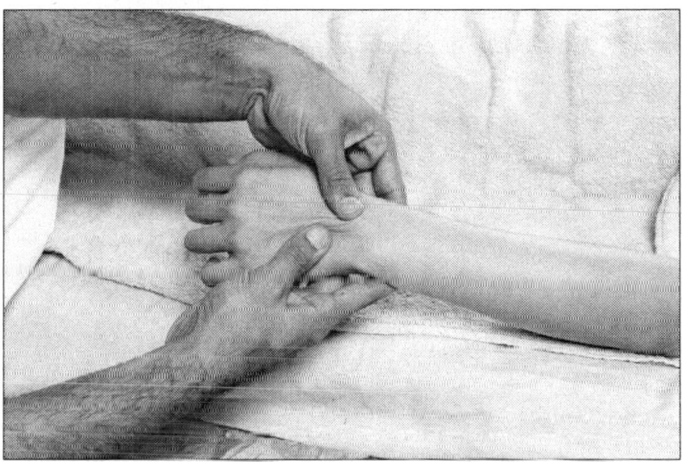

Figure 12-22: Circular rubbing to the wrists.

8. **Use kneading movements on the forearms.**

   These movements, shown in Figure 12-24, are basically a smaller version of the ones you use on the backs of the legs (described in Chapter 11), but that doesn't mean they aren't just as effective. Try to get as much of the muscle tissue between your thumb and fingers as possible, and remember to involve your whole body in the movement, all the way down to your hips.

9. **With your partner's elbow bent and resting on the ground for support, encircle the arm at the wrist with both of your hands, creating a tight seal around the entire circumference; begin pushing up the arm *very slowly* until you reach the elbow, maintaining firm pressure the whole time.**

   This "squeezing toothpaste through a tube" glide, shown in Figure 12-25, is great for tired, achy arms that need some renewal.

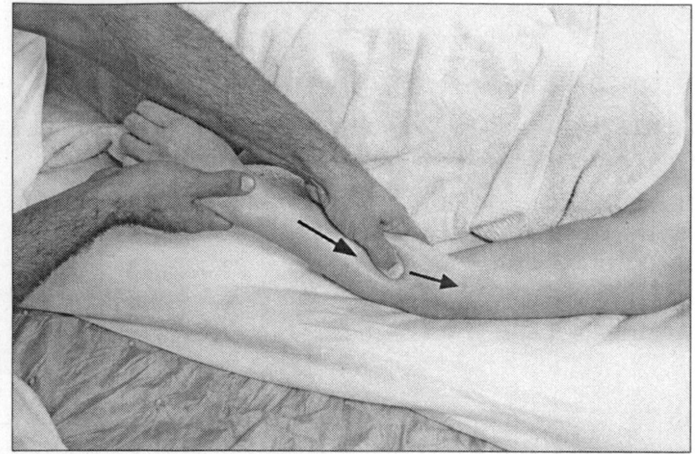

Figure 12-23: Deep gliding to the forearms.

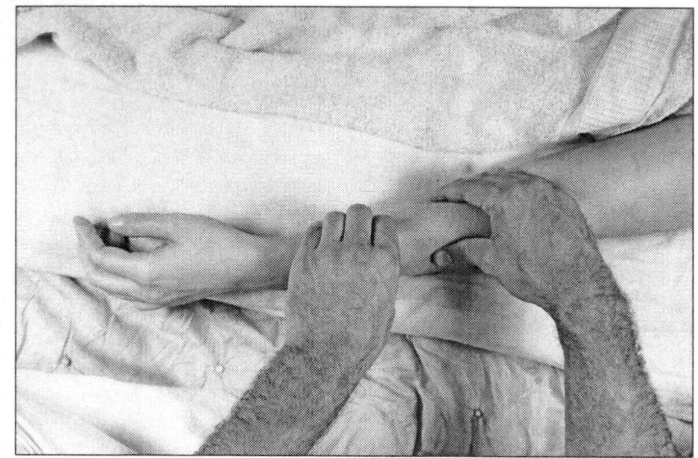

Figure 12-24: Forearm kneading.

10. **Massage the entire upper arm by lifting your partner's arm up, supporting it at the elbow, and allowing her hand to fall back toward the floor near her head; use your free hand to massage the upper arm with a one-hand kneading action.**

    For example, in Figure 12-26a, the left arm is supported by your left hand, allowing the right hand to massage the biceps. In Figure 12-26b, your right hand supports the elbow, leaving the left hand free to massage the triceps.

As you're doing this move, make sure to keep track of where your partner's hand is. If you're banging it against the side of her head, it detracts from the pleasure of the experience.

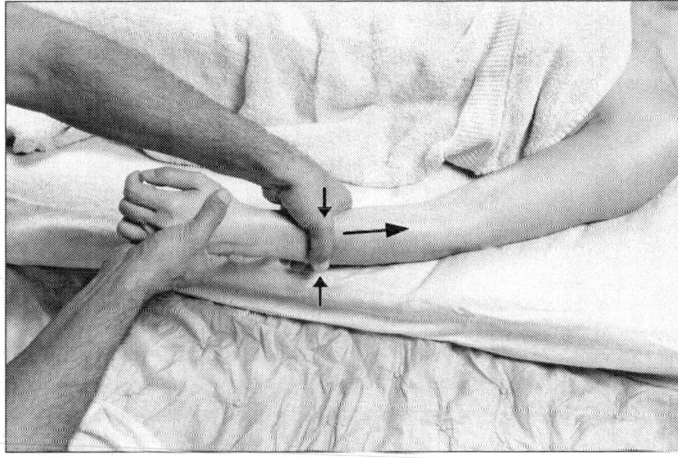

Figure 12-25: Squeezing glide to the forearm.

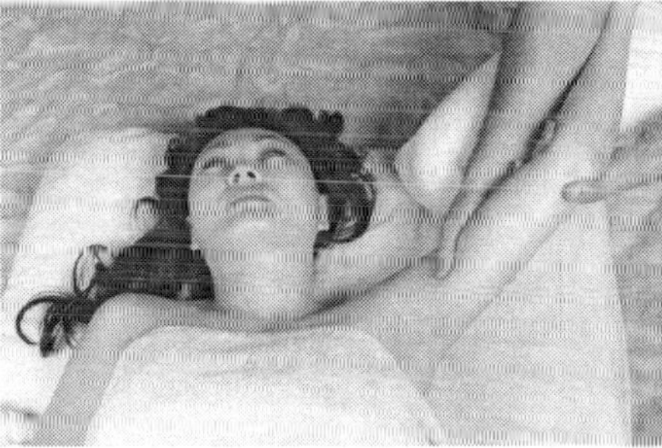

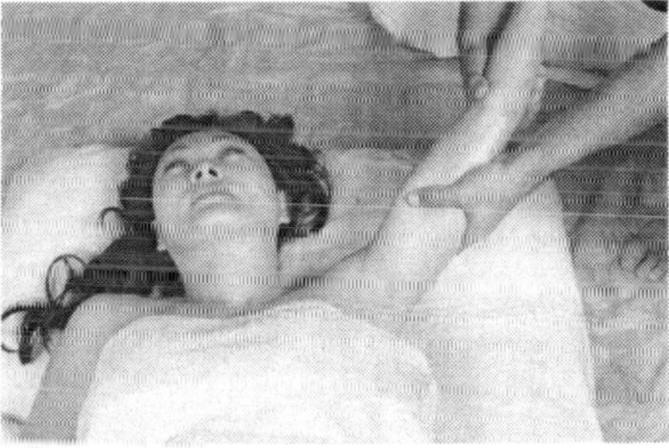

Figure 12-26: Alternate-hand upper-arm kneading.

11. **Grasping your partner's hand near the wrist, shake the whole arm gently until you can see some movement way up at the shoulders, neck, and head.**

    Try positioning her arm at three different angles to achieve a different stretch on the shoulder joint: down by her side, out at a 90-degree angle, or up by her head (as in Figure 12-27).

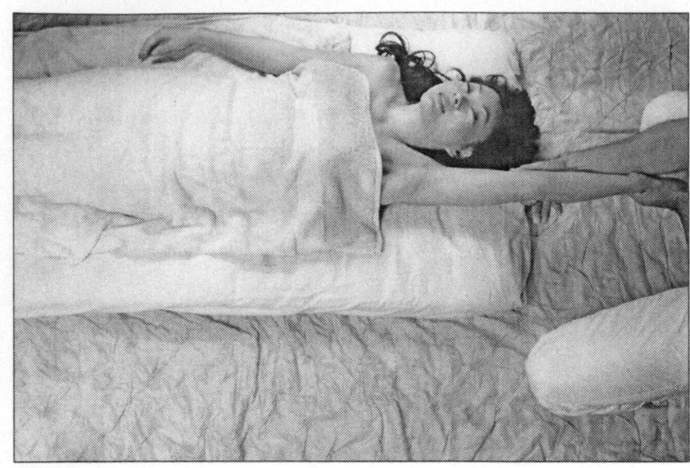

Figure 12-27: Arm stretch.

12. **Finish the arm with a light fingertip glide that floats up over the shoulder to the chest and down onto the other arm (see Figure 12-28).**
13. **Repeat Steps 1 through 12 on the opposite arm.**

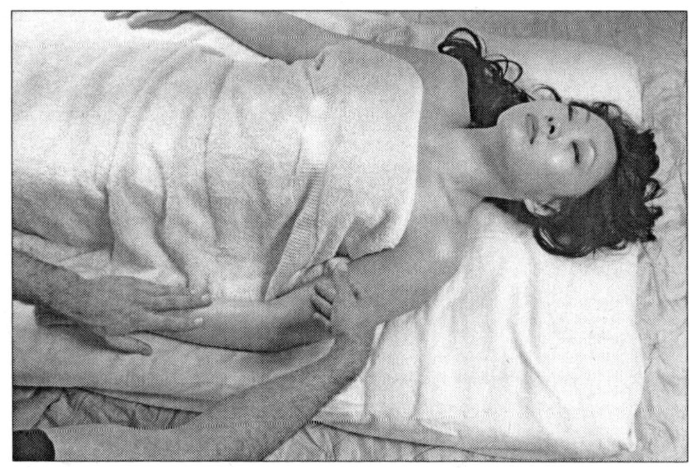

Figure 12-28: Fingertip gliding.

Working Out Tension in the Torso

As a species, we've taken a big collective risk by standing erect on two feet and exposing our defenseless underbellies to the world. The front of your body, especially the abdomen, can be a very vulnerable area, and you have to be extra sensitive when applying massage moves here.

Your abdomen is the physical home of many emotional realities such as fear, anger, and intuition. That's why people say they have a "gut instinct" about something. You're not just massaging a stomach when you place your hands on your partner's belly. You're massaging her soul. This fact has been recognized by many Asian cultures, such as the Japanese, for example, who have even given this soul-in-the-belly a name: the *hara.*

Make your movements on the chest and abdomen gentle at first, until your partner relaxes a little and allows you to massage more deeply. Keep in mind that your touch here penetrates to the deepest layers, both physically and psychologically.

Keeping a need for sensitivity in mind, follow these steps; you can find details on the specific massage moves in Chapter 10.

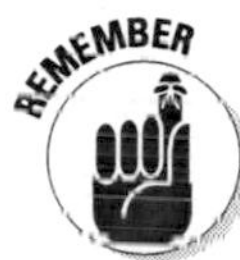

If your partner is a female, keeping the draping towel or sheet securely over the breast area may be appropriate during the chest and abdomen moves in this section. To massage the abdomen, you can place a hand towel over the breasts and then then pull the larger drape down beneath it to the hips, exposing the belly. Of course, if your partner is your wife or girlfriend, draping will most likely not be necessary.

1. **Place your thumbs across your partner's upper chest muscles below the collarbone, with your fingers reaching down toward her sides as shown in Figure 12-29, and begin some kneading.**

   You soon discover that this is a tricky maneuver to perform without causing your partner to squirm and writhe in fits of hysterical giggling. Yes, this area can be quite ticklish. Start out gingerly, like a kitten pawing a pillow, and then gradually intensify, always staying within your partner's comfort level.

   This area can be extremely sensitive, especially on people who exercise a lot or who are overly ticklish. Be careful not to poke your fingers into your partner's ribs or armpits. And make sure to use extra oil if your partner has a lot of chest hair.

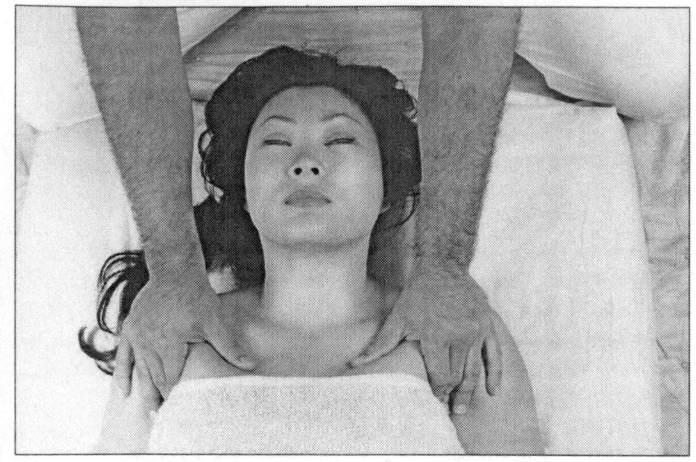

Figure 12-29: Kneading the upper chest muscles.

2. **Lift your hands off the chest just slightly and then press back down by using pinpoint pressure with your thumbs along a line about an inch below the collarbone as in Figure 12-30.**

   This move can have a beneficial effect on your partner's breathing, opening the upper ribcage.

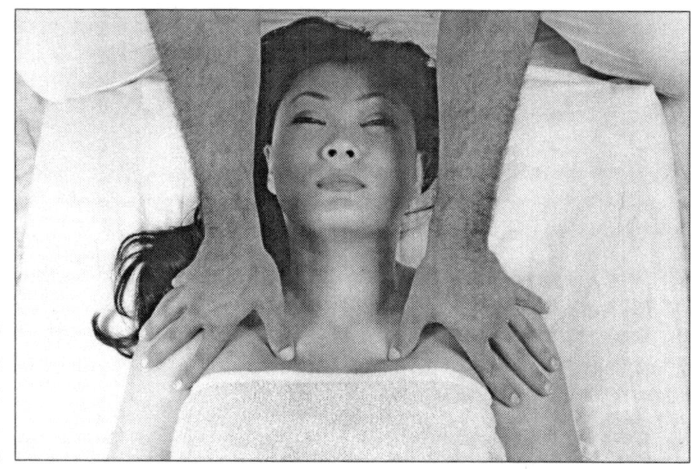

Figure 12-30: Chest pressing.

3. **Placing your fingertips near the top of the breastbone, push in gently and then begin circular rubbing as you move slowly down toward the abdomen as Figure 12-31 demonstrates.**

   As your fingers skim over the edges of the breastbone on either side, you find ridges and valleys where the ribs attach. Make a small circle in each one of these valleys as you move down.

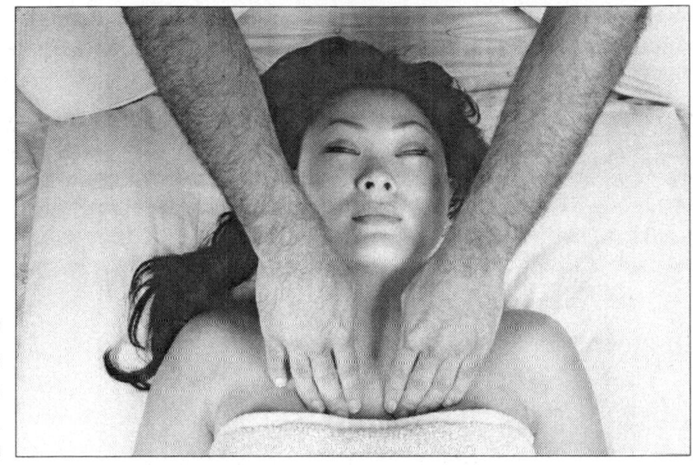

Figure 12-31: Breastbone circles.

4. **Do some gliding on the abdomen to spread oil, relax muscles, and aid digestion.**

   Your large intestine runs clockwise starting on the lower right-hand portion down by your hip bone, up along your side, across the base of your ribs, and down your left side. When you massage in this same direction (clockwise), you're helping the digestive organs do their job. Press in with firm but sensitive pressure so your movements affect these organs as well as the muscles on top of them, as shown in Figure 12-32.

   When you get really good at circling your hands over the belly, try speeding up your movements a little by letting your left hand glide right over the top of the right each time they cross paths, without pausing to lift the left hand up. This technique creates a smoother flow for you and a neat sensation for your partner.

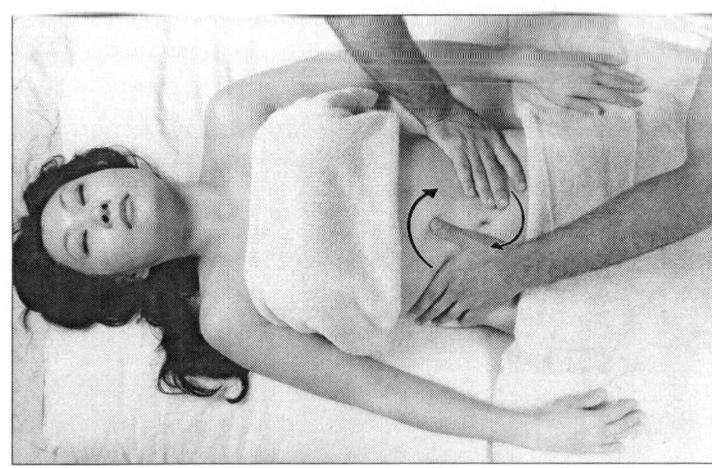

Figure 12-32: Clockwise gliding around abdomen.

5. **Gently touch several points right around the navel, applying just the softest pressure inward, as shown in Figure 12-33, to help coax out emotions.**

   Right around the navel, in the pit of the belly, is where people often store pent-up emotions. Your partner may sigh with relief or even begin to cry when you press here with sensitivity and compassion. This situation is a good time to offer nonjudgmental support and perhaps even suggest a positive image, or visualization, your partner can focus on. (See the sidebar "Visualize whirled peas" later in this chapter.)

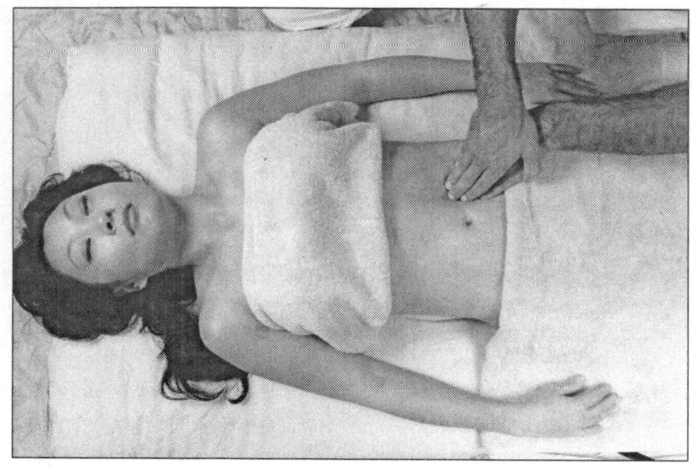

Figure 12-33: Gentle abdomen pressing.

6. **Slide both hands over the waist until the fingertips slip down all the way to meet at your partner's spine and then curl the fingertips up to apply a little pressure as you simultaneously lift the whole lower back a fraction of an inch upwards and glide your hands back toward the abdomen, as shown in Figure 12-34.**

   This move lets you massage the lower back while your partner is lying face up and is a nice stretch. Repeat the move three times.

   During this move, make sure you're not putting too much strain on your own back. Position yourself close to your partner's side and use your legs and hips to do the lifting.

7. **Finish the abdomen with a glide that swoops around your partner's side at the hipbone, onto the front of the legs, and then down to the feet as Figure 12-35 indicates.**

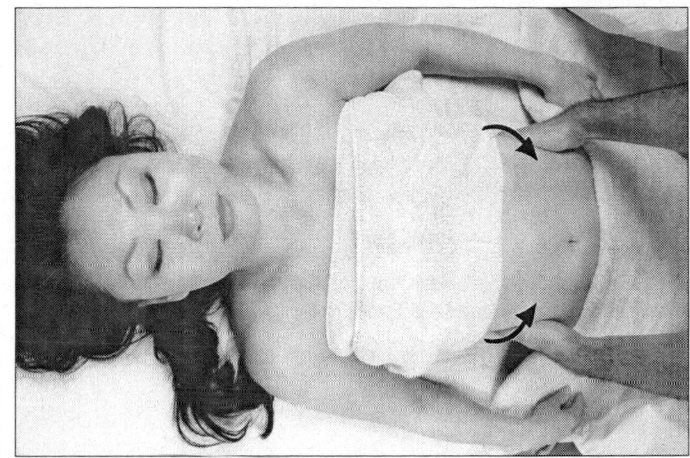

Figure 12-34: Abdomen lifting.

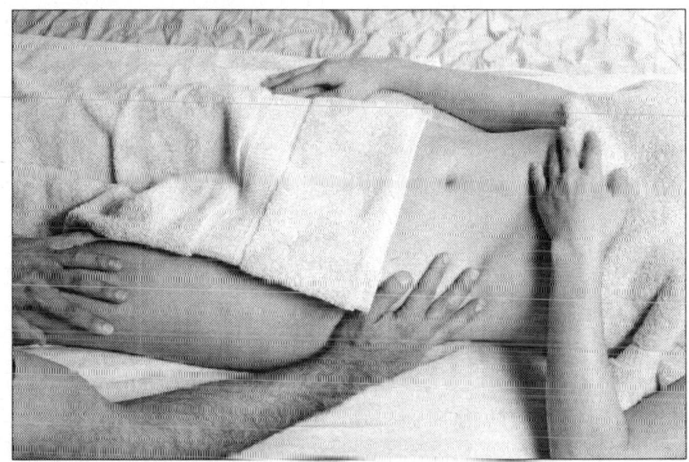

Figure 12-35: Abdomen to leg connective stroke.

Massaging the Front of the Legs and Feet

Think of how many miles your feet and legs have put in for you, selflessly hanging around beneath the rest of your body, taking you everywhere you want to go, seldom asking for anything in return. The average person doesn't realize how great a good leg and foot massage feels, and so you can surprise your partner with the simple, effective techniques in this section. (Check out Chapter 10 for the skinny on the specific massage moves.)

You finish the full body massage on the legs and feet because that's where people stand, literally. Ending here leaves your partner feeling more grounded and down-to-earth.

Feel free to spend some extra time on the feet. Although I describe the full foot massage in Chapter 13, you can incorporate many of those moves here as you work through the following steps:

1. **Begin by pushing in with both thumbs on the bottoms of your partner's foot and then spread open the sole as you move your thumbs out toward the side, as shown in Figure 12-36.**

   Use firm pressure and repeat this move three times.

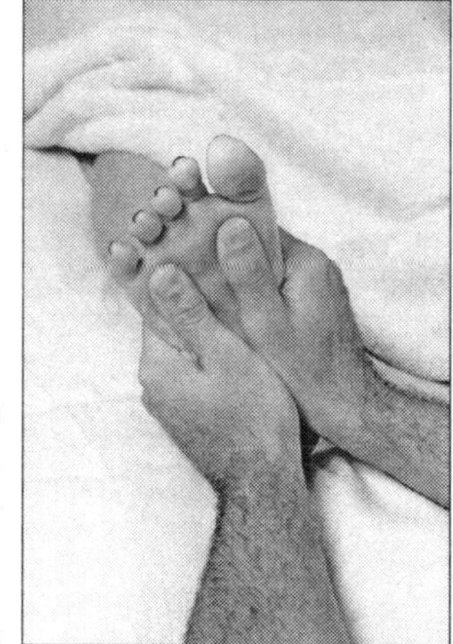

Figure 12-36: Thumb spreading on the soles.

2. **By using the thumb on the sole and forefinger on top of your partner's foot, rub between the long bones of the foot as Figure 12-37 illustrates.**

   You should find a groove between the bones that you can easily slip your finger into.

   Make sure to press sideways, as well as inwards, against the foot bones.

3. **Holding the top of your partner's foot in one hand, use the knuckles of the other hand to rake into the arch of the foot in a continuous, repeated one-knuckle-at-a-time movement, starting with the pinkie finger, ring finger, middle, and then index, as shown in Figure 12-38.**

   Done correctly, this move feels exquisite, but you have to build up considerable finger dexterity to achieve that.

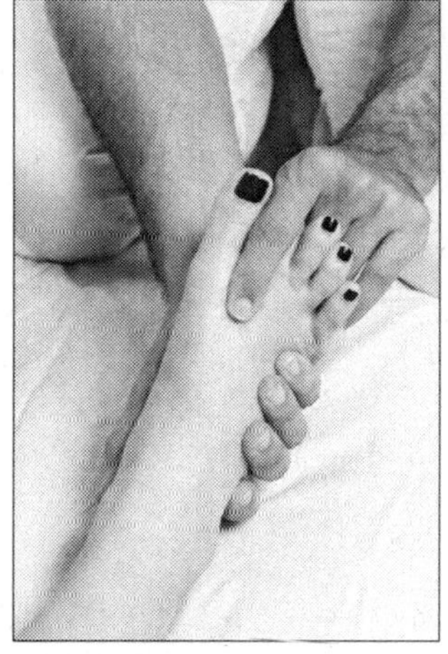

Figure 12-37: Thumb and fore-finger foot squeeze.

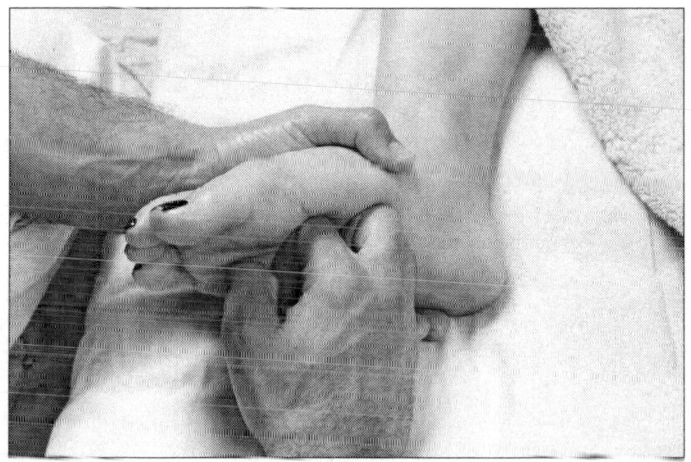

Figure 12-38: Knuckling the arch of the foot.

4. **As if you were squeezing a coin, rub each toe between your index finger and thumb, as shown in Figure 12-39.**

   Start with the little toe and progress toward the big toe, making sure to rub on the sides of the toes as well as the tops and bottoms.

5. **Find the exact location of your partner's shinbone and apply firm pressure with both of your thumbs together along the outside edge of this bone as you glide your way slowly up toward the knee as in Figure 12-40.**

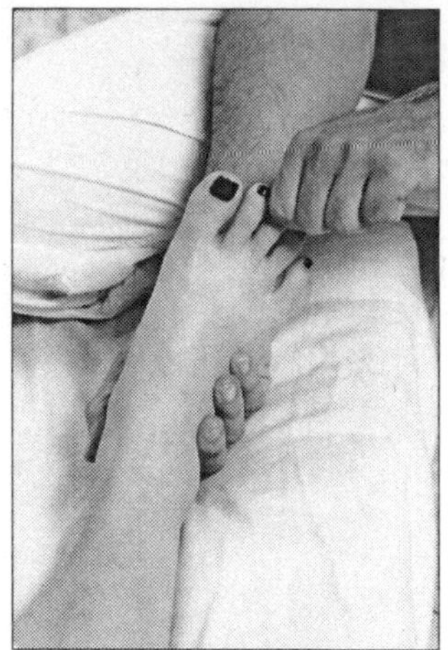

Figure 12-39: Toe rub.

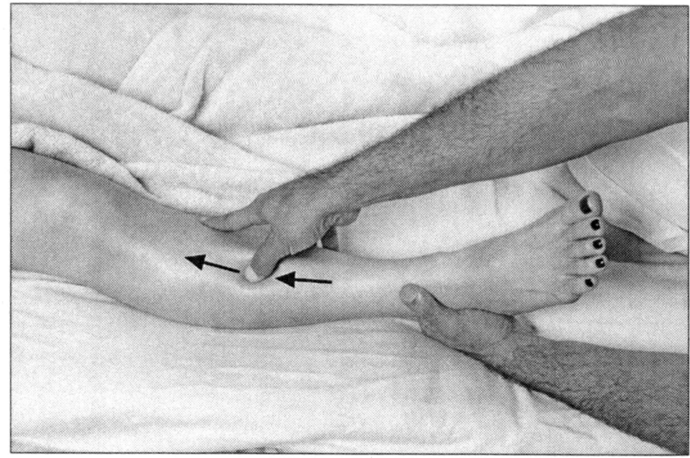

Figure 12-40: Thumb gliding along the shinbone.

7. **Reaching around behind your partner's knee with your fingertips, lift slightly while making circles over the sides of the knees with your thumbs, as shown in Figure 12-41.**

   Use moderate pressure inward against the knee and monitor your partner's response closely; some people are ticklish in this area.

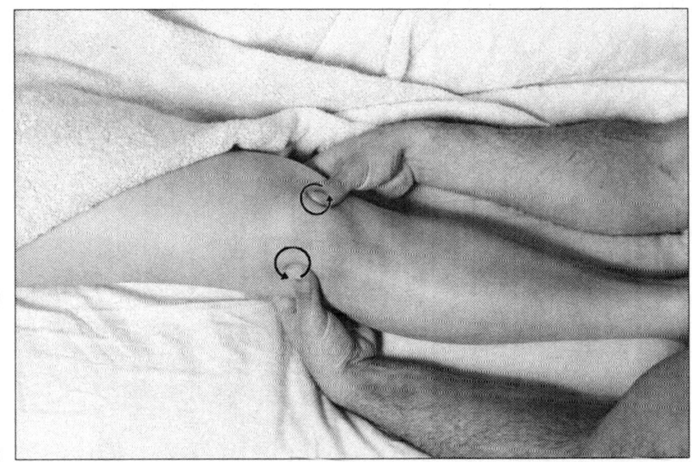

Figure 12-41: Thumb circles around the knees.

8. **Continuing up over the knees, use your palms to glide with firm pressure in an upward direction on the front of the thigh, also known as the quadriceps muscles (see Figure 12-42).**

   Slide back down the thigh with light pressure and repeat four to five times.

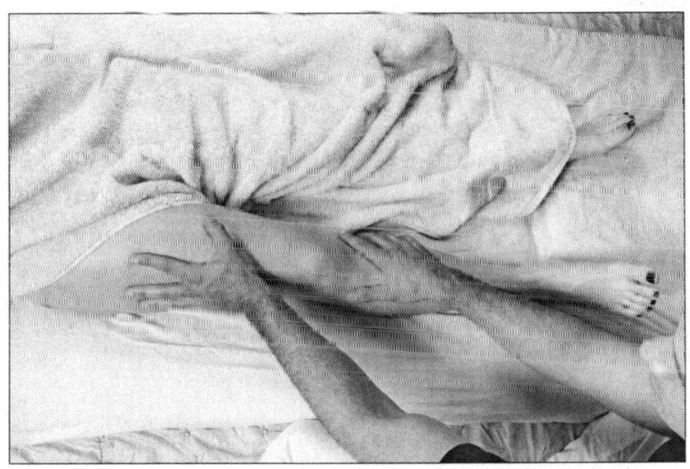

Figure 12-42: Gliding up the thighs.

9. **Positioned at the side of your partner's legs, apply kneading to the front of the thighs as you see in Figure 12-43.**

   This area is where you can use some really big movements, sliding your hands all the way from the inside of the thigh to the outside in a constant motion. Remember to use your whole body to create the kneading motion, not just your arms and hands. And don't be surprised if you work up a sweat during this move.

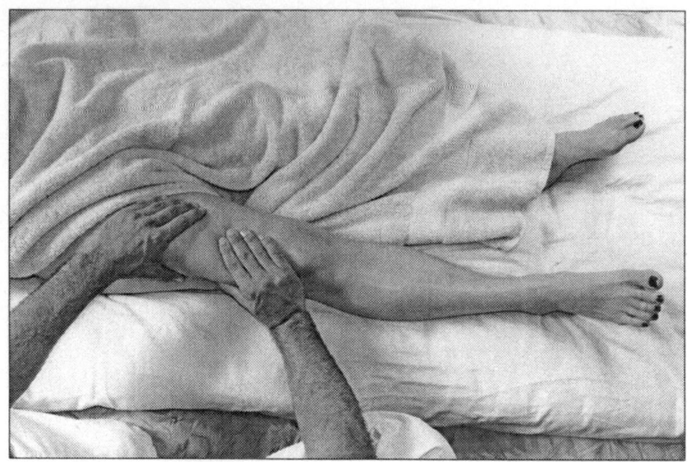

Figure 12-43: Kneading the thighs.

10. **Imagine a line running along the outside of your partner's thigh from knee to hip and, apply pinpoint pressure with your thumbs to a series of points along this line starting at the knee, as shown in Figure 12-44.**

    This line appears where the stripe occurs on many warm-up suits. Hold each point for three to five seconds and then release and move up to the next point. When you reach the hip, slide back down and repeat one more time.

This area is often very sensitive on many people, so you have to be careful when pressing here. Start out softly and increase pressure gradually. You can tell if you push too hard by noticing that your partner tenses her leg. If this happens, lighten your pressure.

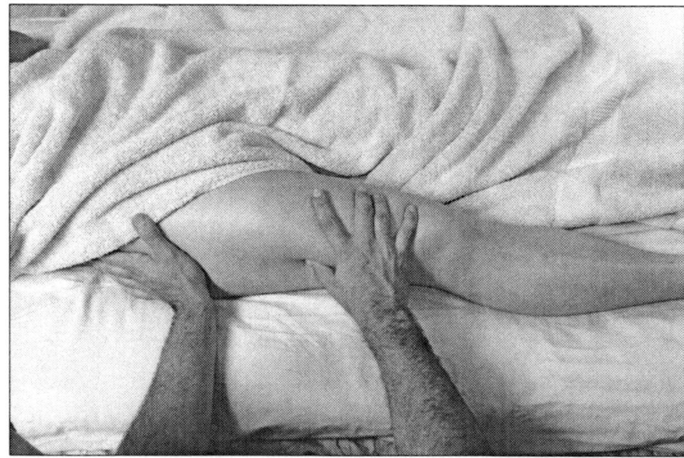

Figure 12-44: Pinpoint pressure to the outer thigh.

11. **Bend your partner's leg at the knee, with the hip open to the side; press down firmly with your palms just above the knee and then glide slowly up toward the hip as Figure 12-45 demonstrates.**

    For even more intensity, use your knuckles instead of your palms. Glide your hands back down to the knee with light pressure then repeat twice more.

    REMEMBER

    This advanced move requires quite a bit of trust on your partner's part. You are putting her in a vulnerable position. Also, make sure the towel or sheet is kept draped securely over your partner for modesty during this move.

    WARNING!

    Lighten your pressure as you approach the upper thigh, which contains many delicate nerves and vessels.

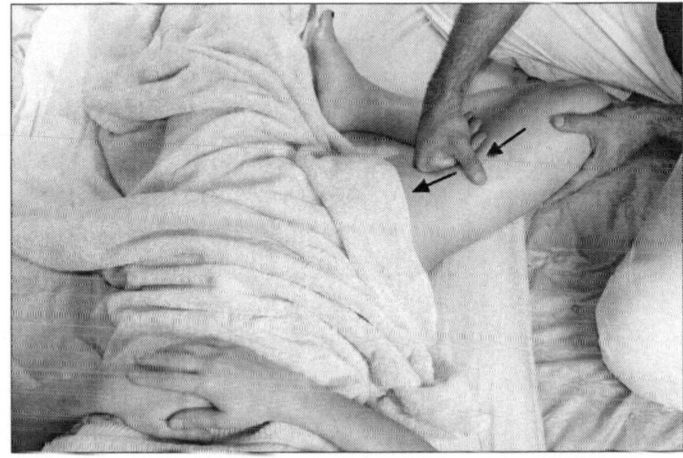

Figure 12-45: Inner thigh gliding.

12. **Lay your partner's leg flat again and then glide your hands upwards over the thigh; when you reach the hip, swivel your outside hand around and slip your fingers toward your partner's lower back, as shown in Figure 12-46.**

    Glide up as far as you can alongside the spine and then press your fingers up into the muscles there as you slowly pull back down toward the hip again, letting some of your partner's weight do the work of pressing. When you reach your partner's leg again, continue gliding down by using both hands on the back of the leg, lifting slightly to get your hands underneath. Finish your glide down at the foot.

13. **Cupping the heel in your palm, lift your partner's leg just an inch or so and shake back and forth with a vibrating motion as in Figure 12-47.**

    Remind your partner to let go if she tries to lift the leg for you.

14. **Finish this sequence with a light fingertip brushing down from the hips toward the feet to leave your partner feeling grounded as in Figure 12-48.**

15. **Repeat Steps 1 through 14 on the other leg.**

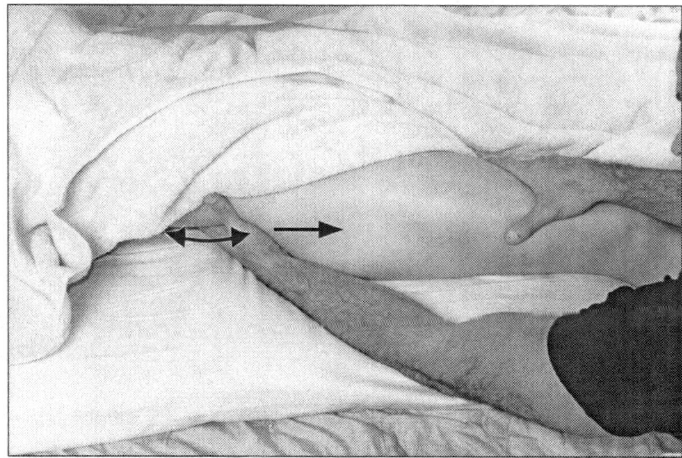

Figure 12-46: Connecting stroke from the leg to the back.

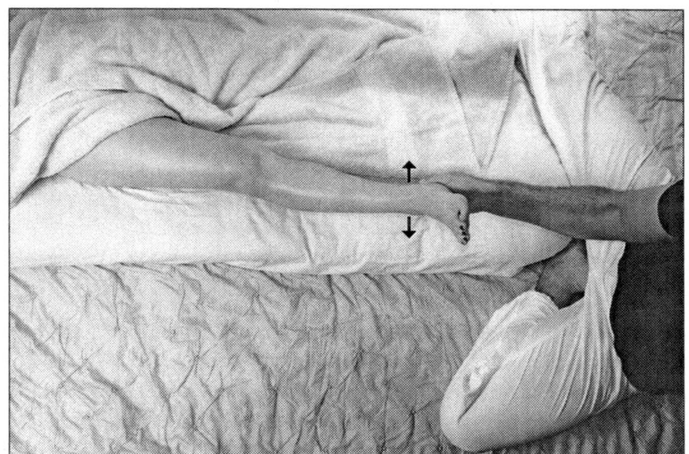

Figure 12-47: Leg vibration.

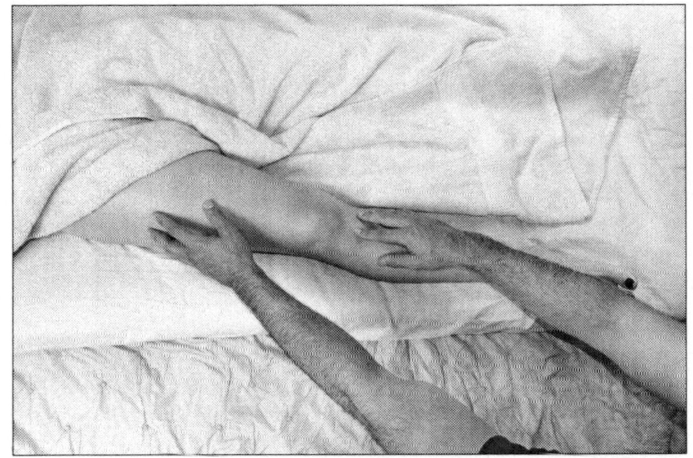

Figure 12-48: Fingertip brushing down leg.

Performing the Grand Finale

As with so many things in life (like fireworks and circus acts), the grand finale is what really counts in massage. Sure, you can apply superlative techniques all throughout the massage, flowing from one bliss-inducing maneuver to the next in seamless perfection, but if you finish with a ho-hum squeeze of the toes and then rush off to grab a cold one from the fridge, you're going to leave a slightly disgruntled partner behind. It's like watching a good movie with a bad ending: All anyone can talk about is how bad the ending was, not how good the rest of the movie was.

The way you end the massage leaves a lasting impression. To make your finish the best it can be, follow these steps (see Chapter 10 for the specific massage moves):

1. **Use long gliding strokes that flow over the entire body, starting at the feet and moving up onto the torso and then down the arms, as shown in Figure 12-49.**

   You can do this long-soft-light gliding because it's not meant to actually affect the tissues beneath the skin but rather to send your partner a message of connection (see Chapter 11).

   You don't have to wait until the end of the massage to use *connective strokes*. In fact, you can use them throughout the entire massage to connect everything together. Starting with an arm? Connect it to the neck you just finished a moment earlier. Go ahead, experiment. Connect away! The point is to make your partner feel that you're treating her body as a whole, not segmenting it into chunks.

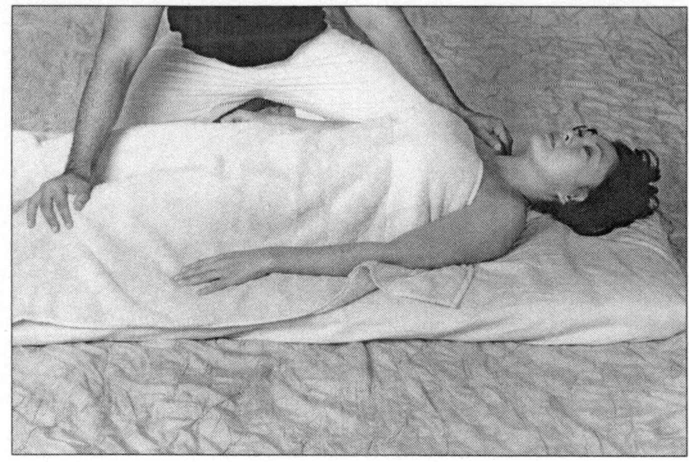

Figure 12-49: Whole-body connective strokes.

2. **To finish your massage, place one hand on your partner's forehead and the other gently upon her belly, letting them rest there in contact but without pressure for 30 to 60 seconds as Figure 12-50 indicates.**

   You may begin to feel her pulse or some warmth emanating from her body. This reaction is good. Just tune in to whatever it is you're feeling and, for just these last few seconds, make sure your partner knows she's the center of the universe.

   This type of intentional hand placement to balance your partner's inner energy is known in some quarters as *polarity.*

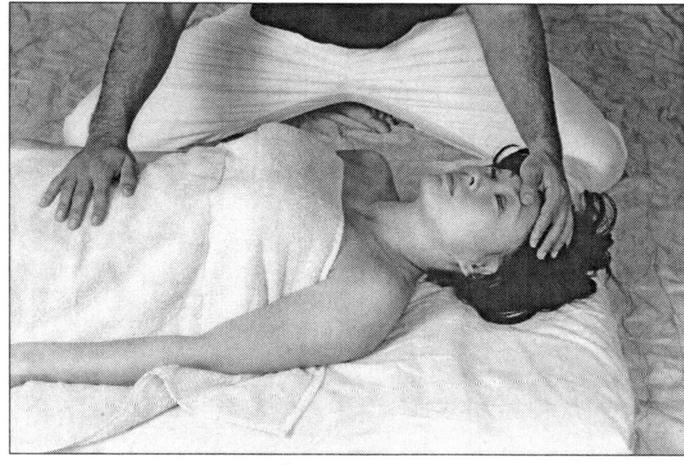

Figure 12-50: The final touch — forehead and belly.

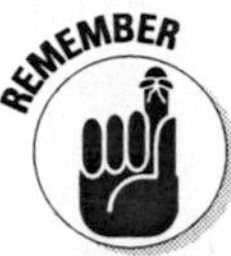

The last moment of the massage is as important as the first. When you finally break contact with your partner for the last time, make it a conscious, gentle letting go.

Visualize whirled peas

At many points during the massage, you can offer a visualization to help your partner relax and melt more fully into the experience. These visualizations usually incorporate three ingredients:

- A reminder about how important it is to breathe during the experience.
- Some guidance about what specifics to think about during the visualization.
- A positive message meant to uplift your partner's state of mind.

I cover breathing pretty extensively in Chapter 6. After you have your partner breathing evenly and deeply, suggest an image to visualize. Concrete is better than vague, so make the images you suggest extremely specific, including textures, colors, sounds, and even aromas.

An example of something vague to visualize is world peace. Plenty of people may tell you to visualize it, but how do you do that? What does world peace look like? What color is it? How big is it? How would it taste? Does it need any salt?

I personally find it much easier to imagine smushed vegetables, which perhaps explains the existence of a well-known bumper sticker that urges us to "visualize whirled peas." It may sound silly at first, but can't you just see them there, swirling around topsy-turvy inside the blender, eventually turning to green mush as the blades increase from chop to blend to puree?

Of course, the image of pureed peas itself is not enough for a fully effective visualization. You have to include the ever-important uplifting New Age message, which in this case may well be, "See the color green as a vast sea of tranquility. Imagine each pea as a grain of green sand on an unending beach of bliss."

Or something like that.

Chapter 13

A Special Treat for the Feet: Reflexology

In This Chapter

- Understanding the theory and benefits of reflexology
- Finding out the key points and basic moves of a fantastic foot massage
- Performing a foot massage routine

One great universal truth exists outside the boundaries of any race, religion, or culture. A truth that has stood for centuries throughout human history, it is so fundamental that most of us take it for granted. That truth is this: Almost nothing beats a good foot rub.

Yes, I'm aware that some people are not big fans of foot rubs and in fact don't want their feet touched at all. In this chapter, however, I flagrantly disregard these people, because the vast majority absolutely loves foot massage. In fact, entire civilizations have been built up and sustained for the sole purpose of giving certain people enough power, money, and influence to be able to get other people to rub their soles.

You may know a certain person in your own circle who is famous for giving "good foot." Some people seem to have a special knack for it, almost as if foot massage were a completely separate entity from body massage. Foot massage isn't really separate from the whole-body massage I discuss in Chapters 11 and 12, but feet definitely deserve a chapter of their own. After all, feet have a massage technique all their own, called *reflexology,* which I cover in this chapter.

High heels and other enemies of the feet

If you're a woman and you wear high heels, you have an especially big problem to deal with. I'll never forget the first woman I saw on my massage table with high-heelitis. She was lying down, relaxed and comfortable, but her legs and feet were still bent into the position they would have been in if her shoes had still been on — feet extended, toes pointed down, calves flexed. Extended wearing of those torture devices known as high heels can actually change the shape of your lower body. The effects reach all the way up into your hips, lower back, and spine.

If you're a man and you wear high heels, you'll have the same problems with your calves and lower back, plus the added problem of seldom finding anything at a clothing store that truly matches your choice of footwear. What a dastardly predicament!

The common problems certain shoes cause are some of the reasons that a large number of massage pros wear Birkenstock-type sandals. We want to give our feet and bodies a little break from the pounding they take on the cruel streets of life.

Part of the reason feet get so sore is the delicate nature of their structure. They sustain your entire weight during walking, standing, running, and so on. Thousands of pounds of cumulative pressure, day in and day out, press on 26 relatively small bones. Add to that the fact that you have approximately 72,000 nerve endings in each foot, making them some of the most sensitive parts of your body, and you can see why keeping your feet happy can be a tough job.

Getting Familiar with Reflexology

The feet deserve massage just for being feet, but another reason exists for concentrating some extra time on the feet and perhaps even devoting an entire session to foot massage. I'm talking about *reflexology*. You've probably heard this strange word somewhere before, right — maybe on the Discovery Channel, or in a magazine with a picture of a New Age MD on the cover? But did you really know what the word meant? Quiz yourself by trying to complete the following sentence. Reflexology is

A. The practice of stimulating certain points on one area of the body (usually the feet) that have an effect on corresponding reflex areas in other parts of the body.

B. The art of developing fast reflexes for use in such real-world situations as gunfights and race car driving.

C. The act of flexing something over again after you've flexed it once already.

D. None of the above.

The answer, as you may have suspected, is A, but just knowing that doesn't do you much good, does it? Not unless you know a little of the background of reflexology and the philosophy behind this unique therapy, as well. For much more extensive information, see that in-depth and wonderful resource, *Acupressure & Reflexology For Dummies* by Synthia Andrews and Bobbi Dempsey (Wiley).

The origins of modern reflexology are rooted in another treatment method called *zone therapy*. In 1917, Dr. William H. Fitzgerald of Boston City Hospital published a book called *Zone Therapy, or Relieving Pain at Home.* In it, he stated that many types of health problems could be helped, or even cured, by applying pressure to various strategic points, mostly on the hands.

This whole idea did not catch on like wildfire, but one of Dr. Fitzgerald's associates, a therapist in his office named Eunice Ingham, took the idea and tweaked it a bit, experimenting with many people, mostly on their feet, which she thought were more sensitive than the hands. Eventually, she wrote her own books, *Stories the Feet Can Tell*, and that follow-up favorite, *Stories the Feet Have Told.* Ingham's work and her books heralded the birth of modern reflexology.

The work of Eunice Ingham is continued today at the International Institute of Reflexology, founded in 1973. You can find more information at `www.reflexology-usa.net`.

But just what is *zone therapy* anyway? According to zone theory, your body can be divided (metaphorically, of course) into long slender pieces. Everything that's going on in any one part of a particular zone can be felt in a distant part of that same zone. You can see, then, how something happening in your abdomen can be reflected, or felt, in your foot. By stimulating a certain point in the foot, you can treat the pancreas, for example.

All of this talk about reflexes and zones may leave you feeling a little zoned out yourself, but don't let that worry you. The whole concept is pretty simple if you just remember that the bottoms of the two feet put together can be looked at like a miniature map of the entire body. So the head is up by the big toe, the spine goes down the middle, and so on. Figure 13-1 shows a reflexology chart.

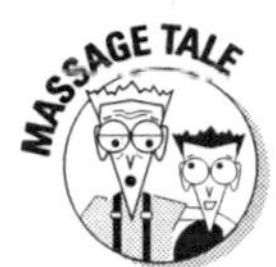

Some people swear by reflexology as a life-saving healing method. In fact, the woman I learned the technique from was diagnosed with a serious form of cancer and not given much chance of survival. None of the conventional treatments seemed to be helping, so as a last resort she turned to a Greek man in his 90s who specialized in reflexology. He also recommended coffee enemas. Within several months, this woman was cured and has been living a normal, productive life for over 20 years. (After the experience, however, she did develop a slight aversion to coffee shops.)

Frankly, nobody can tell you why reflexology works. But the truth is it often does. Reflexology is still a *theory,* but one with practical applications, and it certainly won't hurt you to give it a try. It may indeed help your overall health, but at the very least reflexology is guaranteed to feel darn good on your feet.

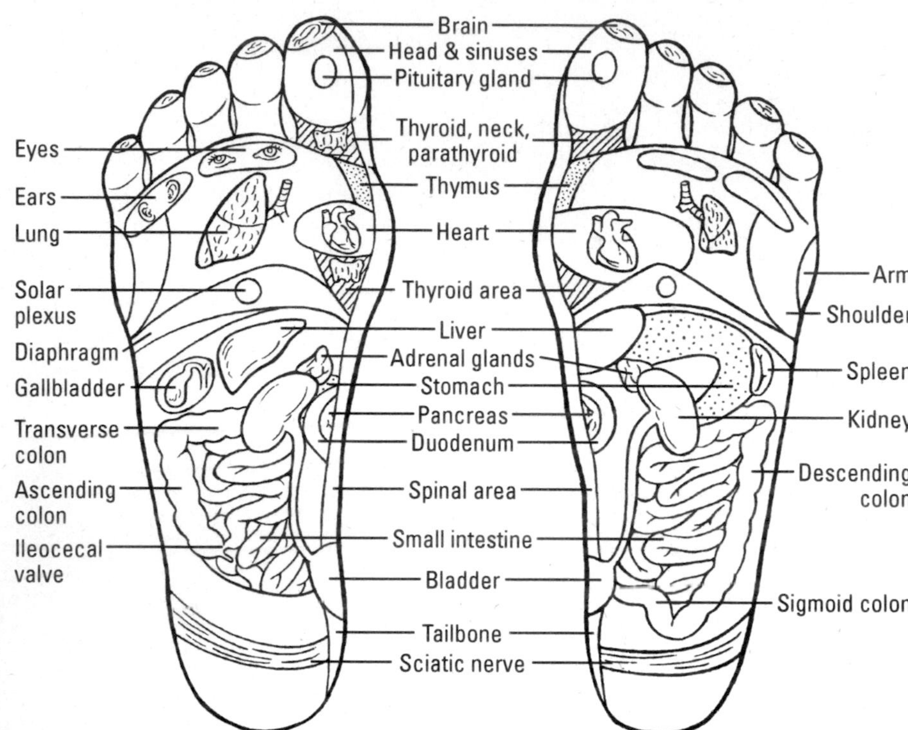

Figure 13-1: A reflexology chart.

Trying Your Hand at Reflexology

This section gives you the moves and pointers you need to give a great foot massage. Take your time getting used to the moves here — you shouldn't have too much trouble talking someone into being your foot guinea pig. Practice the moves a few times first before putting them together into a full routine (which you can find later in the chapter).

Positioning

First, get yourself and your partner in a comfortable position. The partner-reclining position shown in Figure 13-2 is the one favored by professional foot massagers around the world, but you can also position your partner on a bed or massage table so that his feet are just at the edge. Pay attention to the way you're bending over to access your partner's soles and toes, which can cause a serious backache if you're not comfortable. You don't want to hurt yourself while trying to help someone else.

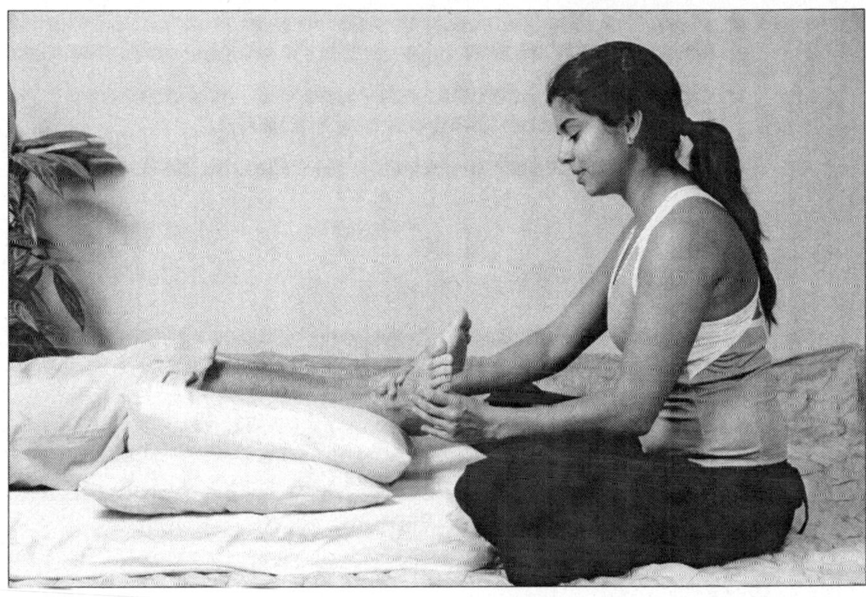

Figure 13-2: An optimal position for reflexology.

You can perform this routine through stockings or socks if you don't want to remove them. So far, though, no method has been devised to perform reflexology through a pair of shoes.

Points to remember

If you want to remain friends with the person you're giving the foot massage to, keep in mind a few things when you're about to dig into his soles:

- **Start on the left foot.** This arrangement complements your partner's natural digestion and circulatory patterns.
- **Don't use oil, because it makes the foot too slippery.** Cornstarch works well to absorb excess moisture, so rub a little on your partner's feet before you begin.
- **Always talk to your partner and ask for feedback.**
- **Don't diagnose any problems or treat someone for serious disorders based on what you feel on someone's foot.** Some over-zealous reflexologists, when they discover a tender spot on someone's foot (say, the spot which happens to correspond to the head) have been known to proclaim, "You have an inoperable brain tumor and have seven minutes to live." Leave the diagnosing to physicians.
- **Don't use any instruments or tools to push against the feet (such as pencil erasers for example, which have been known to get lodged between toes).** Use only your fingers and thumbs.

- **If they're longish, you may want to trim your nails before digging them into the arch of your partner's delicate sole.** Just a suggestion . . .
- **Never push so hard that you cause pain or discomfort.** If your partner is in pain, ease up your pressure a little bit.
- **Finish the left foot completely, and then go on to the right.**

Basic moves

You can make certain basic, time-tested moves on the feet. These moves have been passed down by practicing reflexologists from generation to generation, and now you can use them, too. This section provides you with detailed explanations of these moves and how to use them yourself.

Cradling

Cradle your partner's foot (at either the ball of the foot or the ankle) in both palms, with your fingers pointing straight ahead. Then move your hands back and forth rapidly, just an inch or so (as shown in Figure 13-3). This move is especially good for warming up, and you can also use it in the middle of a foot massage to give your partner a little extra pleasure. Cradling feels so good it was called "dessert" by one of my colleagues who specialized in reflexology at a spa where I worked.

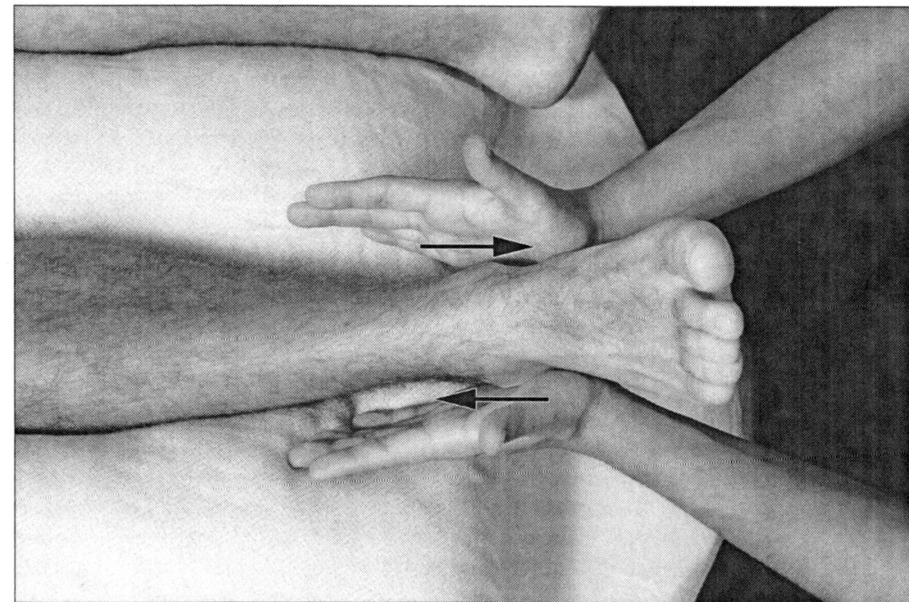

Figure 13-3: This move is called cradling, and it feels most delicious.

Thumb walking

The most basic move of all in foot reflexology is *thumb walking*, which is a lot trickier than it looks. Start by placing the pad of your thumb firmly against your partner's foot (as shown in Figure 13-4a). Then bend the thumb and creep it forward like an inchworm across the surface, pressing in while you do so (as shown in Figure 13-4b). Every time you bend your thumb, move your hand forward just slightly. You may want to practice this technique a little before subjecting your partner to a spastic or weak inchworm movement.

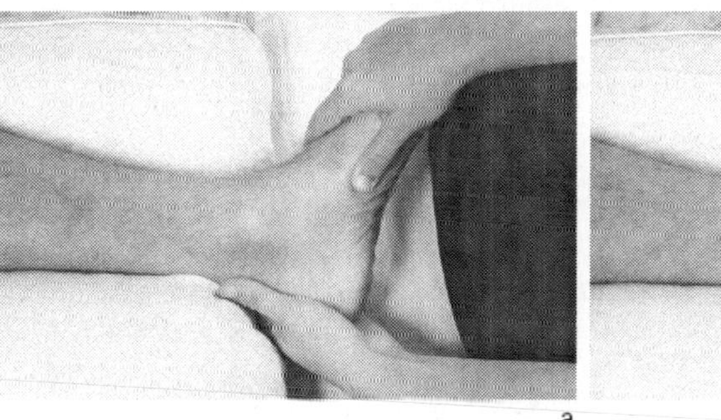
a

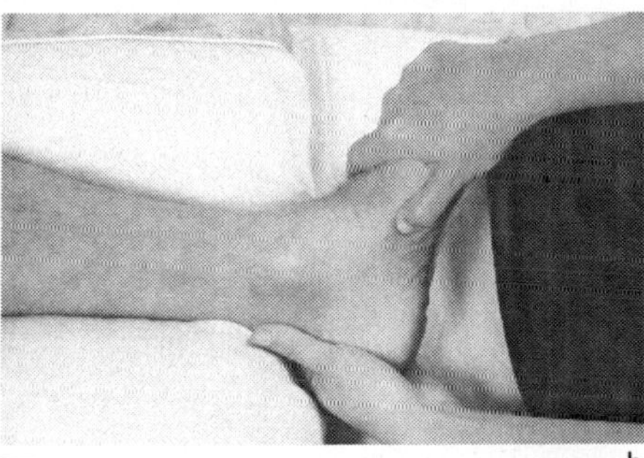
b

Figure 13-4: Start with your thumb in position (a) and inch it forward for position (b).

Index finger techniques

Sometimes (for example, when you're working on the sides and tops of your partner's feet), using your thumbs is just plain awkward. That's when you can use the length of your index finger to slide next to the ankles and between the long bones that run from the heels to the toes, for example, as shown in Figure 13-5.

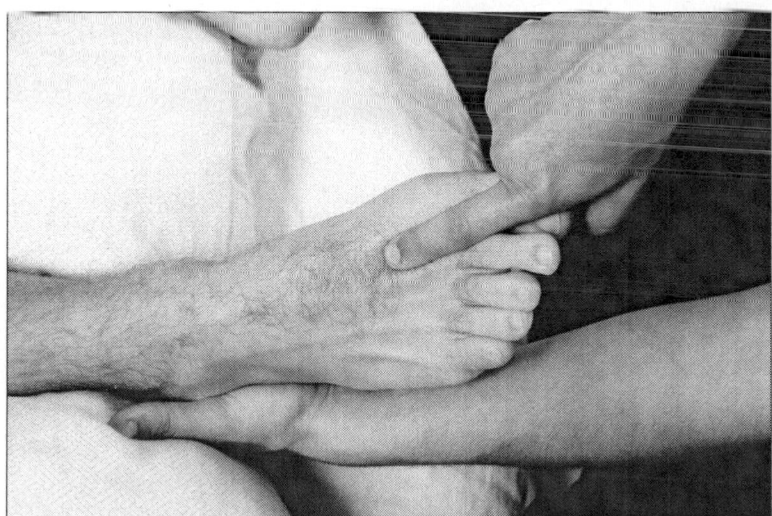

Figure 13-5: Using your index finger.

Hooking in

Using the tips of the thumbs or index fingers, bend slightly at the last knuckle and hook in at the point you're targeting (see Figure 13-6). This technique allows for some pinpoint pressure on the bony, intricate surfaces of the foot.

Wringing the foot

Because the arch of the foot corresponds to the spine in reflexology, this technique is like giving a chiropractic adjustment to the foot. Grasping your partner's toes with one hand and her heel with the other, give a gentle twist in opposite directions as if wringing out the arch of the foot (as shown in Figure 13-7).

Ankle circles

Holding your partner's ankle in one hand, circle her foot around in both directions (clockwise and counterclockwise) for several seconds, stretching the muscles and tendons in the area and warming up the ligaments (see Figure 13-8).

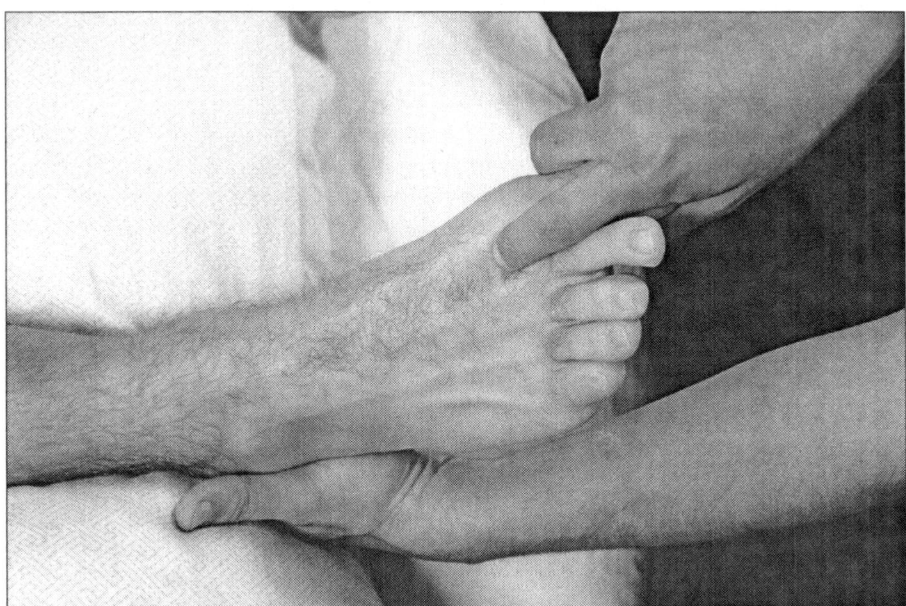

Figure 13-6: Hooking in.

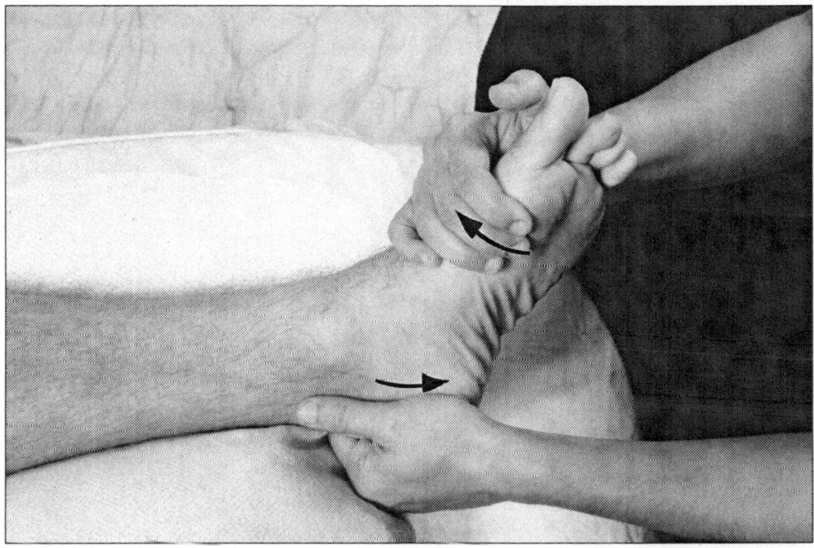

Figure 13-7: Wringing.

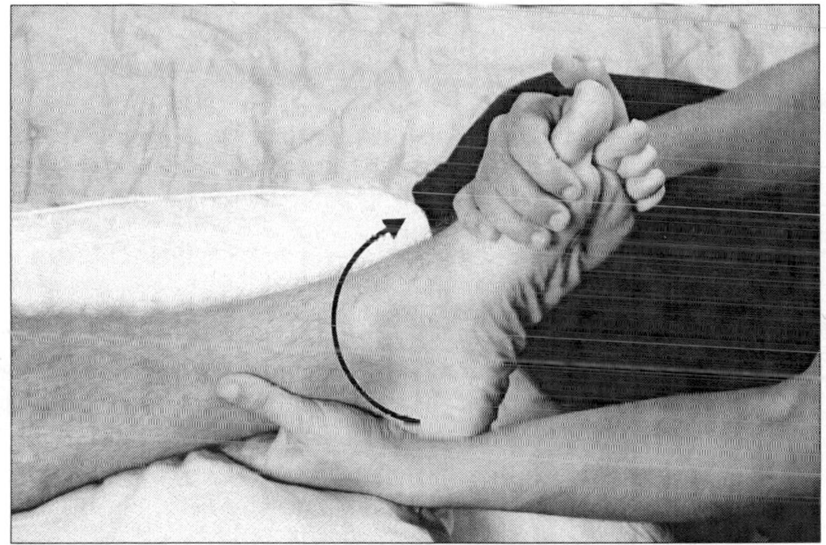

Figure 13-8: Doing ankle circles.

Performing Reflexology Step by Step

This section gives you a 20-minute foot massage routine based on the principles of reflexology. The routine is so easy to do that almost anyone can follow the instructions and perform the entire routine from start to finish the very first time, even members of the U.S. legislature. So, of course, that means you should have no problem at all. But if it all just seems too overwhelming, you can always fall back to the simpler step-by-step foot massage moves from Chapter 12.

You're going to make somebody oh-so-very happy if you offer to give them this quick and easy (yet pleasurable and effective) reflexology treatment.

Warming up

Begin by getting into a comfortable position, as I mention earlier in the chapter, and then do this warm-up:

1. **Cradle the ball of the foot.**
2. **Cradle the ankle.**
3. **Do ankle circles.**
4. **Stretch the toes back and forth.**
5. **Squeeze the foot.**

Getting down to business

After the warm-up, you're ready to move into the 15-step foot massage routine that follows, which is based on the work of reflexologist Claire Marie Miller in North Carolina.

Remember to start on the left foot, complete the entire routine, and then repeat the process on the right foot. Refer to Figure 13-1 if you need help remembering where specific points are located.

1. **Head.** Your head is filled with lots of important anatomical highlights, such as the brain. Spend a few extra minutes here as you begin your reflexology routine.

   To affect the reflexes of the head, do some small, focused thumb walking in three lines down the big toe as in Figure 13-9.

2. **Neck.** The neck can be an area of nagging pain. Sometimes working the reflex areas for the neck can help bring relief.

   Do thumb walking back and forth along the base of the big toe, right where it attaches to the foot (see Figure 13-10). To specifically treat the region at the base of the back of your skull, hook in with your thumb on the lower, inside part of your big toe, between it and the second toe. This point is key for relieving headaches and neck tension.

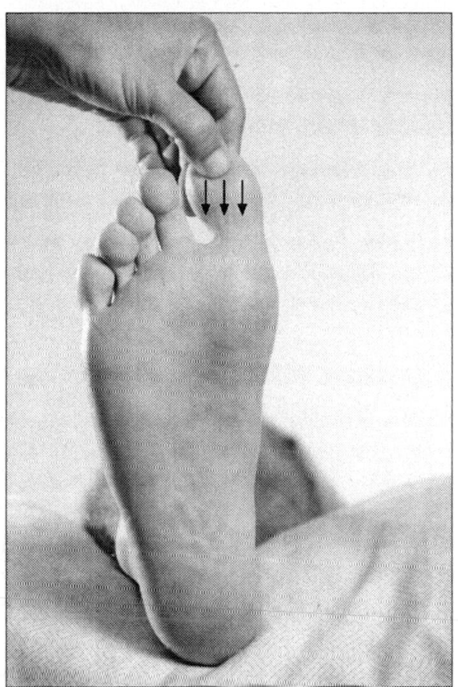

Figure 13-9: Reflexology points for the head.

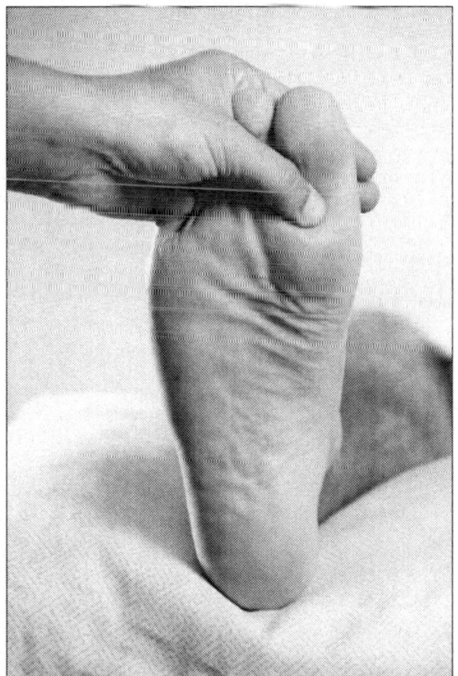

Figure 13-10: Points that target the neck reflex.

3. **Face.** Yes, even the face has a reflex on the foot, which is perhaps why it seems so easy to put your foot in your mouth.

   Do thumb walking across the top of the big toe, as shown in Figure 13-11, then hook in right at the base of the toenail.

4. **Sinuses.** The sinus cavities are hollow areas in your head behind your face. Keeping them clear and healthy helps you breathe more easily.

   The points for the sinuses can be found on the bottoms of all of the little toes. To stimulate them, use thumb walking down the bottom of each toe, and hook in right in the center of each toe for a couple seconds as in Figure 13-12.

5. **Ears/eyes.** The ears and eyes have reflexes by the base of the middle toes.

   Using your knuckles or both thumbs, press in on the spots on the bottom of the foot between the second and third toes (for the eyes) and between the third and fourth toes (for the ear reflexes), as in Figure 13-13. You can press both areas at the same time. The spots are on the very edge of the bottom of the feet, almost on the webbing between the toes themselves.

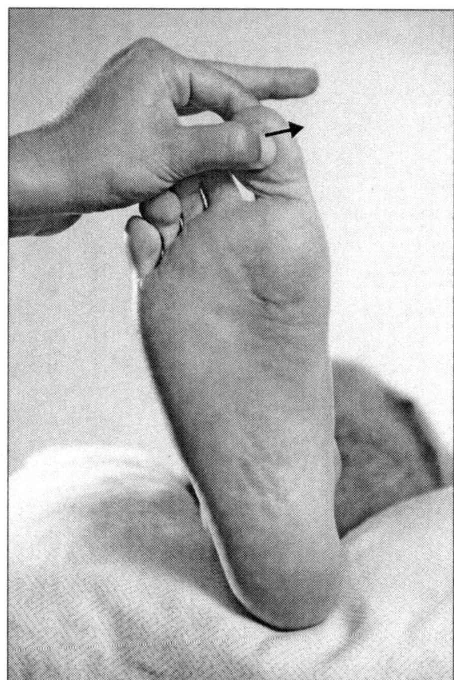

Figure 13-11: Face reflex points atop the big toe.

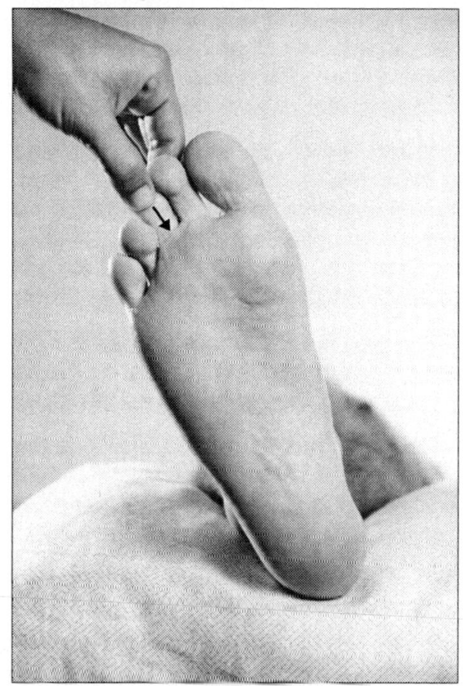

Figure 13-12: Sinus points along the bottoms of all the little toes.

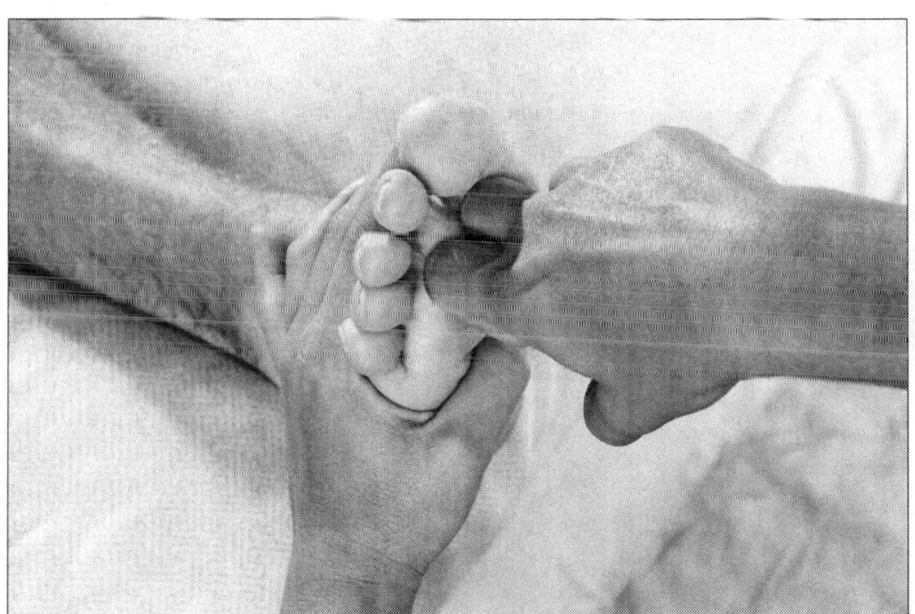

Figure 13-13: Targeting the ear and eye reflex points.

6. **Lungs/chest.** The area around the balls of your foot reflects your air passages, bronchial tubes, lungs, and chest muscles. If you stop breathing, you may run into some serious problems, so you benefit by paying attention to the healthy functioning of your lungs.

   Use the index finger technique for this reflex, sliding the length of your finger between the long metatarsal bones on top of the foot and pressing in against them while squeezing up with your thumb from below, as in Figure 13-14. You can also switch your hand around and slide your finger between the same bones from the bottom. After you have the right position, twist your hand back and forth while maintaining the pressure.

7. **Diaphragm.** The diaphragm (discussed in more detail in Chapter 6) is the muscle at the bottom of your lungs that is responsible for keeping you breathing. So, if you like breathing, try to keep this muscle happy.

   Pushing the toes up toward your partner's head with one hand, use the thumb of the other hand to walk back and forth along an imaginary line across the base of the ball of the foot, approximately two inches from the toes, as shown in Figure 13-15.

8. **Spine.** Many people experience back pain, and many of those same people have pain in the arches of their feet as well. A coincidence? Not when you know that the arches of the feet correspond in reflexology with the spine.

   Do thumb walking up and down the reflex for the spine, which is basically the arch of the foot (see Figure 13-16). You may want to switch thumbs when you're moving up the arch and back down, which makes this technique less awkward.

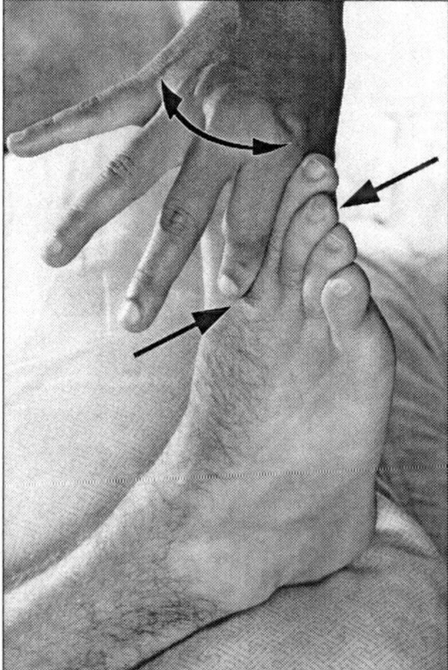

Figure 13-14: A squeezing twisting move for the lungs and chest reflex points.

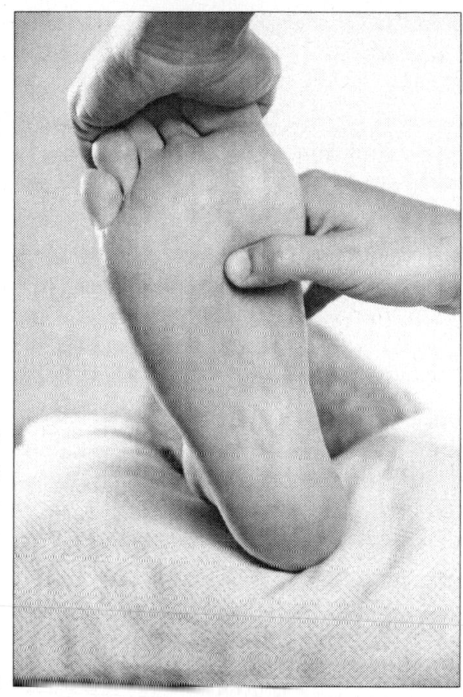

Figure 13-15: The diaphragm line is at the base of the ball of the foot.

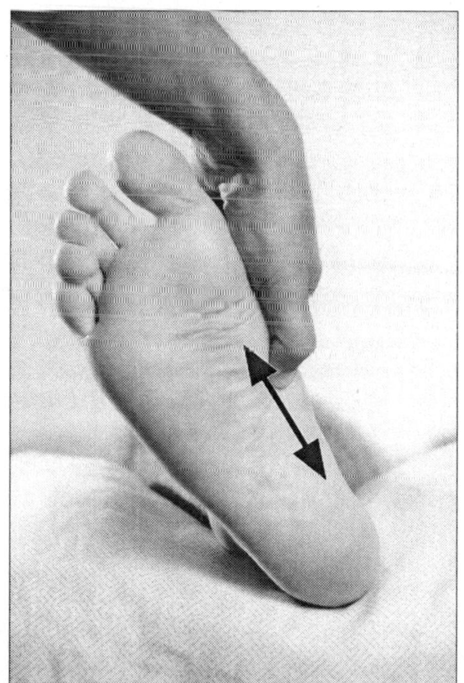

Figure 13-16: Spine reflex area along arch of foot.

Then "wring" the spine out by twisting the arch of the foot. Hold the heel with one hand and the toes with the other, while twisting gently in opposite directions.

9. **Inner organs.** The center of the bottoms of the feet correspond to several of your internal organs, and this is the area where you can easily get confused. You may want to study the chart in Figure 13-1 quite closely as you go about stimulating the reflexes here.

   When you're working on the left foot, do thumb walking in the center below the lung and diaphragm reflexes, where you'll find the areas corresponding to the stomach, the pancreas, the spleen, and the heart. Then walk your thumb from left to right across the center of the foot and down the outside, which corresponds with the last half of the large intestine.

   When working on the right foot, walk the thumb in the same area, but as you do, you'll be stimulating the liver and gallbladder instead. Then walk your thumb up the outside edge of the heel and across the center of the foot to stimulate the first half of the large intestine.

   Understanding the large intestine reflex is easier if you consider both feet together. Picture the large intestine going up the right side of the abdomen, across the upper abdomen, and down the left side (because this is what it actually does). Now you can imagine how you're affecting this reflex by walking your thumb up the outside of the right foot, across the center of both feet, then down the outside of the left, as in Figure 13-17.

10. **Small intestine.** "A man is only as happy as his digestive tract." This ancient saying, which I just made up this minute, highlights the importance of healthily functioning intestines.

    Using your thumbs or knuckles to walk helter-skelter in all directions, crisscross back and forth over the bottom of the heel like in Figure 13-18, which corresponds to the lengthy loops of the small intestine.

11. **Hips/knees.** Your hips and knees are your foundation, and stimulating these reflexes can help keep you in balance.

    Walk your thumbs along the upper part of the foot toward the outer edge, midway between the toes and the heel, moving in all directions around the general area of the *cuboid bone,* which is the little protuberance that sticks out the farthest in the middle of the outside edge of the foot, shown in Figure 13-19.

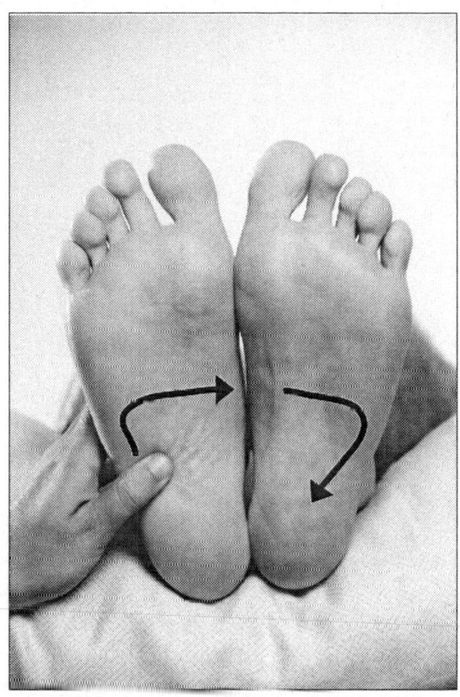

Figure 13-17: Reflex points for the large intestine.

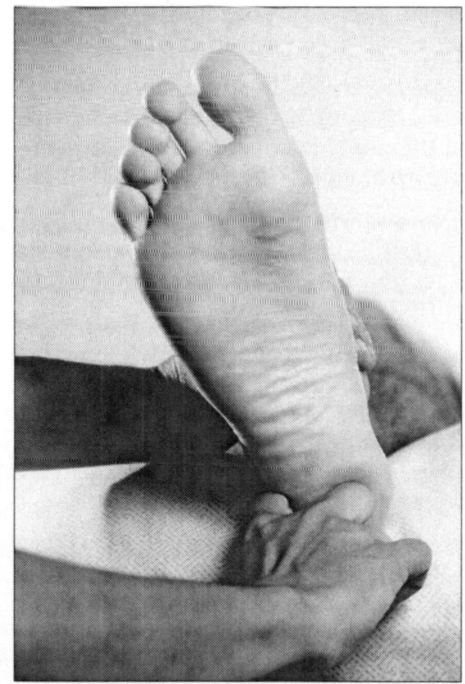

Figure 13-18: Small intestine reflex points on the bottom of the heel.

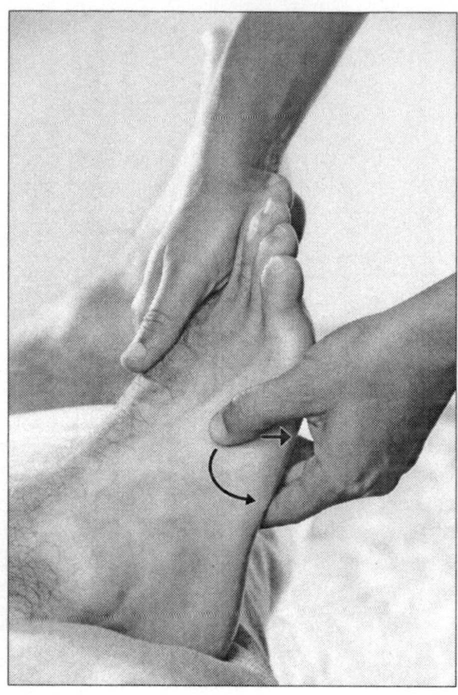

Figure 13-19: Hip/knee reflex points.

12. **Sciatic.** The largest nerve in your body, the sciatic can be the unfortunate victim of a proportionally large amount of pain.

    Sciatic points run from the back of the heel up the bottom of the Achilles tendon. Using the thumb and index finger, pinch all along the back of the base of the heel and then up a couple of inches along the Achilles tendon toward the calf, as in Figure 13-20. Repeat several times.

13. **Reproductive organs.** Men and women, as you've undoubtedly noticed by now, have different reproductive organs. But, as it so happens, the associated reflexes are located on the same areas of the feet for both sexes.

    Halfway down from the center of the ankle bones, toward the bottom of the heels, you find the reflexes for the reproductive organs. The inner ankle points correspond to the uterus or prostate, and the outer ankle points correspond to the ovaries or testicles. Use your thumb or the tip of your index finger to hook in for a few seconds on these points, as in Figure 13-21. You can also walk your thumb up over the top of the ankle from one point to another, which stimulates the fallopian tubes.

Stimulating the reproductive organ reflex points for pregnant women is said to help induce labor. Although I've never heard of a woman going into premature labor due to a massage to the foot, just to play it safe, stay away from this area completely if your partner may possibly be pregnant. Some people skip foot reflexology altogether on potentially pregnant people for this reason.

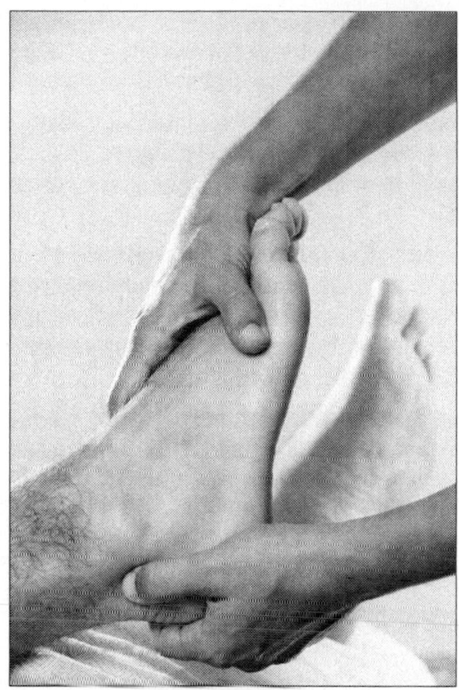

Figure 13-20: Sciatic reflex points.

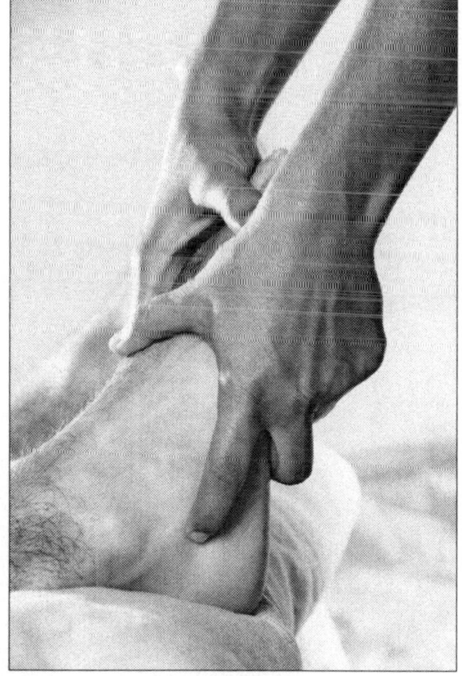

Figure 13-21: Reproductive organ points.

14. **Bladder and kidneys.** Save these reflexes for the end of the routine, because they're organs of elimination, and stimulating them promotes a cleansing reaction, which may involve a trip to the restroom.

    Starting near the heel, use thumb walking up and back along the arch of the foot, almost up to the ball of the foot, as in Figure 13-22. This line is a little more onto the bottom of the foot than the spine reflex (explained in Step 8). Repeat twice.

15. **Overall squeeze of the foot.** Never finish a foot without saying goodbye to it first. You may want to reapply some of the warm-up moves from the beginning as a cool-down here. Reflexology can be rather intense, and leaving your partner with some nice, pleasurable sensations at the end is a good idea.

    Finish with an overall squeeze of the foot, very quickly touching all the areas you've worked on before, cradling a little bit, and generally being nice. Some people like to apply a soothing skin cream at this point. Cooling mint preparations feel especially good, and you can find plenty of mint cream options at popular bath stores.

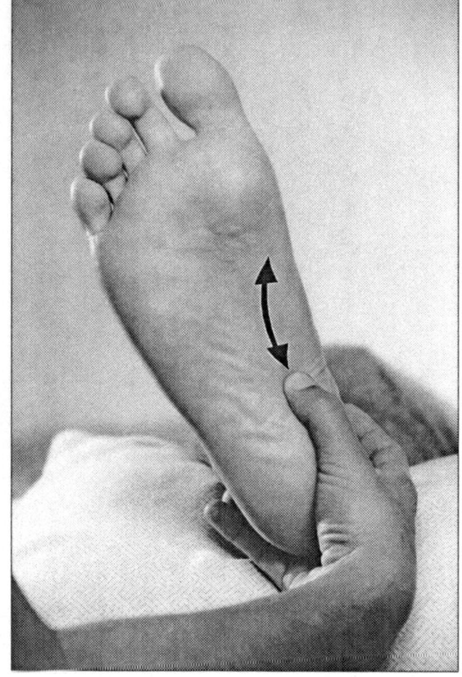

Figure 13-22: Bladder and kidney points stimulated at the end of the routine.

Chapter 14

Have Hands, Will Travel: Doing Massage for a Living

In This Chapter

- Exploring whether a career in massage fits you
- Tracing the massage career path
- Understanding the future of professional massage

After practicing your massage techniques and discovering the incredible benefits of massage, you may be thinking to yourself, "Hey, all this massage stuff is just *too much fun*. I want to find out how I can spend a large percentage of my own time making others feel better like all those fantastic professional massage therapists I've been reading about. And besides, it may help to pay the rent."

Right here in this chapter, you get enough information to make a preliminary decision on whether massage therapy may be the right career choice for you. You also find several tips and connections to get you going in the right direction.

May I also shamelessly take this opportunity to suggest to you a fantastic book on exactly this subject, a book that was, coincidentally, written by me? The book is *Massage Therapy Career Guide for Hands-On Success* (Milady) and is packed with over 300 pages of essential information for anybody who is seriously considering a walk down the massage career path or has already begun that journey.

Determining Whether Massage Is the Career for You

The first thing you should do when considering a career in massage is ask yourself a series of tough questions (found in the following sections) to determine your true motivations and chances for success.

The twelve traits of a born massage therapist: A questionnaire

Answering the following questions, excerpted from *Massage Therapy Career Guide,* may give you a good preliminary idea about how well suited you are to this profession. Keep track of how many times you answer "yes" and compare that to the list at the end of the survey.

1. Do people swoon and tell you that you have "great hands" when you simply place them upon their neck and shoulders and squeeze a little?
2. Do you feel sympathetic pain someplace in your own body when someone else tells you about their own pain?
3. Do you feel comfortable with your own and others' bodies; are you free from excess inhibition and body image hang-ups?
4. Do you have the ability and desire to work several hours a day at a very physical endeavor requiring significant stamina?
5. Can you easily remain in silence for an entire hour (or several hours in a row), without indulging in conversation if a client doesn't want it?
6. Have people ever told you that your presence makes them feel peaceful or calm?
7. Do you take your own health seriously by exercising, watching what you eat, and using moderation?
8. Does the idea of changing your lifestyle and livelihood seem exciting rather than horrible?
9. Is the human body a source of wonder and intrigue for you, making you want to learn more about how it works through intensive study?
10. Are you willing to invest a significant amount of time and money for schooling, supplies, association memberships, and equipment?
11. Is helping other people more important to you than making tons of money right away?
12. Are you willing to go through some potential ups and downs financially as you become established as a professional therapist?

Count up the number of "Yes" responses and compare your total with the following:

- **10–12:** Head to the nearest massage school to enroll.
- **7–9:** Begin serious investigation about the possibilities; send away for more information from massage schools.

- **4–6:** Seek the advice and inspiration of established massage therapists in your area who may be able to give you some insight about what daily life in the massage field is really like.
- **0–3:** Consider more deeply what your needs and motivations are for looking into massage as a career.

An honest look at yourself

Even if you have the traits of a massage therapist (see the preceding section), before you take the plunge you really need to stop and ask yourself, "Am I really into touching all those strangers all day long for the rest of my life?"

This career isn't for everybody. It takes a certain kind of person to be a massage therapist. And if you're that kind of person, what you may discover, after a short while, is that those "strangers" you may be touching aren't really strangers after all, but fellow human beings whom you can relate to on a meaningful level through your newfound skills.

Massage provides an acceptable avenue for empathy. Practicing professionals can touch others in a caring, compassionate way, helping them with their problems, easing their stress, and letting them know they're not alone. Massage therapists are paid to *be there* for people. That's no small thing.

So take an honest look at yourself. Does that deep desire to help and empathize with others outweigh whatever reservations you may have regarding the nitty-gritty reality of dealing with the not-always-wonderful public? If so, maybe you have quite an adventure ahead — a massage adventure, which I discuss in the following section.

Pursuing the Massage Adventure

After you make this fundamental choice and decide to pursue your career in massage, you have to prepare yourself for your new role in society. Yes, people may look at you with different eyes when they see you carrying around one of those big massage tables that look like padded suitcases. How will they react? What will the neighbors say?

Thinking of yourself as becoming a new person is strange, isn't it? It's almost like becoming a police officer or ship captain or any other profession that involves wearing a uniform. You're on display as what you are, and it may be uncomfortable at first.

These sensations gradually fade away, though, as you begin to associate more and more with other people who make a similar career decision. The first place you begin to meet your fellow travelers is usually in massage school. The following sections let you know what to expect from that training, as well as getting licensed and venturing out into the world of professional massage therapy.

Getting trained

Chances are that you already know somebody or know somebody who knows somebody who has taken up massage as a career. It's increasingly popular, with people from many different backgrounds.

The United States boasts over 1,200 massage schools, and training lasts about 6 months on average. In some areas you can get certified in as little as 100 hours, and in others you need more than 1,000 hours, which can take up to a full year. Other countries can require significantly more training; Canada has schools that have 2,000- or even 3,000-hour programs lasting up to three years. Most schools offer part-time classroom hours for those students who work another job, and some even have Saturday classes for extended periods.

Here are some of the subjects you explore in massage school:

- Anatomy
- Physiology
- Massage (of course)
- Applicable history, law, and so on
- Hygiene
- Allied therapies, such as hydrotherapy
- Professional conduct and ethics
- And much more

Sounds like an actual academic program, doesn't it? That's because it is. Massage school isn't just rubbing and relaxing all day, but that doesn't mean it isn't fun. Most graduates have very fond memories of their massage school days. And, just like in other schools, you establish new friendships, possibly spark romance, and change life paths.

Choosing a school

All massage schools aren't created equal. And the one you choose may play an extremely important role in your overall experience of massage. Some schools have a very grass-roots feeling, and attending them makes you feel like a part of the massage revolution as it unfolds across the globe, touching people's spirits as well as their bodies in many important ways. Other schools are more interested in providing their students with a no-nonsense, technically oriented approach to massage based more strictly on a medical model.

All schools let you attend an open house or a class to see whether the school's personality is the right match for you. Take advantage of this opportunity, and make sure to ask plenty of questions when you meet past and present students.

Another way you can check the standards of a school is to see whether it's accredited by an official organization. In the States, for example, schools accredited by the Commission on Massage Therapy Accreditation (COMTA) have to meet some very strict guidelines, and you can rest assured of their quality. Information about this accrediting organization is available at `www.comta.org`.

The prospect of attending a massage school may excite you, but you have no idea how truly valuable the experience is until you go through it yourself. Some of the high points include

- Camaraderie
- Increased knowledge and self-confidence
- Exposure to new techniques and systems
- A return to the stimulating, youthful lifestyle of the student
- Credentials you can travel with
- Self-transformation (see the sidebar later in this chapter)

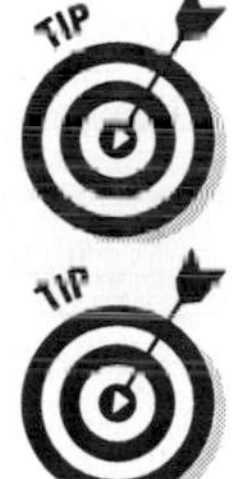

`Naturalhealers.com` is an information-packed Web site about massage schools and more. The site showcases schools from many health and healing traditions in addition to massage, including acupuncture, chiropractic, nutrition, and more. If you're on the lookout for a good massage school, check it out.

Chapter 18 lists ten of the best places to study massage.

Determining cost

Massage school may cost anywhere from a couple of thousand dollars a semester at a vocational technical school up to around $15,000 at some of the top schools, with the average seeming to hover in the $7,000 to $8,000 range. Schools in countries outside the United States, based more on a medical education framework, can cost quite a bit more.

Transformation through massage school

It's a rare person who can go through massage school and not be transformed on some fundamental level. What makes this so, you ask? Several things:

- Everybody there is making a life change of some sort, which makes for a lot of very open people, ready to share themselves with you and to have fun!
- People enrolled in massage school are there to take charge of their own lives in an entrepreneurial sense and a health sense, too, so you're likely to do some important networking with kindred spirits. Many business relationships have been forged in the classroom.
- Many students are often scared out of their wits that they won't be able to support themselves after they graduate; this fear makes them feel vulnerable, and vulnerability is a very endearing quality in most people. It lets you all communicate on an honest level.
- School offers you a time-out from the race you've been running in your life up to now. It gives you time to take stock of what's most important, where you've been, and where you truly want to go.
- When you begin literally touching people on a daily basis, as you do in school, you quickly get back in touch with what's real and what matters. Life matters. Health matters. People matter. What you're doing is important, and as you realize this fact more and more each day, your life may transform.

Attending massage school is no guarantee for a changed life, but it's a pretty good bet that you may come away with some insights and direction that you never even considered before you began. Just stay open.

As you can see, massage school usually entails a substantial investment. And that doesn't include the equipment and supplies you need to get started after you finish school. You need things like a massage table, business cards, and so on. So you need to think long and hard before plunking down that much dough for an education in touch therapy. This thought process is good. Think of it as a filtering system that keeps the less-than-serious from getting into the profession. Even with the costs, many tens of thousands of new massage therapists enter the worldwide market every year; 58,000 new massage students enter school in the United States alone!

Obtaining licensing and certification

After you graduate from school, you receive a certificate stating that you passed the course. Then, in many areas, you have to take that certificate and apply to take yet another exam to get your license. The license legally allows you to practice massage in your area. You never thought it would be so complex, did you?

The laws regarding licensing can indeed be confusing, and they're different everywhere you go, so the best advice I can give you is to do some thorough research into the regulations in your own area. Ask a local massage therapist, inquire at a local massage school, or call the local department of professional regulation. Get the license you need. Just one little accidental slip-up can turn you into an outlaw massage rogue, which isn't good for your professional reputation.

Discovering your new lifestyle

Freedom at last! After you make it through schooling, certification, and licensure, you're out there in the real world massaging real people — for real money. This new lifestyle you create for yourself is nothing like the boring 9-to-5 routine at your old job. But with your old job, you knew when you were working and you knew when you were off. Now, it seems like you're always either coming back from giving a massage, just about to give a massage, or thinking of ways you can get more people to sign up for massages.

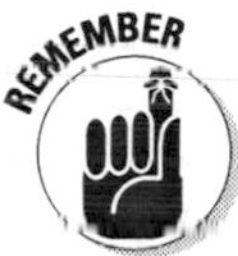

When you decide to pursue a career in massage, you may discover some things about life and about yourself that you never would have guessed otherwise. You literally get in touch with your own existence in a new way. You change. You grow. This transformation is the most valuable gift you receive, and it comes to you when you start to dedicate yourself to giving to others. What a concept.

When you work for yourself doing massage, you have to create some new rules and boundaries, like any self-employed person, so that your work life doesn't swallow you whole. Whether you work in a spa, a clinic, a doctor's office, or in your client's homes, you're going to need new boundary rules (see the sidebar about boundary rules in this chapter).

So how much will you make? The real story

Many would-be massage therapists add up the numbers. "Let's see, $70 per massage, doing just 5 massages a day, 5 days a week, makes $1,750 per week, times 50 weeks . . . oh my god! I'm going to be rich. Rich, I tell you!"

As a result of such calculations, many unsuspecting people have found themselves several months later sitting in a classroom studying the function of the gluteus maximus muscle. They bide their time, going through the motions, just waiting for their chance to graduate and become massage millionaires.

Well, the money doesn't always work out exactly that way. In fact, it seldom ever does. The average annual salary of a massage therapist in the United States is under $20,000 per year, according to one association's statistics, and the number of massage school graduates who end up not working in the field at all is surprisingly large as well. Fifty-eight thousand new massage students may enter school each year, but 50,000 folks drop out of the massage profession each year, too. Sobering, isn't it?

Boundary rules

The rules you come up with for yourself as a massage therapist are completely personal. No two massage therapists need follow the exact same guidelines. The important thing to remember is to stick by whatever rules you set. This firmness increases your self-esteem, makes life a lot easier for you, and lets your clients know that you're serious about your business.

The following are just a few suggestions of potential boundary rules. Yours may be much different. Practice saying your new rules out loud in front of the mirror a few times to yourself, as if you were talking to a client. Eventually, they seem natural.

- I don't work on weekends.
- I don't work after 8 p.m.
- I only take new clients by referral.
- I don't accept tips/I do accept tips.
- I have a 24-hour cancellation policy or the massage must be paid for in full.

The truth is that, like any field, the massage business is a hard business. It may be a little more "romantic" than some other fields, but the day-to-day reality of it includes an awful lot of good old-fashioned hard work, combined with many things you may not have thought you'd need, like marketing savvy, business plans, self-promotion, and managerial skills.

You can, indeed, make a very good living doing massage, and that may continue to be the case as more and more people worldwide realize the benefits that massage offers. But don't do it just for the money. You need to have another, deeper, reason, too, or you may end up like certain old rock-and-roll stars and massage therapists, eventually burning out.

The "tip" of the iceberg

You may have heard stories about massage therapists who get incredible tips from wealthy clients, and you may have wished that you, too, could receive such large gratuities. This desire is very natural. Yet some people say that if you receive tips for massage, you do a disservice to the industry. They say tipping turns massage into a service (like a waiter serving food to your table) rather than a treatment (like a doctor helping you find relief from a particular problem). You wouldn't consider tipping your doctor, would you?

The problem here is just the tip of the iceberg, so to speak, of a larger underlying issue about how we massage therapists want others to perceive massage. In the end, whether to receive tips or not is up to you. Turning down that cash staring you in the face as someone hands it to you isn't easy. Believe me, I've accepted a few whopper tips myself over the years. Nothing is really wrong with it, in the right circumstance, but you also want to be aware of the larger issue. (See the discussion on tipping in Chapter 5 for more information.)

Becoming a real pro

After you're out there and actually making a living giving massage, you may soon find more to the job than just the hours spent working hands-on. In order to become a real pro, you need to network your way into the industry and become a part of it, just like you'd become a part of the telephone industry, say, or the music industry. And that means . . . going to parties!

That's right. You have to go to some organized massage parties, also known as conventions, that are held every year in various locations. Another great idea is joining a massage professionals' organization, at least for a year on a trial basis, to see how the contacts, information, and sense of community can help you get going with your new career.

Make sure to subscribe to an industry magazine or two, and read each issue from cover to cover. This step may help you feel like an insider as you become familiar with all the people, places, and history that make massage what it is today.

Moving forward as a massage therapist

If you spend the time to gain some expertise in massage, people may eventually seek you out for your services rather than the other way around. Believe me, this flip feels very good — it's the exact opposite of sitting in your underwear on Saturday morning searching through the want ads and hoping someone out there can appreciate your abilities.

After you work to establish yourself as a massage therapist, you may be at an entirely different place than you have ever experienced up to now. A good place. It's a place that often leads to other places because those who gain success turn around and teach their skills to others in a variety of ways

Many massage therapists compound their success by turning to teaching at massage schools, at weekend workshops, and in books and videos that they create for other massage therapists. Some massage therapists even go on to become consultants, speakers, and sought-after health experts.

And just think, it all starts when you make that simple, profound decision to reach out and touch other people. Through massage, you can do just that.

Predicting where the Profession Is Headed

In a nutshell, up. And I'm talking on a worldwide scale here. If you're looking to get in on a growth industry, you really can't pick a better one than massage, because the number of human bodies out there available to be massaged is growing at a tremendous rate. Since the publication of the first edition of this book, for instance, world population has grown by nearly another billion people. So the number of potential clients is growing by leaps and bounds. And, although wealthier people will continue to pay top dollar for massages given in luxurious environments, a new trend has started in the past few years toward more affordable massage offered in storefronts across the land, as evidenced by the meteoric success of the Massage Envy chain of massage shops, where a massage costs as little as $39 (though the lowest rates typically require membership). Also, insurance companies have become more willing to pay for massage because the fact that massage can lower overall healthcare costs through stress reduction and preventative wellness is increasingly obvious.

That's right — in the future, as a massage therapist, others may respect you as a part of the evolving medical field, and your services may be paid for through insurance billing. This scenario is already happening, and it may soon become more common.

And in addition to the respect and success that you can claim, there's a certain something that makes massage special, too. It's in the simple human act of touching — of contact. That's our true specialty, and let's hope it never changes, no matter how successful we become.

Part IV
Massage for Every Body

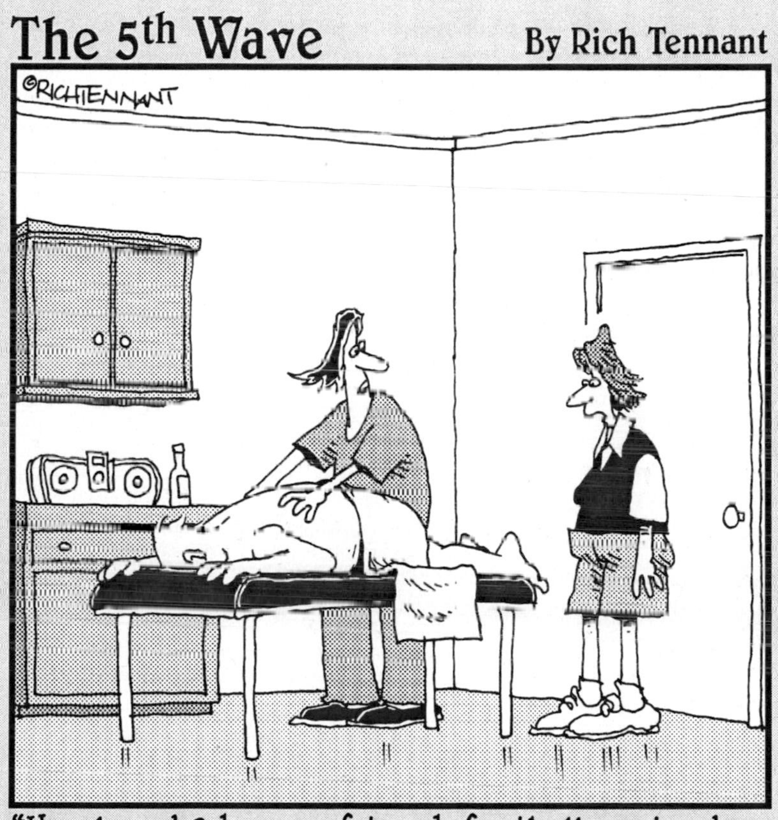

"He played 3 hours of touch football yesterday, and I think he strained his ego."

In this part . . .

All right, you can confess. You're reading Part IV with a nagging little voice in the back of your head saying something silly like, "Massage really isn't for me, at least not on a consistent basis. Sure, maybe as a novelty once or twice it's great, but how am I supposed to take advantage of it in real life? Isn't it just for the rich and famous, after all?"

No, no, no! Don't get so down on yourself like that. You can enjoy massage in many areas of your life, areas that perhaps you hadn't thought of before. That's what this part is all about.

Say you're a weekend warrior looking for a way to stay limber and uninjured while pursuing your part-time passion for sports. The massage moves and stretches in Chapter 15 should be perfect for you.

If you're "in the mood" and you're with that special someone, you can use massage as a sensual prelude to your encounters, as I explain in Chapter 16. And how about if you have a new baby? Or if you're pregnant? Or you're 7 months old? Chapter 17 provides easy-to-use tips and techniques made exactly for you. Chapter 18 is for those of you who spend too much time at a desk in front of a computer and need to de-stress ASAP.

Whether you're an athlete, an infant, a road warrior, a hedonist, a cubicle dweller, or an expectant parent, you can find something here that can provide many levels of enjoyment, pleasure, and health in your life. Massage truly is for every body.

Chapter 15

Higher, Faster, Stronger: Sports Massage

In This Chapter

- Understanding the techniques of sports massage
- Tackling pains specific to certain sports

Hey . . . you there . . . do I see you getting ready to put this book down and rush out to the local schoolyard for an impromptu ballgame? Yes, you. Are you planning on stretching much before you jump into that game? If you're like most part-time athletes, you're probably not guilty of over-stretching. Am I right? It's just such a hassle. Well, this situation is another arena where massage can come in handy. What's better than having someone stretch your muscles for you? That, and much more, is precisely what you can do with sports massage. And you get the lowdown on it in this chapter.

Heading to the Starting Line: Sports Massage Basics

When the going gets tough, the tough get massaging. If you're a serious athlete, chances are pretty good you probably understand the benefits of massage already. Most competing athletes think massage is valuable to athletic performance. Just look at Lance Armstrong, who won the Tour de France bike race seven times while making the color yellow famous. He received 200 massages a year. Also, a large percentage of Olympic competitors have used massage for years to gain an extra edge. In fact, beginning in 1996, massage became an official part of the services offered to all athletes in the Olympic Village itself.

Athletes utilize massage in a number of ways:

- To rehabilitate after getting injured in their sport
- To recover from intense workouts and competition

- To maintain optimal muscle tone and flexibility on an ongoing basis
- To appear relaxed and cool getting their massages in front of the competition at big events

The following sections give you the skinny on when sports massage can be helpful and guide you to finding a sports massage therapist.

Knowing good times to use sports massage

You can use sports massage any time you want, even right before church on Sunday morning or at midnight after drinking margaritas all evening at the annual company party. But using sports massage right around the time you're going to be engaging in sports just plain makes more sense, don't you think? And that basically boils down to three different occasions:

- **Pre-event massage:** As the name implies, athletes use this type of sports massage directly before the event. And, contrary to popular belief, a massage at this time doesn't zone the athlete out to a state of zombiehood but rather invigorates her further in preparation for competition.
- **Post-event massage:** Directly after an event (like just past the finish line at the Boston Marathon), is a place and time that athletes almost universally appreciate a good massage. Massage helps the muscles, not to mention the psyche, recover more quickly.
- **Ongoing training massage:** Getting massaged throughout the training cycle is becoming more and more popular with many athletes. Some even receive massage every day.

Finding sports massage

If you live in a large metropolitan area, chances are good that you have a sports massage clinic somewhere close by. If you live in a small town, try inquiring at your local osteopath or chiropractor's office. They may know someone who offers sports massage.

Massage pros go through a special advanced training in order to become certified sports massage therapists. You won't offend anyone by asking about their certification and where they got it. So if you're really looking for a qualified person, check out their qualifications. Makes sense, doesn't it?

Athletic trainers are quite often also sports massage therapists, or they can at least recommend one. Beware, though, of the trainer who thinks he's doing sports massage just because he knows how to give a few karate chops to your back. He may be doing you a disservice, and he probably doesn't understand that true professional sports massage is becoming a highly evolved discipline.

The days of Rocky Balboa's coach giving him a shoulder rub along with a motivational speech before the big fight are over. "And if he gets up, hit him again!"

Call the American Massage Therapy Association (AMTA) toll free at 877-905-2700; it may be able to provide you with the name of a qualified practitioner in your area who offers sports massage.

Examining Sports Massage Techniques

Sports massage, when applied by skilled practitioners, is an advanced form of massage therapy with several specific techniques. The instructions in this chapter obviously aren't meant to make you an expert. They simply suggest a couple of moves that can help ease the strains of the weekend warriors in your life, including you. In other words, after reading this chapter, don't go out and announce yourself as a special trainer for Olympic marathon runners — leave that to the pros.

Sporty moves

This section provides you with some basic sports massage moves. You may notice that they're similar to regular massage moves; they're just bigger and often deeper, and certain moves are used much more frequently during sports massage than, say, during a relaxation massage.

Compression

Often in sports, overworked and overtired muscles have to be pressed into submission. With this move, shown in Figure 15-1, you can apply enough direct pressure to help relieve muscle spasms and provide a calming effect to the area.

Cross-fiber friction

You may recognize the term cross-fiber from Chapter 10 (and then again, you may not). What the heck is cross-fiber friction anyway? *Cross-fiber friction* is simply the use of some relatively intense rubbing in the opposite direction that the muscle fibers run in any particular area (rubbing against the grain, so to speak), as you can see in Figure 15-2. This technique is especially good for muscle fibers that are put under strain during sports.

Deep pressure

People who work out a lot often end up creating some really sore spots along with the improved tone in their bodies. Pinpointing these sore spots can be tricky, but after you do, treat them to some direct deep pressure, as shown in Figure 15-3, to help release knotted, cramped, and contracted muscle tissues.

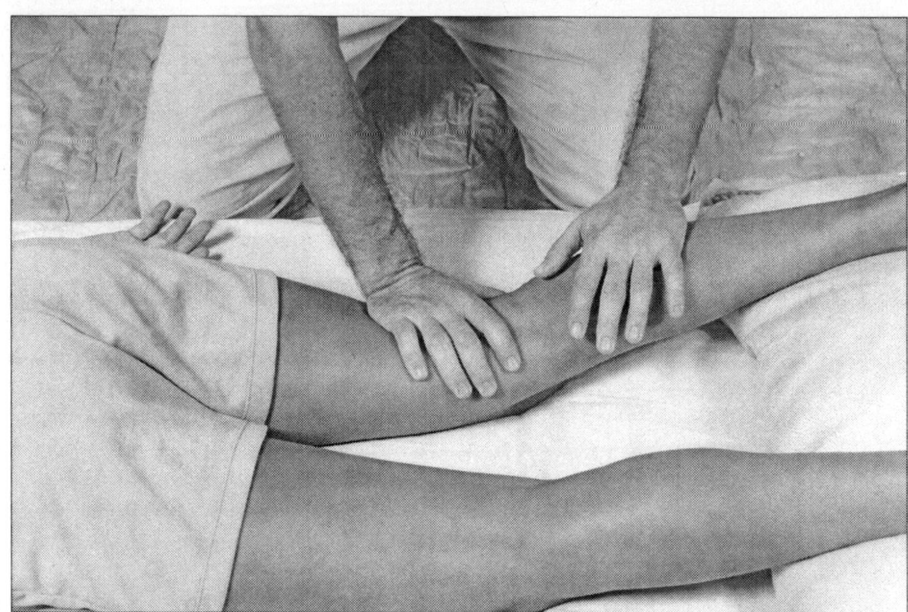

Figure 15-1: Compression to the hamstrings.

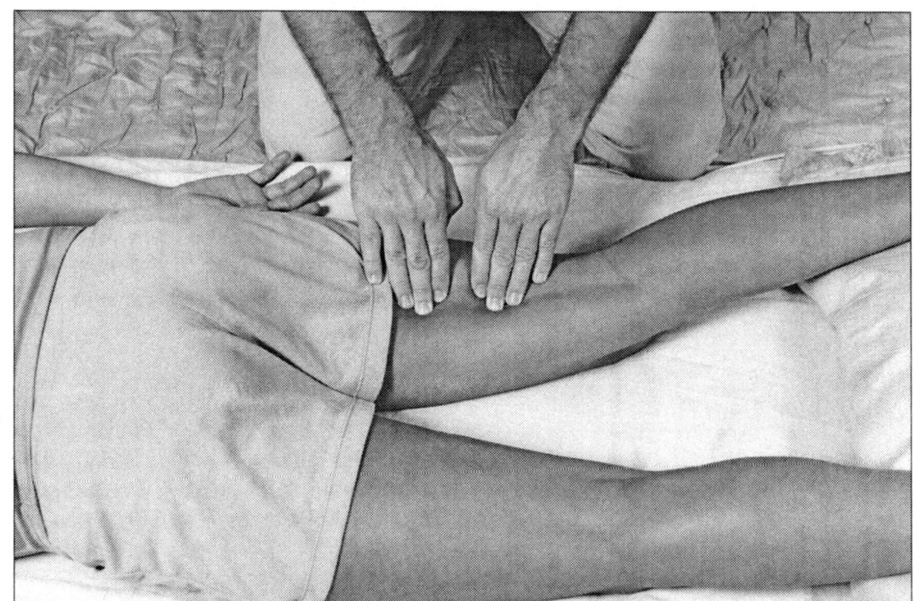

Figure 15-2: Cross-fiber friction to the hamstrings.

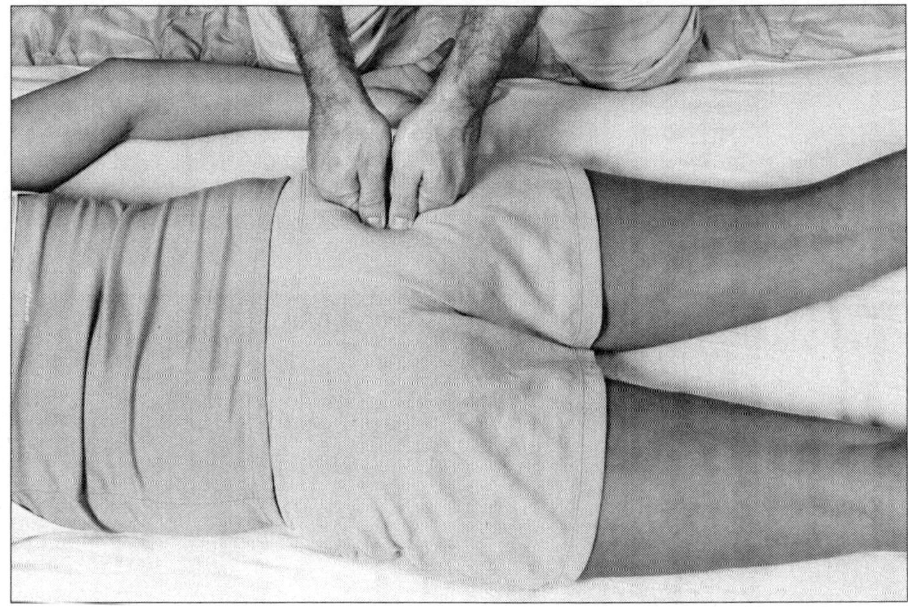

Figure 15-3: Deep pressure to the gluteus maximus.

Kneading

When you're kneading an athlete, you want to make sure your motions are big and strong and that your hands grasp as much muscle tissue as possible. See Figure 15-4, and refer to Chapter 10 for more on the three steps of kneading (squeezing, rolling, and pushing)

Stretches

This section walks you through some basic stretches that are part of sports massage. The moves are a great way to help a partner warm up before an activity or cool down afterwards.

Stretches feel really good to people who've been using their muscles a lot in sporting activities, but be careful not to overstretch people and possibly injure them. Always ask for feedback from your partner while you're performing the stretch, and always err on the side of not enough stretch instead of forcing it toward too much.

Hamstring stretch

With your partner lying on her back, lift one of her legs up, supporting it firmly at the ankle and on the hamstrings themselves as you push the leg slowly and steadily back toward her head. Don't lock the knee during this maneuver but rather leave it slightly flexed. Hold the stretch for 5 to 10 seconds, and then release (see Figure 15-5). You can add more impact by having your partner push back against your hands for 5 to 6 seconds at first and then releasing while you stretch her leg a little farther for about 30 seconds. This über-stretch is known by the important-sounding name *proprioceptive neuromuscular facilitation* (PNF), and it should be applied only if your partner is already warmed up and if you feel confident about supporting the leg sufficiently. Don't overstretch in this technique. In other words, take it easy!

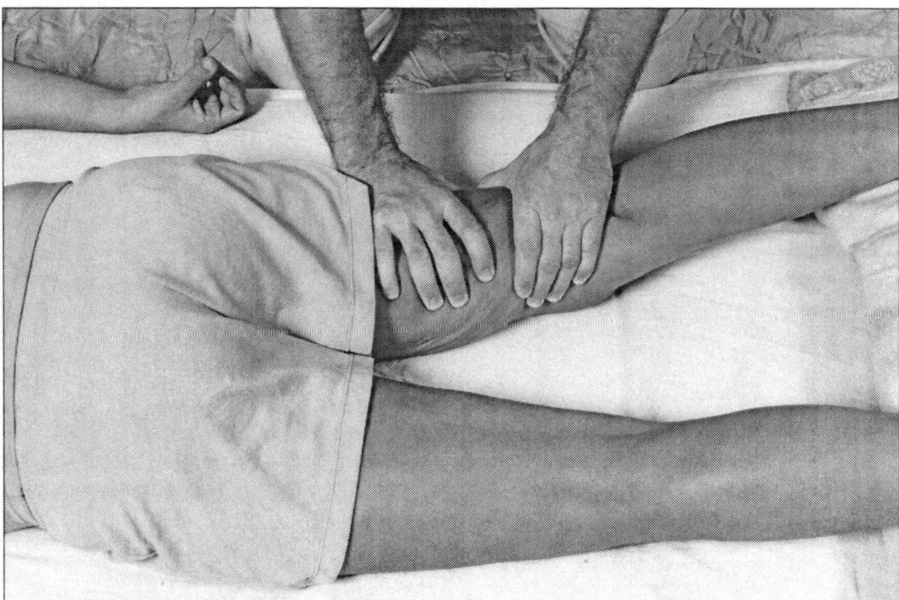

Figure 15-4: Kneading the hamstrings.

Quad stretch

The quadriceps muscles in the front of the thigh get especially tight on runners and other athletes. A good way to stretch them is to have your partner lie face down, bend her knee 90 degrees and then lift her foot straight up while also lifting beneath her knee with your other hand. Only lift until you feel the natural resistance of her muscles. For an extra stretch on limber partners, bring the foot closer to the buttocks at the same time, as shown in Figure 15-6.

Calf stretch

When you stretch the calf, you stretch the Achilles tendon, too, which is extremely strong. So don't be afraid to give a deep stretch here by cupping the heel and pressing your forearm firmly against the bottom of the foot, moving the toes toward the head, as shown in Figure 15-7.

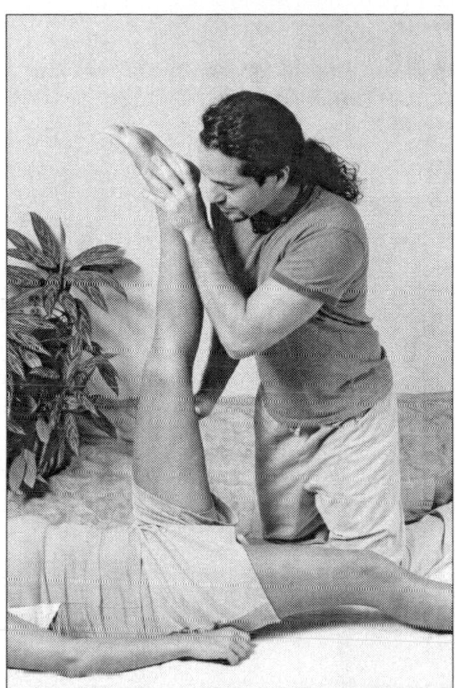

Figure 15-5: Hamstring stretch.

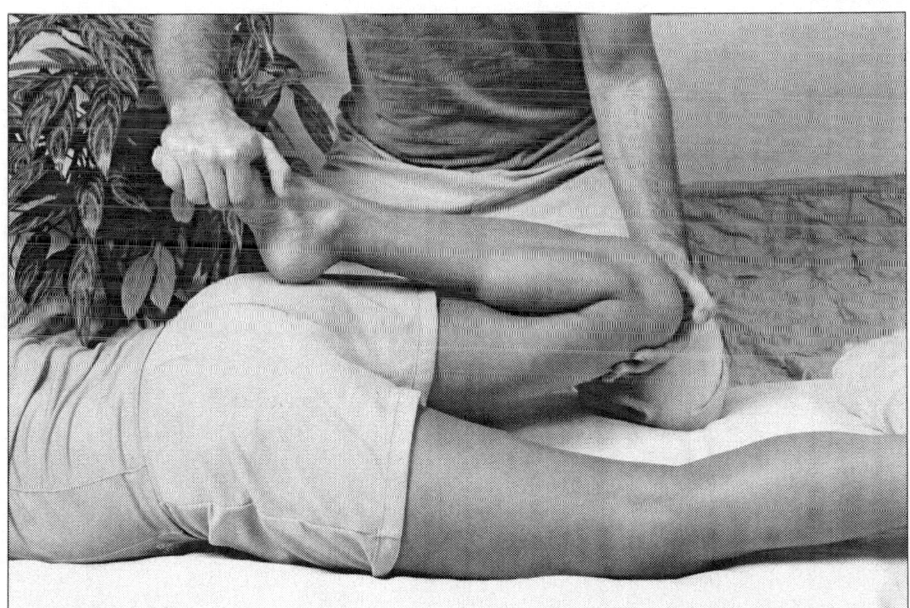

Figure 15-6: Quadriceps stretch.

Arm stretch

With your partner face down, lift her hand up over her head and position her hand palm down with fingers pointing toward her feet and pull up slightly on the elbow, as shown in Figure 15-8.

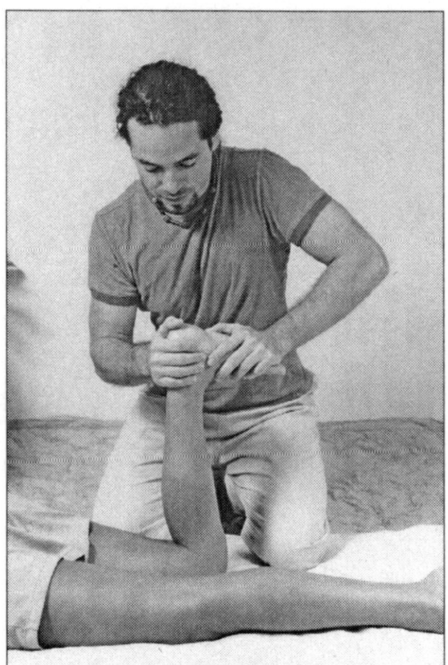

Figure 15-7: Calf stretch.

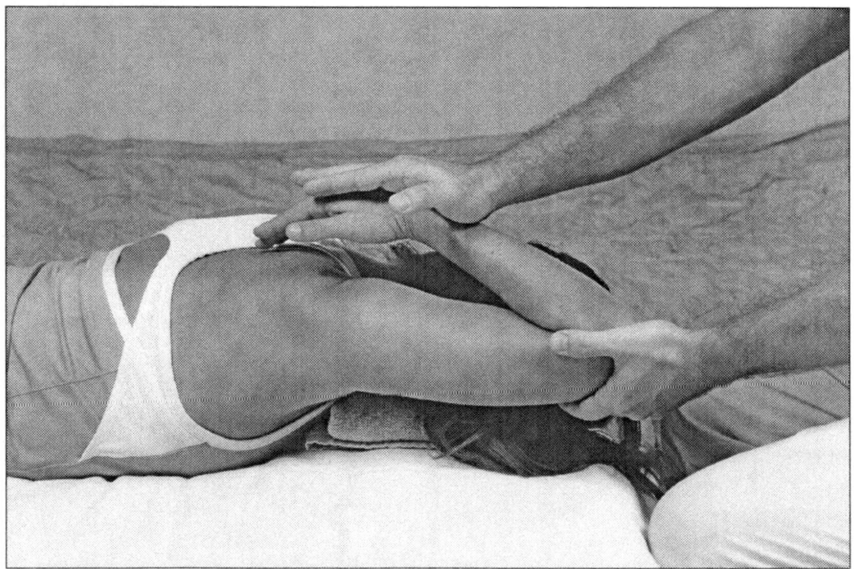

Figure 15-8: Arm stretch.

Routines

You can perform an entire sports massage routine, which is going to look similar to the regular routines I cover in Chapters 11 and 12, except that your partner will be wearing an athletic outfit rather than a towel! But that's not the only difference. You also use a lot more cross-fiber friction, compression, and deep kneading, focusing on the muscles that have done the exertion. And you add some extra stretching to aid in recovery, too. Other than that, though, don't be too surprised if sports massage looks amazingly similar to non-sports massage.

A Pain in the Elbow, a Pain in the Butt

Athletes run into all kinds of problems because they push their muscles to the limits, and certain sports are famous for causing certain pains. You've probably heard of tennis elbow, for example, and runner's cramps, both of which are problems that sports massage can help.

Tennis elbow

Tennis elbow is a slow, creeping, debilitating condition that can really make you unhappy over a long period of time. This condition is a swelling of the tendons in the forearm near the elbow and an irritation of the muscles there caused by repetitive use. Of course, the best thing to do when you start noticing this type of pain is to stop doing what's causing it (namely, playing tennis). Some people don't want to stop playing tennis, though. In that case, try taking a break just for a few days and using ice to reduce soreness in the area. Also, a physician may be able to help by prescribing anti-inflammatory drugs, so check with your doctor.

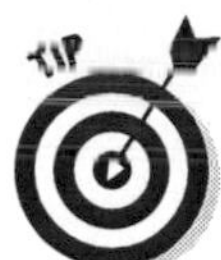

A little sports massage can help tennis elbow, too. Remember to do some gradual warm-up massage moves first before digging straight in with these two rather intense maneuvers. Also, apply ice for 5 to 10 minutes beforehand to reduce inflammation. Then follow these steps:

1. **Supporting the arm at the wrist, with the elbow resting on the floor or massage table, grasp your partner's forearm and slide your hand down *slowly* from her wrist toward her elbow, pressing in with your thumb as you do so, as shown in Figure 15-9a.**

   Repeat this move several times with your hand in different positions so your thumb presses against the entire forearm.

2. **Using the tips of your fingers or thumbs, apply cross-fiber friction to the muscles on top of the forearm (straight up from the back of the hand) near the elbow, as Figure 15-9b illustrates.**

   This area is most directly affected in tennis elbow, so take it easy on your partner, using more ice if necessary to lessen discomfort. Apply more squeezing, gliding, and a little kneading afterward to help smooth things out.

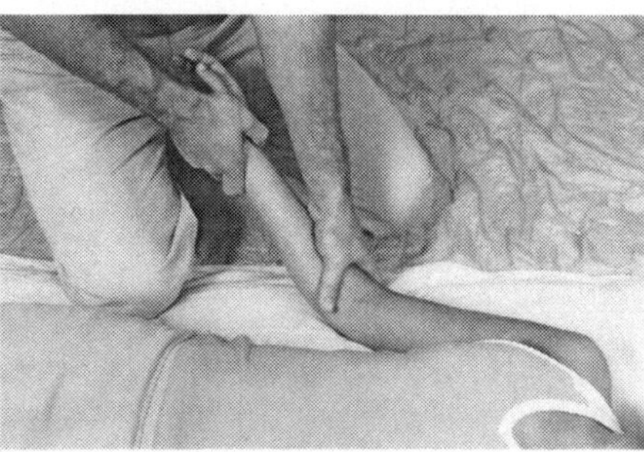
a

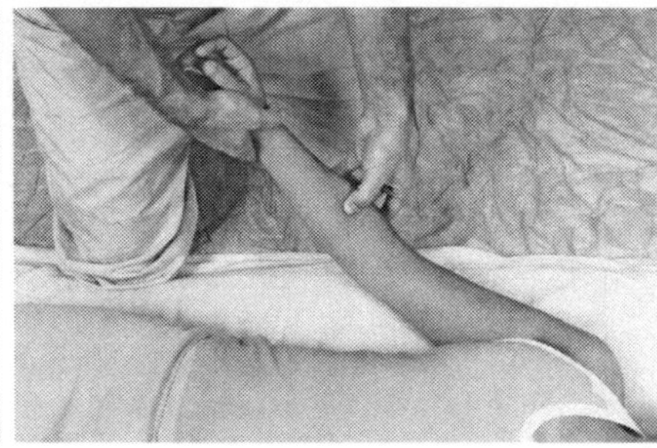
b

Figure 15-9: Squeeze the forearm muscles (a) and apply deep friction near the elbow (b).

Runner's cramps

Runners often get muscle cramps in their calves, hamstrings, quads, or buttocks after pushing themselves to the limit. If you've ever been the victim of runner's cramps, you know that they aren't fun at all. These cramps take over your leg like an invading alien on *Star Trek,* and they show no mercy. If you're standing at the time the cramp starts, you begin limping around and screaming like a maniac. And if you're lying down, the cramp is even worse. The following techniques may help the next time someone you know falls victim to a charley horse.

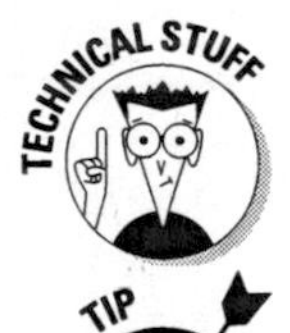

For over a century now, runner's cramps have also been known by the term *charley horse,* which originally came from the world of baseball. No one knows for sure who Charley was, or why he had a lame horse, though some people say he was a groundskeeper at a Sioux City ballpark.

Make sure the athlete drinks plenty of fluids to counter the cramping effects of dehydration. And after the massage, try placing some ice on the area for a few minutes to further reduce soreness.

When a cramp strikes, follow these steps to help ease the athlete's pain:

1. **Get the person to lie down comfortably and apply direct compression to the area, as shown in Figure 15-10.**

2. **After a few seconds, release the pressure and apply a stretch to the muscle that is cramping, as in Figure 15-11.**

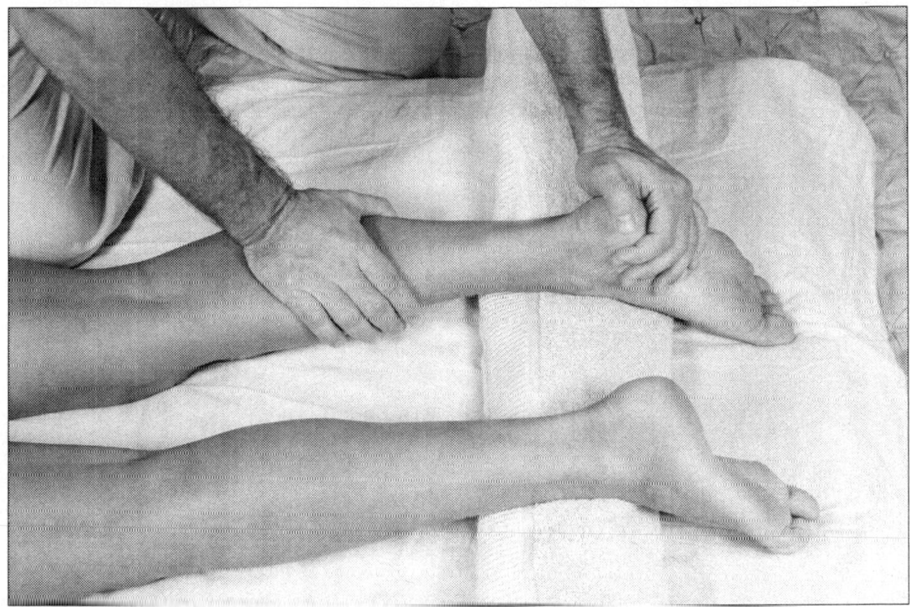

Figure 15-10: Compression on cramping area.

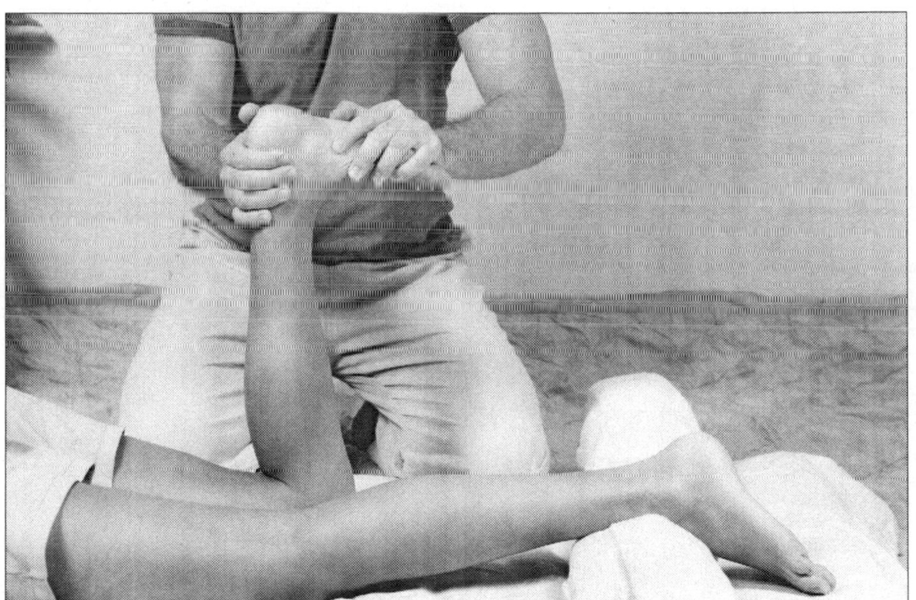

Figure 15-11: Stretch for the cramping area.

3. **Grasping at the far end of the muscle on either side of the spasm itself, push the muscle fibers in toward the middle as Figure 15-12 demonstrates.**

   Hold for several seconds.

4. **Have your partner contract the opposing muscles, which in Figure 15-13 are the muscles in front of the lower leg, by trying to pull her toes up toward her head as you resist the movement.**

   This technique has the effect of further loosening the cramping muscle.

5. **Stretch gently one more time.**

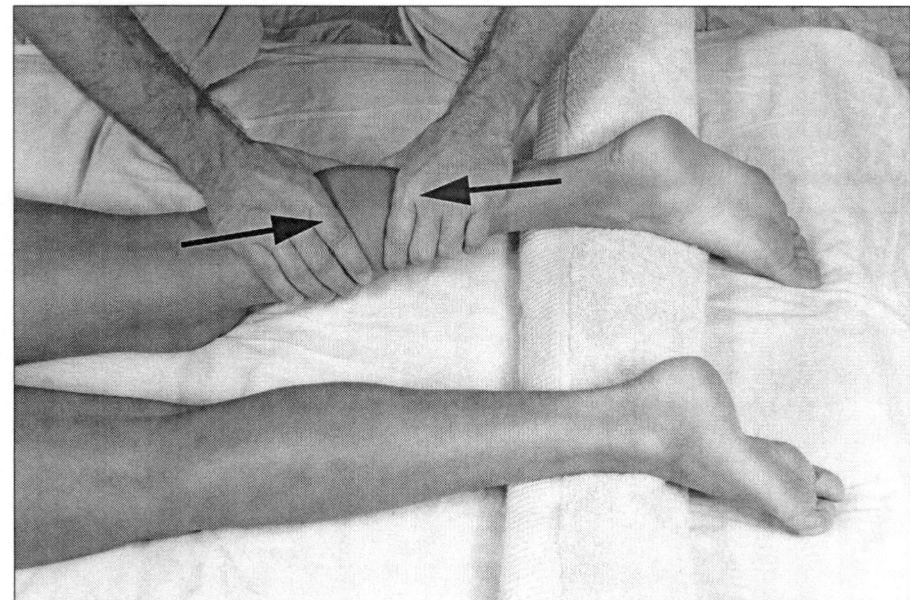

Figure 15-12: Bunching the muscle fibers of the cramping area together.

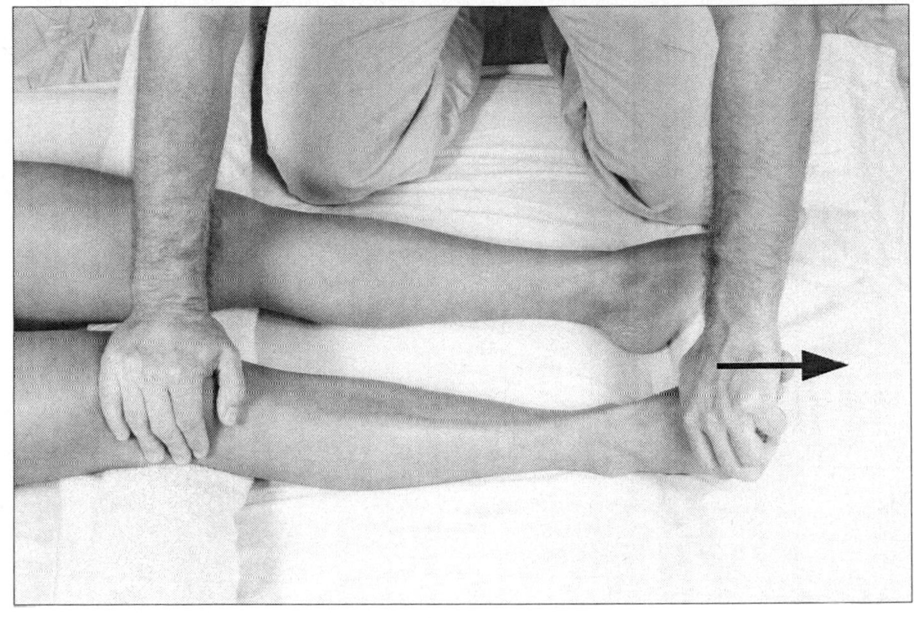

Figure 15-13: Contract muscles that oppose cramping muscle.

Chapter 16

Sensual Massage

In This Chapter

- Preparing to use sensual touch with your partner
- Getting into the sensual mood
- Trying out sensual moves

Sometimes, massage can just plain be sexy. Regardless of how therapeutic it is. Regardless of how favorably many physicians think of it today. And regardless of the way it's used by superstar athletes in smelly locker rooms.

As a practitioner of therapeutic massage myself, I am among those who want to convince you of the *big* difference between sensual touch and therapeutic massage. Hundreds of thousands of professional practitioners help heal millions of people through their nonsexual touch. But that doesn't mean sensual touch can't be therapeutic. In fact, the famous musician Marvin Gaye sang a song on that very topic. You guessed it: "Sexual Healing."

This chapter offers a few basic ideas to get you started with some sensually oriented massage. You can take many of the suggestions from the rest of this book, too, and add a little spice to them. Be careful who you use your sensual healing techniques on, though, because they can be quite powerful.

Exploring Sensual Touch

You need a few important ingredients in order to create a great sensual massage. These include the following:

- A naked supermodel
- A gallon and a half of musk-scented massage oil from ancient Persia
- Any CD by Barry White

Just kidding! Actually, having any of those ingredients on hand may indeed improve your chances of experiencing the ultimate sensual massage, but they're certainly not necessary. The following are the three things that you definitely need for a good sensual massage:

- The right intention
- Spontaneity
- Sensitivity

The right intention

So how do you go about being sensual with your chosen partner after you've decided you want to share a sexy massage together? The trick is to change your *intention.* You can tell the difference instantaneously when someone has a sensual intent with their massage moves. You may be surprised how the very same moves performed on the very same part of the body can have incredibly different effects, depending upon who's giving the massage, and what his or her intention is. You can feel it in the touch.

A fine line lies between sensual and sexual massage, and believe it or not, sometimes sensual is better. Sensual massage is more relaxed. It doesn't expect anything. Sex is something that gets done; sensuality just *is.*

Once in a while, simply enjoy the touch without thinking about where it may lead. Relax there in the arms of sensuality for a time, taking some pressure off of you and your partner. You may like what you find.

Spontaneity

Perhaps the most important rule for sensual massage is, "Go with the flow." If you feel like the most appropriate place for the massage is on the beach at midnight, take your bottle of oil and head outside. Then again, the kitchen floor can become an exotically sensual environment when you lie down on it with your partner. Wherever you are, look around for items that can enhance your experience. You're bound to be able to use something that you have on hand — a texture, a sound, or a taste — like a big, juicy, ripe strawberry, for example.

Sensitivity

With sensual massage, you have to be especially sensitive to your partner's emotions during the session. Envelop him in a sense of warmth, caring, and safety. You don't have to beat your partner's tension into submission or accomplish anything at all really. Just *be there* with him.

A massage called Tantra

You may want to know about a special, sensual, energy-raising technique called *Tantra* that combines meditation and lots of interesting activities you can use to change sexual energy into sensual/spiritual energy. You and your partner can engage in sensual massage, for example, to heighten your experience of togetherness instead of rushing straight into the whole sex thing and then rolling over and falling asleep afterward.

If you're into enhancing your sensual life, you can choose among many workshops, videos, and books on Tantra. Pick up one of the books by Mantak Chia, for example, which you can find on the Web at `www.universal-tao.com`. Also, `www.tantra.com` has a treasure trove of information on sensual subjects, including massage. While you're there, you can have fun discovering other aspects of Tantra, such as art and instructions from the *Kama Sutra,* an ancient text on sensuality. Plenty of couples' workshops on the subject are available, too.

Have fun!

In sensual massage, the idea isn't so much to soothe your partner's sore muscles but rather to enchant him. So you don't need to use as much pressure or strength as you do in a regular massage. Practice using *soft hands,* letting your fingertips and palms drift over the surface of the skin without trying to achieve any therapeutic purposes. This technique changes the massage mood, making it more sensual.

Setting the Sensual Mood

Sensuality is all about creating a sensual mood, right? So, it follows that your inner chamber, as I describe in Chapter 8, is especially important during a sensual massage. But just how exactly are you supposed to make it sensual? You can use candles and incense, but how about something a little more daring?

You may want to check out a few of the items listed below to help you and your partner get into the appropriate sensual mood. After all, you don't have all day to lie around waiting for the proper mood to strike. You're a busy person, and you have lots of other things on your mind. If you're feeling adventurous, try the following suggestions, and see what happens.

Flavored massage oils

Okay, I admit it . . . flavored massage oils are a little on the hokey side. But you can't knock it till you try it, right? These days, you can find flavors for every taste, including, believe it or not, a cappuccino-flavored massage oil, which must be for those times you need a quick pick-me-up and don't want to suffer the extreme embarrassment of falling asleep with your tongue in your partner's navel.

Of course, the idea here is to enjoy the flavor of the oil while you're licking it off, but be careful not to get addicted to this pastime. Don't swallow whole pints of the stuff, because it may jeopardize your health. Like all oils, edible ones have a lot of cholesterol and fat, too. And nothing would be worse than gaining weight by licking your mate, which can lead to the worst of all excuses for not giving your honey a sensual massage: "I'm on a diet."

If edible oils interest you, a Web search turns up dozens of options that can be sent directly to your home in a matter of two or three days, most of them "discretely packaged." How convenient!

Little devices

Little devices that buzz and vibrate can be quite a pleasurable addition to a sensual massage experience. You can purchase such devices guilt-free at trendy shops in cities around the world these days, or you can order them online or through catalogues. Certain items you already have around the house may come in handy here as well, such as feathers, soft brushes, scarves, strawberries, chocolate syrup, or whipped cream. Let your imagination take you where it wants to go with these items during a sensual massage and see what happens.

Videos

All kinds of sensual massage videos are out there for you to use to help get you in the mood, but they share one big problem: The models are too good looking. For most people, watching one of those videos without feeling a little inadequate is difficult. If you do watch them, just keep reminding yourself that those people spend ten hours a day exercising, seven days a week. When they're not exercising, they're at the tanning salon, or the local health food restaurant having a bowl of lettuce for lunch, dressing on the side.

Discovering Sensual Moves, and Other Sensual Massage Tidbits

Here are a few moves that you can use when you're creating your sensual massage together. You may notice that some of these moves aren't really moves at all but rather attitudes. In a sensual massage you take more liberties with your partner. You drape yourselves over each other more, coming closer and dissolving the giver/receiver barrier.

Creating fuller contact

In therapeutic massage, you usually bring just your hands and arms into contact with your partner, for the most part. In sensual massage, on the other hand, it doesn't matter how much of your body comes into contact with your partner. In fact, the more contact the better, as shown in Figure 16-1. For massage maneuvers you apply to the back, the neck, and the head, sit right down on your partner's tush. Just make sure not to rest all your weight on him, though, because you may cut off his circulation.

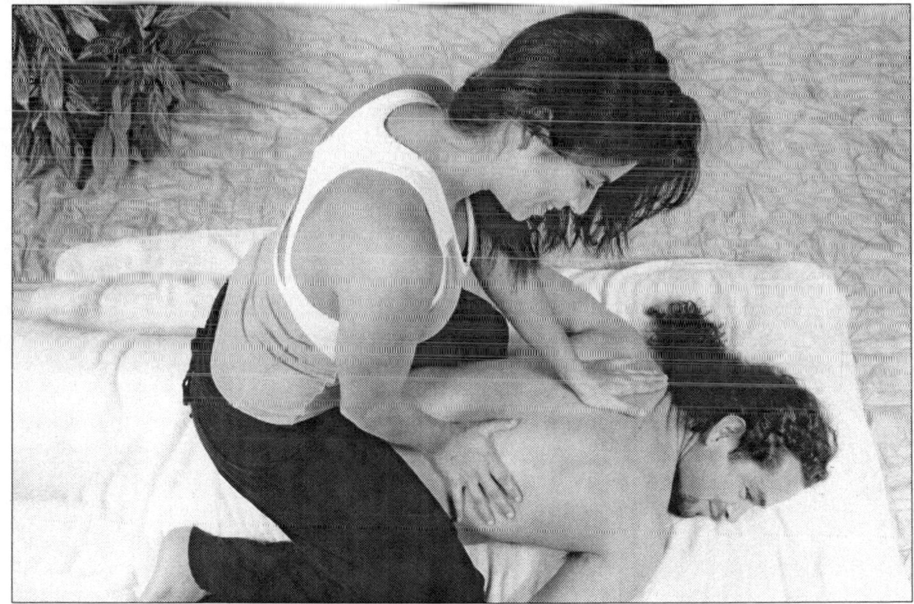

Figure 16-1: Sitting on top of your partner is great in sensual massage.

Limb draping

When you're massaging your partner's limbs, let the entire leg or arm rest across your body. This positioning creates a sensation of support and intimacy, especially when you combine it with light, lacy moves with your fingertips on the inner thigh area as Figure 16-2 demonstrates. Ooh la la!

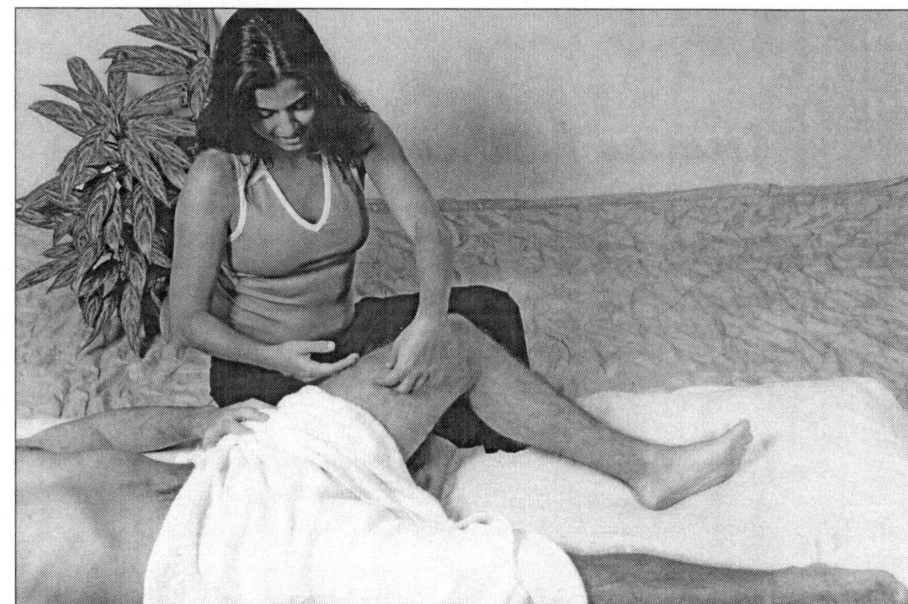

Figure 16-2: Draping your partner's limbs over your body adds to the experience.

Hair gliding

The fine ends of your soft, silky hair can be instruments of exquisite pleasure. Simply let your hair hang down and brush lightly across your partner's skin anywhere on his body while you're giving the massage, as shown in Figure 16-3.

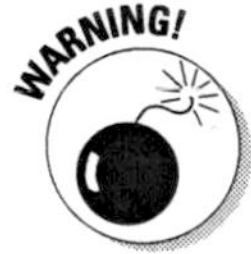

Don't attempt this move if you have a shaved head with just a few days' growth of spiky nubs on it or an extreme Mohawk hairstyle with 12 pounds of gel in it because you can inflict serious damage.

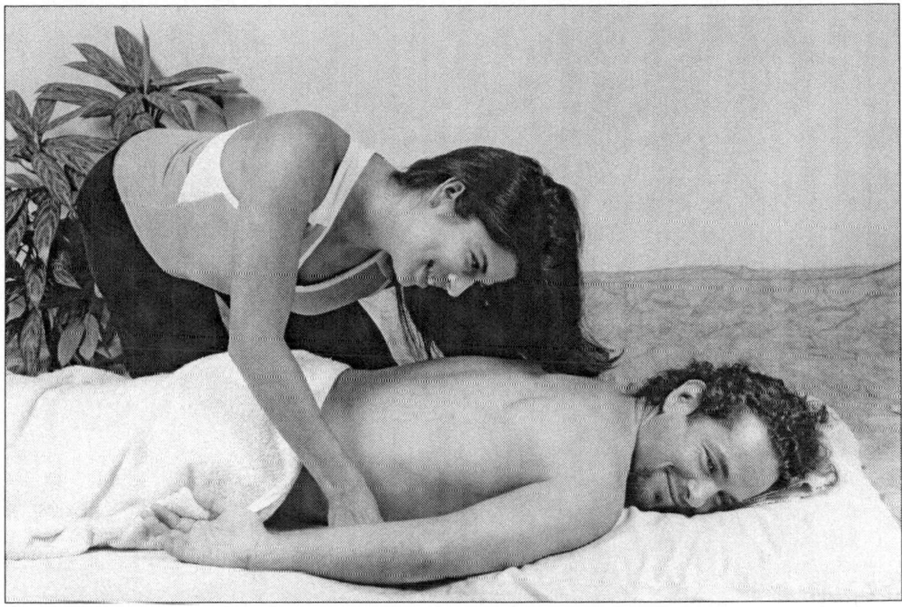

Figure 16-3: In sensual massage, using your hair is part of the fun.

Belly touching

Ever notice how you instinctively cringe and protect your chest and abdomen when danger is present? You do it because the front of the human body is incredibly vulnerable and sensitive. This vulnerability is bad for self-defense from attacking wolverines, but it's great for sensual massage. Simply use a series of light, gliding strokes all up across the abdomen and chest, as shown in Figure 16-4. These moves aren't meant to affect the muscles, as the chest massage moves in Chapter 12 are, but rather just to stimulate the skin (and the mind) of your partner.

The most sensual organ of them all

Simply rubbing your hands and fingers over a person's erogenous zones can be, well, erotic, but it's not the only game in town. If you've been with your partner for a long time, you may want to explore some newer, less obvious zones.

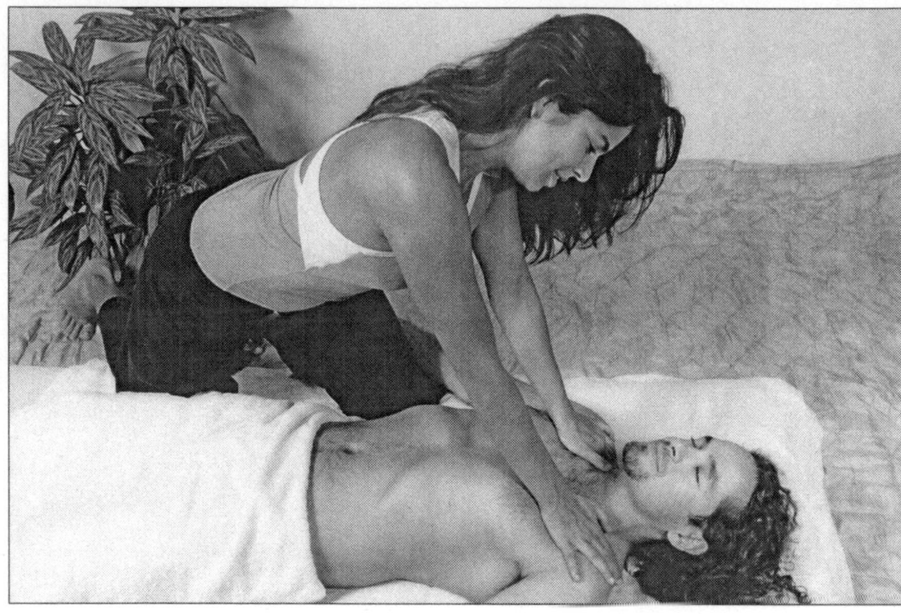

Figure 16-4: The chest and abdomen are perfect for sensual touch.

One particular organ is too often neglected, and it can be the most sensual one of all. On all humans, it's found in the same area. Everybody responds to stimulation there in a different way, though, making seduction and sensuality an endless surprise.

Of course, I'm talking about the brain. If you can get inside your partner's imagination, you can lead him on an infinite number of new erotic experiences without ever leaving the safety of your house. Try it the next time you're sharing a sensual massage together.

Fantasizing is okay

If you find yourself repeatedly imagining that you're receiving your massage from a naked movie star on a beach in Tahiti, don't worry. That's normal. In fact, you may even use the fantasy to make the sensual massage more sensual.

Encourage your partner to share a few juicy morsels from his fantasy life while you're applying these sensual moves. You may be surprised how the combination of your familiar touch and the fantasy of an exotic, unfamiliar situation adds to your experience.

The ultimate aphrodisiac

I once had the pleasure of massaging Dr. Ruth Westheimer, and I'll never forget what she said to me at the end of the massage. Still lying on the table, she glanced up at me with her trademarked mischievous grin, and said, "Don't you want to ask me a question?"

"A question?"

"Yes, you know, about love, or sex?" Her eyes twinkled.

I couldn't pass up the opportunity for some free expert advice, so I asked Dr. Ruth what the most powerful aphrodisiac in the world was. Oysters? Ginseng? Bark from the yohimbe tree in Africa?

"Whatever works for you, works!" said Dr. Ruth, and the phrase has rung true all the years since she spoke it. You and your partner can create the ultimate, personalized sensual massage experience that's right for you. Just remember Dr. Ruth cheering you on from the sidelines, which should put a smile on your face, and then go for it!

Chapter 17

A Massage for Baby (and Mommy Too)

In This Chapter

- Massaging your baby
- Enjoying massage during pregnancy and beyond

Welcome to the chapter that focuses on those super important people — mothers and babies. Without mothers, there would be no babies, and without babies, the human race would become extinct. Perhaps you yourself are a mom or mom-to-be, and you want some specific information about what it takes to feel your best during this special time in your life. Or perhaps you're a mom of grown children who have long since left home but you just plain feel like getting a massage. Well, why not!

This chapter starts with babies first. Babies are extraordinarily sensitive beings, and massage can play a vital role in their early lives. After that, moms and moms-to-be get the focus.

Baby Massage

"Where touching begins, there love and humanity also begin — within the first minutes following birth."

—Ashley Montagu

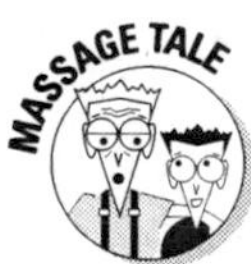

My wife and I were waiting in line at the grocery store one day with our 4-month-old son sitting in his stroller. Suddenly, the woman behind us reached over and started massaging his toes. "Massage is very good for babies," she said, "especially here on the big toe. If he's depressed or angry, this will make him feel better." We were amazed, and it must have shown on our faces, because she looked up at us and smiled reassuringly. "Don't worry," she said, "It really works. I saw it on TV!"

Regardless of how you feel about strangers touching your child's feet in supermarkets, this story does point to the widespread acceptance of baby massage and child massage by people everywhere. Cultures from around the world embrace the concept of baby massage:

- People from India have massaged their babies for centuries.
- Eskimos and people from East Africa have long histories of using baby massage, too.
- In Bali, children have traditionally been held in constant physical contact for the first six months of life, and only then are their feet first allowed to touch the ground.

Touch is part of the fabric of life, from the moment a baby first emerges from the womb into its parents' arms. Unfortunately, the more "civilized" and technologically advanced humans become, the less time they seem to have to touch their babies, and that's why spending some quality time massaging babies is so important.

Why baby loves massage

If you spend a little time around babies, you may start to think to yourself, "Hey, babies are different than normal humans. They seem hyper-sensitive. Every little touch is magnified a hundred times. Is it just me, or do babies feel things differently than we do?"

Babies do indeed feel things more intensely than adults. This discrepancy is caused by an abundance of special touch-sensing organs in the skin called *Meissner's corpuscles*, which are four times more prevalent in children three years old and younger than they are in adults. Babies have 80 Meissner's corpuscles per square millimeter of skin versus 20 per square millimeter for adults and 4 per square millimeter for seniors.

Meissner's corpuscles are especially good at detecting light, fleeting movements across the skin, so this type of movement is especially effective on babies.

Also, researchers at the Touch Research Institute (TRI) in Miami have found that massage can actually help premature infants grow faster and leave the hospital sooner. Touch is a lifesaver for infants, who crave it as deeply as they crave oxygen or light. So, when you add to that the pleasure it provides, it's no wonder babies love massage.

Baby massage tips

One thing about babies: They're really, really small. You can tell how small they are when you try to massage them and one of your hands covers their entire back. Besides, most of the time they're either squirming around like tadpoles or lying fast asleep. So, what techniques are you supposed to use on such tiny, wriggling creatures?

Here are a few pointers to get you started:

- **Choose a time when the baby is tranquil to give the massage, perhaps after a bath, shortly after waking up, or right before bedtime.**
- **Use light touch to stimulate the Meissner's corpuscles in your baby's skin, providing extra pleasure that makes him want to stay in one place longer.** You can read about Meissner's corpuscles in the preceding section.
- **The massage may only last one or two minutes before the baby squirms away, but that's okay.** Just give as much as you can.
- **Don't be afraid to make firm (but not hard) contact.** Babies are more resilient than they look and like a nice, solid, reassuring touch. If you use only very light, tickling touch, the baby misses some of the benefits of massage.

Baby massage routine

The following moves are easy to do, as you can see from the figures in this section. The hardest part is probably getting your baby to sit still for them.

1. **With the baby lying face up, run your fingertips lightly up over his abdomen, chest, and face and then bring them back down again as shown in Figure 17-1.**

   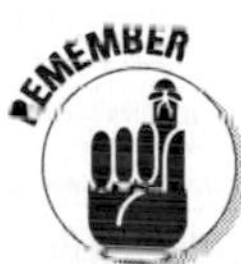

   This move is just to stimulate the Meissner's corpuscles (covered earlier in the chapter), so it doesn't need to be firm at all. You can add some extra fun and effectiveness to this move by saying "Whoooosh!" as you bring your fingers up over the baby's body. After a little practice, your baby begins to anticipate this deliciously pleasurable move and smile when you approach him with outstretched fingers.

2. **With your hands on the baby's sides, sweep your thumbs up over his abdomen, moving them outwards, and then lightly brush them back over the skin and repeat four to five times.**

   This calming stroke is good for the internal organs. ***Note:*** This move (shown in Figure 17-2) requires relatively firm pressure, and you may need some oil or lotion as well.

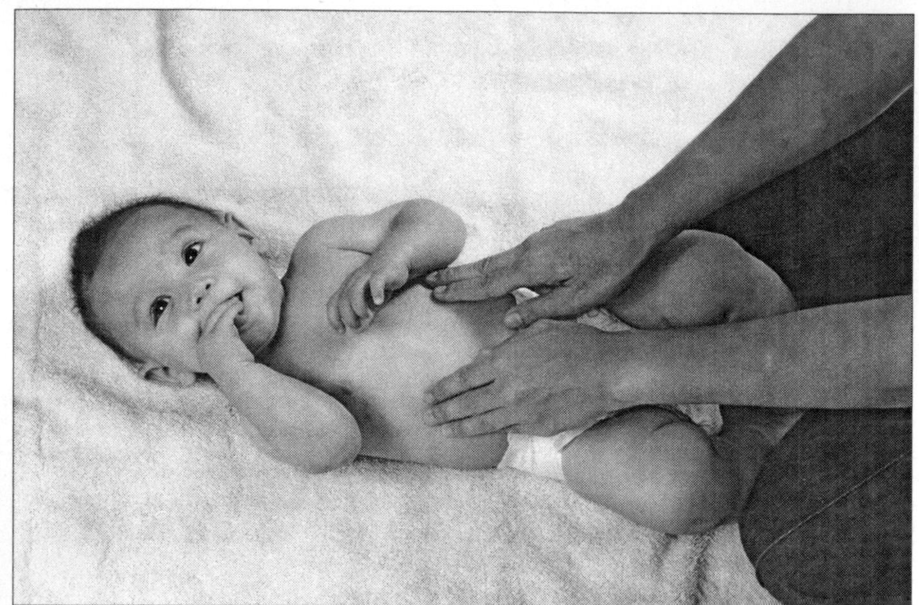

Figure 17-1: Fingertip brushing for baby.

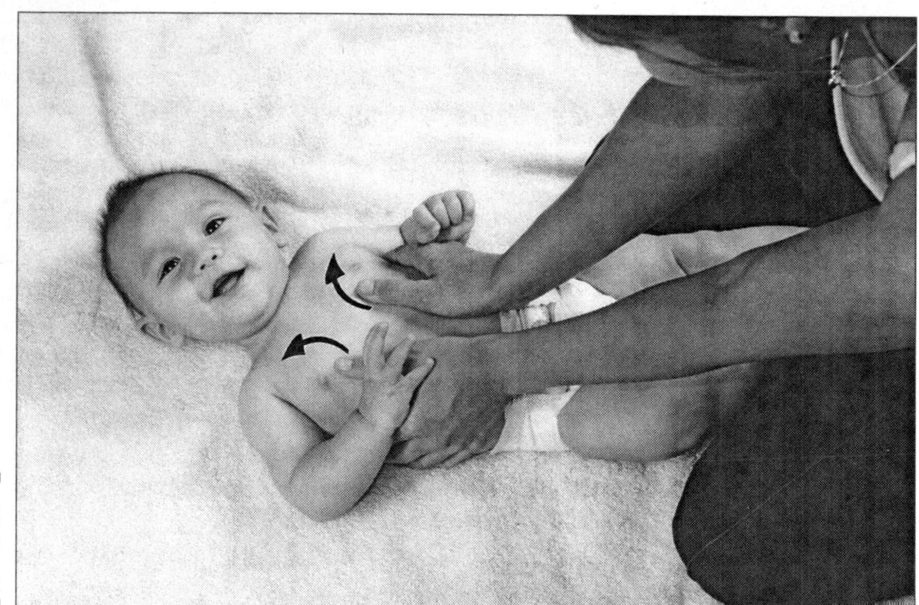

Figure 17-2: The baby belly rub.

3. **Help your baby stretch his legs by grasping his lower leg, pushing his knee up toward his chest, and then gently stretching the leg out straight toward you (see Figure 17-3).**

   Repeat this move three to four times. Support his opposite hip with your other hand to keep him steady while you do the move. Babies naturally love to stretch, just like dogs and cats, so this move feels especially good.

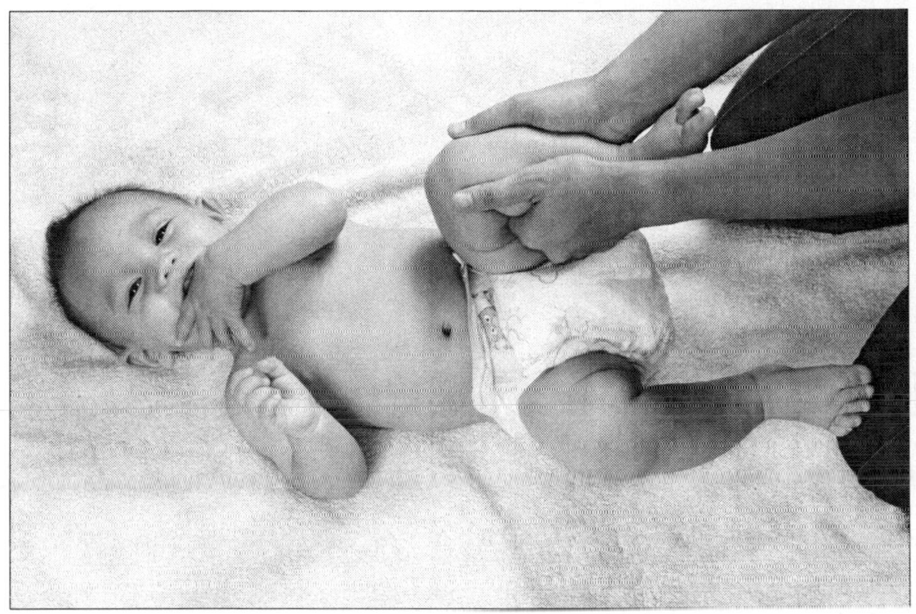

Figure 17-3: Baby leg stretches.

4. **If you can get him to sit still long enough, you can apply a light (and very quick) version of the reflexology moves from Chapter 13 to your baby's feet.**

   Babies are born with a complete set of reflexology points on their feet, and, in general, they love to have them stimulated, especially those little toes (see Figure 17-4).

5. **Using your thumbs, make little circles with moderate pressure into the fleshy area of baby's little tush as shown in Figure 17-5.**

   He may try to squirm away from you while you're doing this move, but you may catch him smiling as he does so. This move feels great.

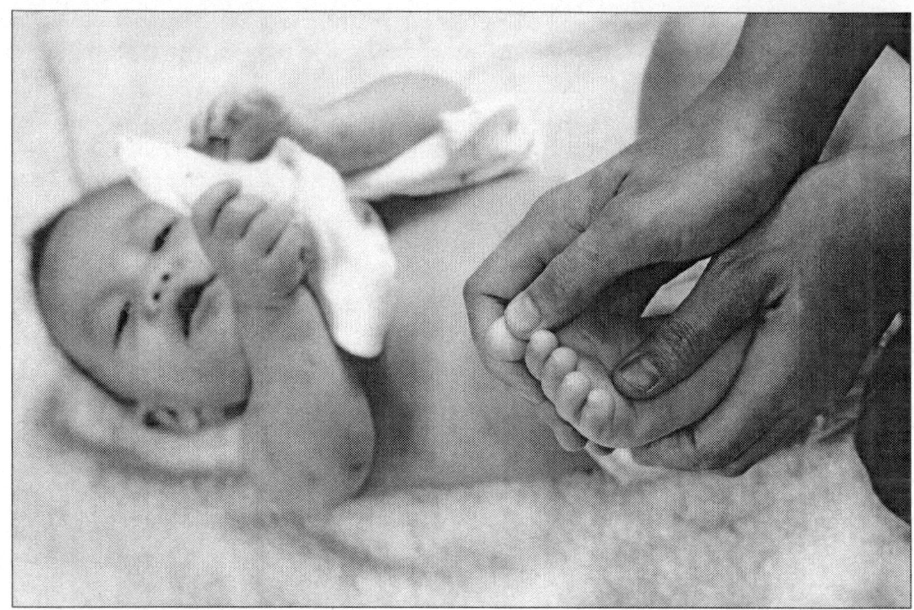

Figure 17-4: Baby reflexology.

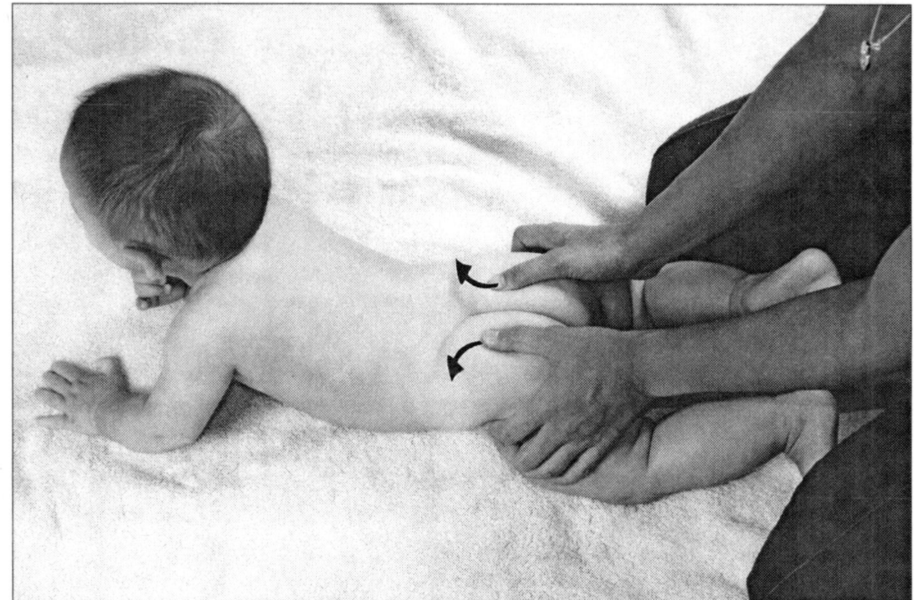

Figure 17-5: Baby tush massage.

6. **Apply an itty-bitty version of kneading (see Chapter 10) to the baby's chubby little thighs as Figure 17-6 illustrates.**

   Babies appreciate a little attention to these muscles, especially as they become more active and stand on their legs longer.

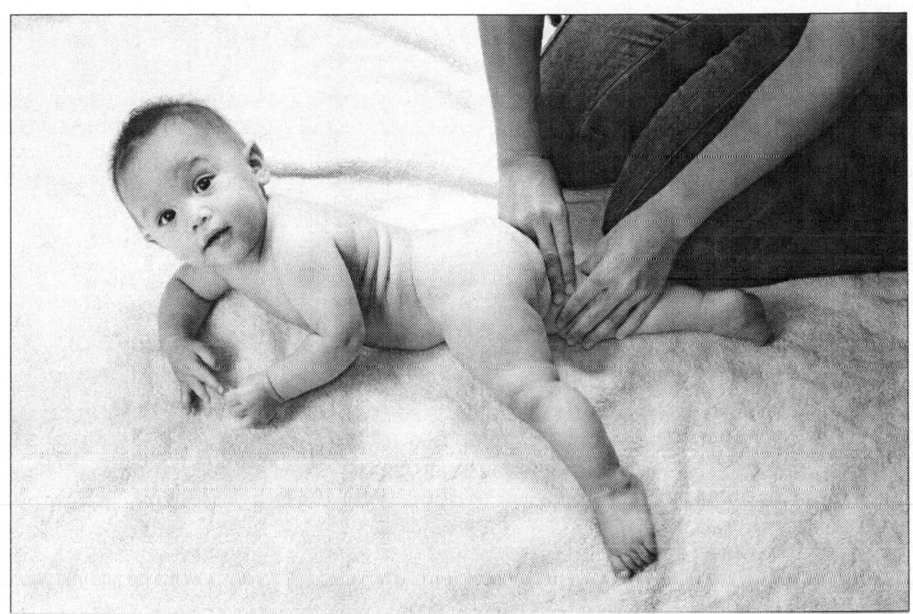

Figure 17-6: Kneading baby's thighs.

Baby massage training

Babies don't need any special training to begin enjoying massage, but mommies and daddies can certainly benefit by learning a few tips from baby massage experts. Check out *Baby Massage For Dummies* by Joanne Bagshaw and Ilene Fox (Wiley) for more information on baby massage. Some good videos are also available on the subject, and you can find classes in many areas for parents, foster parents, grandparents, and anyone else interested. The massage techniques taught aren't just for newborns either. Toddlers enjoy massage, too.

If you really get into it, you can become a certified baby massage instructor yourself. Some good training programs in the U.S. are offered by a woman named Vimala Schneider McClure, who experienced baby massage first-hand in India and brought it back to the U.S. She founded the International Association of Infant Massage, which now has thousands of members in 38 countries, and she wrote *Infant Massage: A Handbook for Loving Parents,* (Bantam Doubleday Dell Publishing Company).

If you're interested in baby massage, contact the International Association of Infant Massage at Heidenstams Gata 9, S-422 47 Hisings Backa, Sweden; Web site `www.iaim.net`; phone 46 (0)31-528980.

Massage for Pregnancy and More

Massage can be enjoyed equally by men and women, of course, but women definitely receive a little something extra from the experience under certain circumstances. I'm talking about specifically female conditions:

- Pregnancy
- Postpartum
- PMS
- Menopause

When a woman receives a massage during any of these times in her life, it benefits not only her but also all the people she lives with as well. Who are the women closest to you? Usually they're related to you in one way or another. Mothers come to mind right away, for example. Massage is one of the best things you can do for your mother, whether it comes directly from your hands or as a gift. Wives and girlfriends deserve special massage attention, too, because they have the ability to instantaneously cut off a man's supply of something that he loves very much indeed — his happiness.

If a lot more women received a lot more massage, there would be a lot less strife in a lot of families. Think about it.

Massaging mommy-to-be

If you're living with a pregnant woman, you can't do too many things for her that would make her happier than a nice massage. In fact, she'll absolutely love you for even offering.

Some women blend the lines between working as a massage therapist and a childbirth assistant. In many countries, women calling themselves *doulas* go through the process of labor with a woman, offering encouragement, support, and often touch. If you want more information or are interested in becoming a doula or childbirth assistant yourself, contact The Organization of Labor Assistants for Birth Options and Resources (toLabor) at `www.tolabor.com`. You can also try the International Birth and Wellness Project at 877-334-4297 or `www.alace.org`.

Labor day massage

I was once asked by a client to accompany her into the labor room and assist with some massage during delivery. It sounded like a good idea, so I read up on the subject and consulted with several experienced colleagues. When the big day came, however, things didn't turn out exactly the way we all expected.

A few minutes after arrival in the hospital birthing suite, I reached down to massage my client's feet between her rather powerful contractions.

"Don't you touch me!" screamed my normally demure client in a voice that reminded me of Linda Blair in *The Exorcist*.

Perhaps I was the wrong gender. For centuries, women have stuck together at the crucial time of labor, offering each other the support and understanding that only they know how to give. A man, even with the best of intentions, often just can't seem to get the touch right at moments like that.

About half an hour later, standing a respectful few feet away, I watched with amazement as my client's daughter made her appearance in the world. The massage could wait for another day.

Pregnancy massage pointers

Giving massage to a pregnant woman is perfectly safe, but keep a few points in mind for safety's sake:

- A pregnant woman should not lie facedown on her abdomen but rather faceup or on her side unless you're using a special table with big holes in the center (so she can lie down on her stomach) made especially for that purpose.
- After the first trimester of pregnancy, she should not lie face down or faceup, but only on her side, because the extra weight of the fetus can put pressure on the major blood vessels of her torso and cut off circulation when she's on her back.
- Make sure that she's comfortably supported at all times, using pillows and other cushions beneath her legs and head.
- Use only very light and soothing touch directly on the abdominal area.

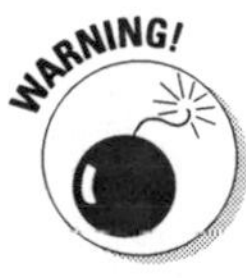

- Stay away from the reflexology points near the heel that correspond to the reproductive organs because they're supposed to help induce labor. Refer to Chapter 13 for the location of these points.

With these guidelines in mind, you can confidently offer massage to your favorite pregnant person. A high percentage of pregnant women report back pain, sciatic pain, leg cramps, swelling of the ankles, and other problems that massage can help ease. So, she will definitely appreciate your efforts.

To find out more, a good book on the subject is *Mother Massage: A Handbook for Relieving the Discomforts of Pregnancy* by Elaine Stillerman (Delta Books).

Pregnancy massage techniques

Here are a few techniques for massaging your favorite pregnant person. First, make extra sure to follow the guidelines in the preceding section. You need to treat expectant mothers with extra caution when dealing with massage. If you're at all nervous about touching your pregnant massage partner, skip it altogether. But if you feel confident that you can follow these few easy steps to offer some safe and much-appreciated massage during this special time, by all means go right ahead.

After you make sure mama's comfortable, follow these steps:

1. **A great way to massage the back, at any stage of pregnancy, is to position the woman on her side, facing away from you, with a pillow between her knees and another supporting her chest and upper body, as shown in Figure 17-7; apply stroking and kneading as in the regular massages you can follow in Chapters 11 and 12.**

   Pay special attention to the lower back during this technique because that's where many pregnant women report having the most discomfort. This discomfort is due to the extra weight in the torso tipping the pelvis forward. Just remember to be gentle and to keep communicating with your partner.

2. **Place your partner in a side-lying position and knead the calves and upper legs (see Figure 17-8), which are also working harder during pregnancy.**

   You can move all up and down the legs in this position, but it's a little trickier to maneuver with a side-lying partner. You can have mommy roll slightly forward and then slightly back in order to make more of her calves, thighs, and hamstrings available for massage. Kneading is the best move to use here.

3. **With mom thoroughly propped up on pillows behind her back and under her knees, apply some delicious foot massage movements like the ones in Chapter 13, being careful to avoid particular reflexology points as mentioned earlier; this move is shown in Figure 17-9.**

4. **Use some kneading into the tops of the shoulders, as shown in Figure 17-10.**

   With all that thinking moms-to-be do about their soon-to-arrive off-spring, the tension is bound to build up around the neck and shoulders. Use the kneading and pressure point techniques you learned in earlier chapters to massage this area.

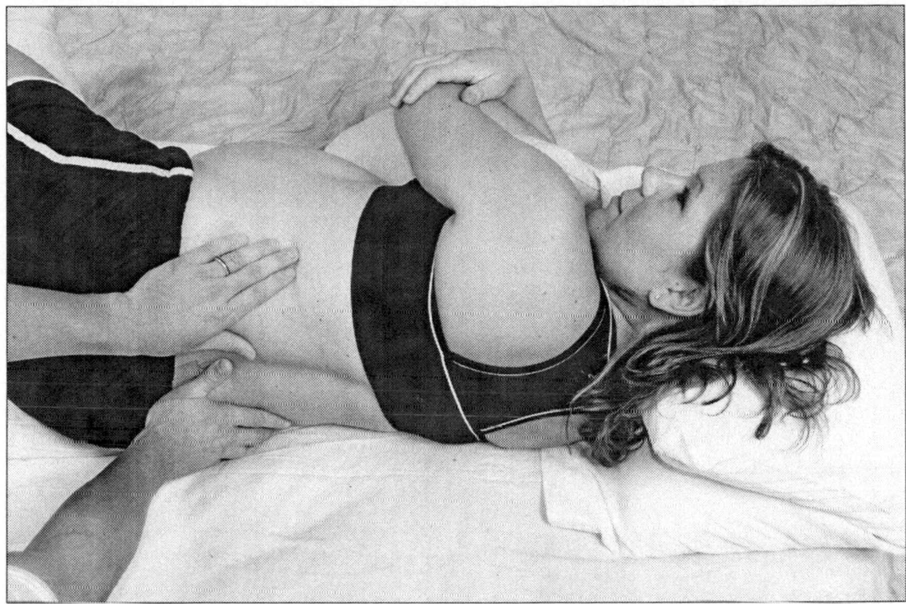

Figure 17-7: Back massage for Mommy.

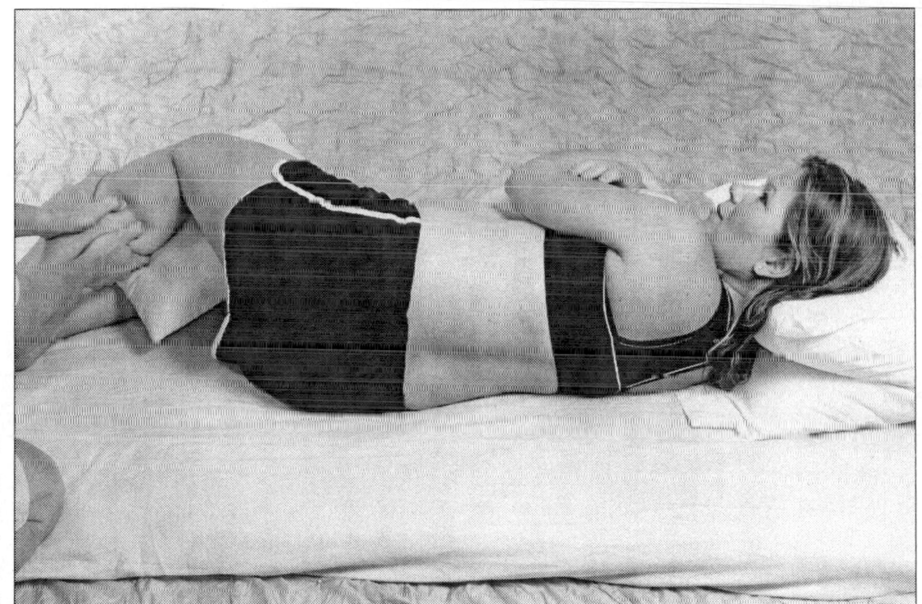

Figure 17-8: Leg massage for Mommy.

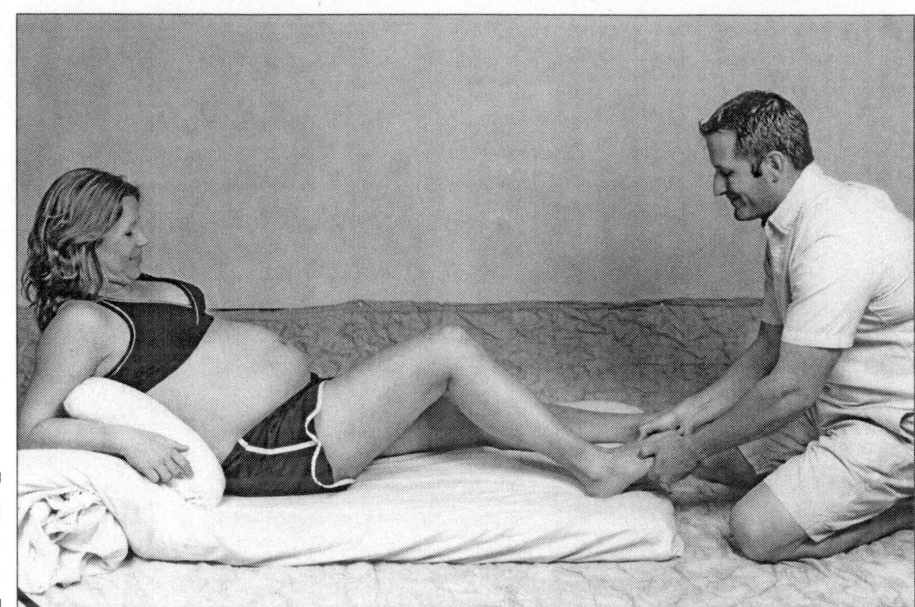

Figure 17-9: Mom-to-be reflexology.

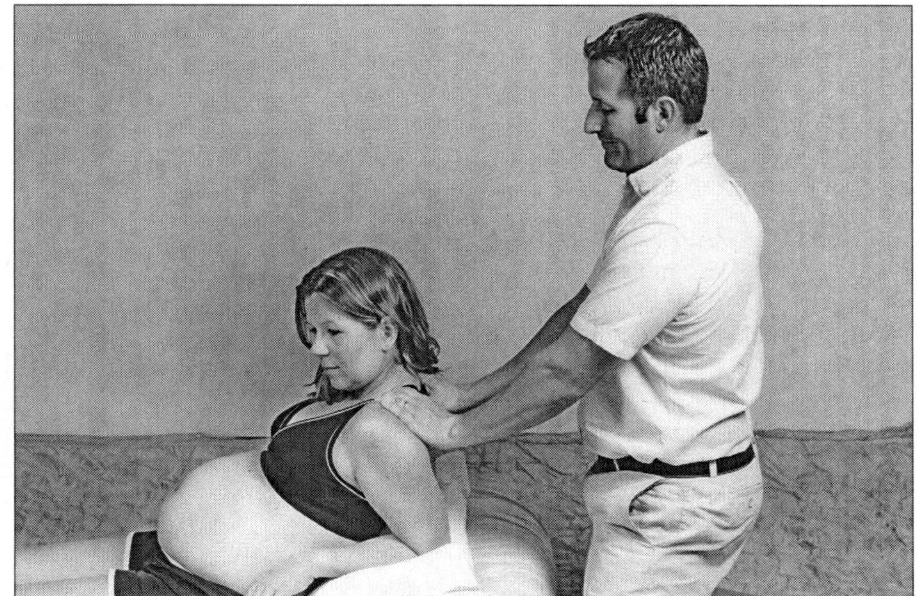

Figure 17-10: Shoulder kneading during pregnancy.

Massage beats the postpartum blues

Women sometimes report feeling a little down after giving birth. This (very common) experience can be a mild case of the "baby blues" to an intense bout of postpartum depression, which, according to Mayo Clinic experts, occurs in approximately 10 percent of women after their babies are born. The causes for this condition vary widely, sometimes stemming from the physical changes that take place in a new mom, such as a drop in estrogen and other important hormones, plus all those other obvious bodily changes. Emotional factors can also come into play, especially in overwhelmed sleep-deprived women faced with all the stress of a whole new person that needs to be taken care of 24/7 for the next 18 years. Of course, it doesn't help if hubby isn't there in full-support mode the way he ideally should be.

What can be done? Can massage help? Well, as a matter of fact, yes it can. Of course, receiving a massage can help bring a smile back onto a new mom's face, but it can be equally as therapeutic for moms to massage their babies. Sometimes moms can literally get out of touch with their newborns, especially if the little ones are experiencing any health issues. Massage puts mother and child back in touch. Massaged babies have been shown to grow stronger and develop more quickly, too.

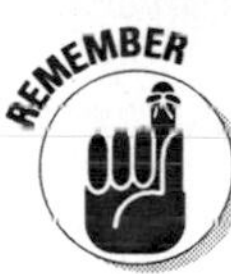

Keep mom propped up sufficiently during all massage moves. If she's ever uncomfortable, discontinue the massage and let her rest.

PMS (please massage soon)

Few people realize that the real words behind the acronym PMS are "please massage soon." The phrase was coined back in the 1970s when some men started noticing that their wives or girlfriends periodically seemed to need an especially large share of love and attention. Massage was the perfect answer, and so many a man offered his sweetie some tender touch at those times when she seemed to need it the most.

If your honey comes to you looking stressed-out or on the verge or tears for no apparent reason and asks you for a massage, don't ask any stupid questions. Just start massaging. Immediately.

Meno-possiblities

All kinds of crazy things start happening with a woman's hormones about the time she's going through menopause. Many of these things have an effect on the way she looks and the way she feels.

Massage can help create continued possibilities for health, good looks, and pleasure as a woman enters this stage of life. Massage is extremely beneficial at this time because the increased circulation and the actions of the oils and creams used are good for the delicate collagen and elastin fibers that are beginning to break down, causing wrinkles. You're not going to rub away the wrinkles, but you can definitely add a healthy glow to gracefully maturing skin. The emotional reassurance and comfort given through caring touch do a lot to renew a woman's balance, too.

The face treatment and the full day of spa pleasures I outline in Chapter 7 are sure to be appreciated by menopausal women in addition to massage.

Chapter 18

Self-Massage Techniques to Use at Work

In This Chapter

- Utilizing self-massage
- Trying out some self-massage moves at work

You're not always going to be able to convince somebody else to give you a massage, especially when you're on the job. Like it or not, at times you're sore, achy, tired, emotionally needy, and just plain crying out for a massage, but the people around you are much more interested in office gossip or in going to lunch.

Don't despair. You can use some simple massage techniques on yourself without the need for anyone else's participation — or sympathy. With the moves you find here, you can move straight into a ten-minute mini-routine right at your desk. You can do this on a sofa or a stool just as easily as you can on your desk chair. In fact, you can do these moves anywhere you can sit down, although you may look a little funny massaging your own feet on a city bus.

Even though these moves work equally as well in many places, I'm including them here in the massage-at-work chapter because that's where so many people end up all stressed-out with no outlets to relax. Sure, you can stand up in your cubicle and sing the Frank Sinatra line "I did it *my* way" to take a slight edge off the tension, but wouldn't quietly engaging in a few self-massage techniques be easier — and a little more discreet?

Some of these moves not only feel good but can also actually make quite a difference in your productivity level, which should make your boss happy, too. Happy, relaxed workers can save their employers some expensive worker's comp bills in the long run, so if any supervisors begin questioning your self-massage habits, tell them it's all for the greater good of the enterprise.

Self-massage: The basics

Say you're sitting at your desk. Your neck is killing you, but you don't want to ask a co-worker to massage it because the other people in your office may get nervous, jealous, or both. What're you gonna do? Well, sitting right there in your chair, you can give yourself an entire mini-massage, get some good relief, and be relatively discreet.

Here are the basic rules for self-massage:

- **Keep breathing:** This rule holds true whether you're massaging a partner or yourself.
- **Focus on the sore spots you find and be willing to experience a little "pleasurable pain":** At the same time, don't overdo it — self-inflicted black-and-blue marks are hard to explain to co-workers.
- **Be intuitive:** Nobody knows better than you where that tight spot is. Use the techniques in this chapter as a template; follow your own inner guidance.

So, limber up those fingers (use the massage-muscle building tips from Chapter 9 if you want) and get ready for a treatment from one of the most talented and reliable massage masters around — you.

When you finish self-massage, take a couple of deep, relaxing breaths before you dive into whatever activity you have lined up next. And you may want to wash or sanitize your hands afterward, too, especially if you apply a little self-foot massage (see the "Foot Rub" section later in the chapter).

Irrigating Your Head

One of the biggest causes of all of your problems, whether you know it or not, is a nonirrigated head. Think about it. All day long you're walking, standing, or sitting, and your head is the highest point on your body. Your heart has to pump the blood against gravity to supply your brain, which can leave you feeling foggy-headed at times. Have you ever experienced that in the middle of a long day at work? Why not help your brain stay sharp by irrigating it with extra oxygen-rich blood?

A great way to start any self-massage is to simply lean forward in your chair, getting your head somewhere in the vicinity of your knees. Keep your feet flat on the ground and clasp your hands behind your back, as shown in Figure 18-1. If you feel limber enough, raise your hands up toward the ceiling for a nice stretch.

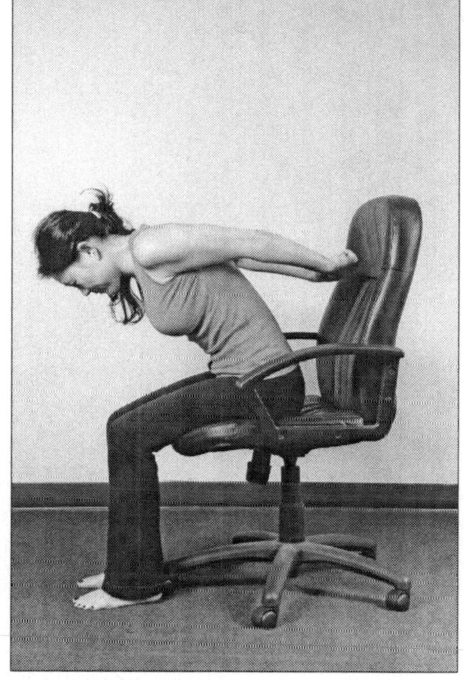

Figure 18-1: Lean forward in your chair and bring some fresh blood to your brain.

Stretching Your Arms and Upper Back

For a good self-massage warm-up, sit upright, reach across your body with one arm, and grasp it at the elbow with the opposite hand. Pull the elbow in against your chest (see Figure 18-2), which should create a stretching sensation across your shoulder. If you don't feel a stretching sensation, you're either super limber or you're not pulling on your elbow firmly enough. Repeat with the other arm.

Then reach around to the back of your neck, grasp your elbow once again behind your head, and pull to the opposite side (as shown in Figure 18-3), which stretches your upper arm and further opens your shoulder joint. For an extra stretch, bend your body toward the side you're pulling with at the same time. Repeat with the other arm.

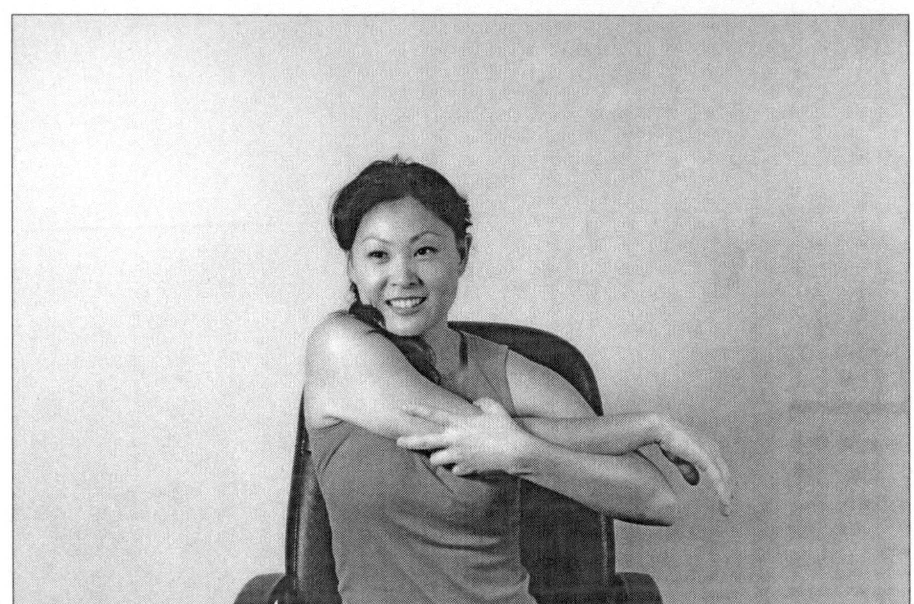

Figure 18-2: Stretch your arm.

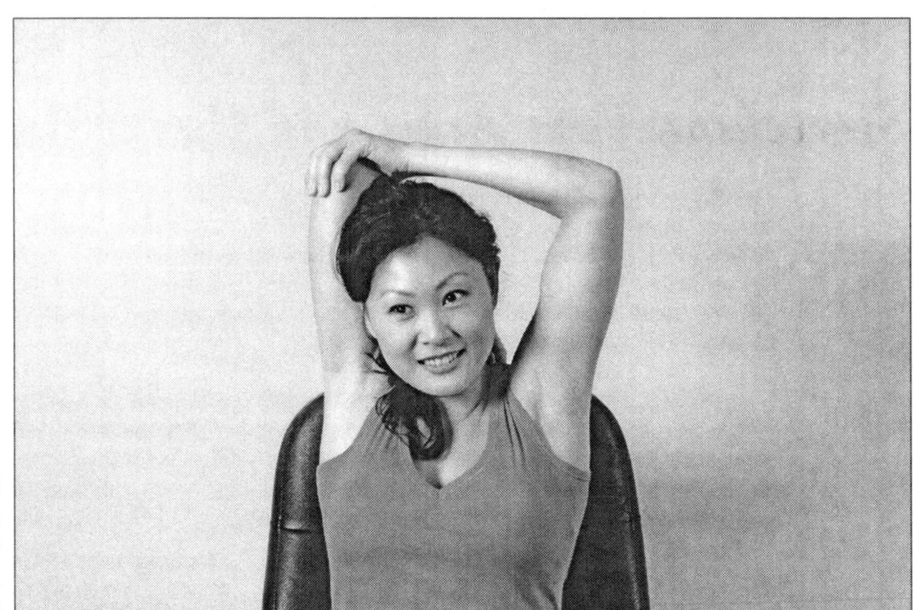

Figure 18-3: Stretch your upper back.

Using Scalp Circles

Place your fingertips firmly against your scalp and make little circles while pressing down, as in Figure 18-4. Make sure your fingers don't slip across your hair but rather remain firmly pressed against your scalp as you move the skin and thin muscles below. Then, after a few seconds, lift your fingers and repeat the circles on another spot on your scalp, being careful not to totally mess up your hair so that you look ridiculous afterwards and your co-workers think you've gone Einstein on them.

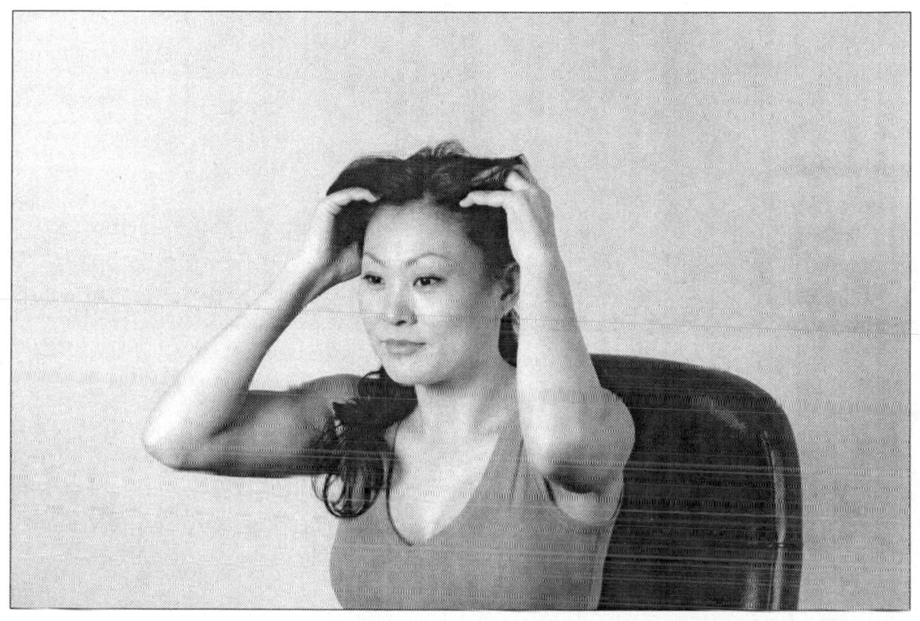

Figure 18-4: Self-scalp massage feels really good.

Massaging Your Temples, Face, and Jaw

This move is a good way to combat tension headaches. Just follow these steps:

1. **Reach up and apply circular rubbing — see Chapter 10 — to your temples, as Figure 18-5 shows.**

   Make your circles slow, deliberate, and firm, staying in contact with one area on the skin while you move over the bones below.

2. **Sliding your fingers up onto your forehead, continue the circular rubbing until your fingers meet in the middle above your nose (see Figure 18-6); push in with your fingertips and glide back toward your temples again, keeping firm pressure against the skin the whole time.**

Repeat two more times.

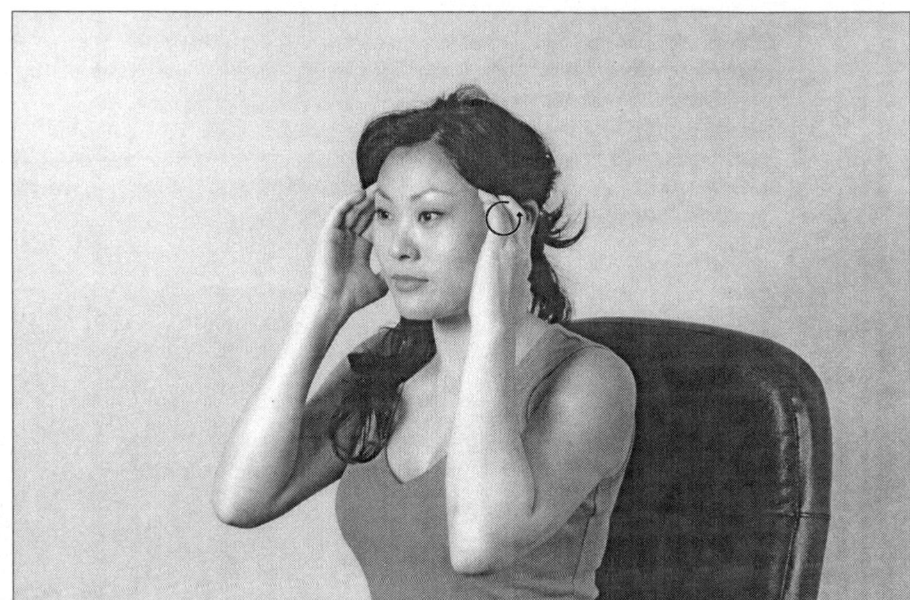

Figure 18-5: Rubbing your temples.

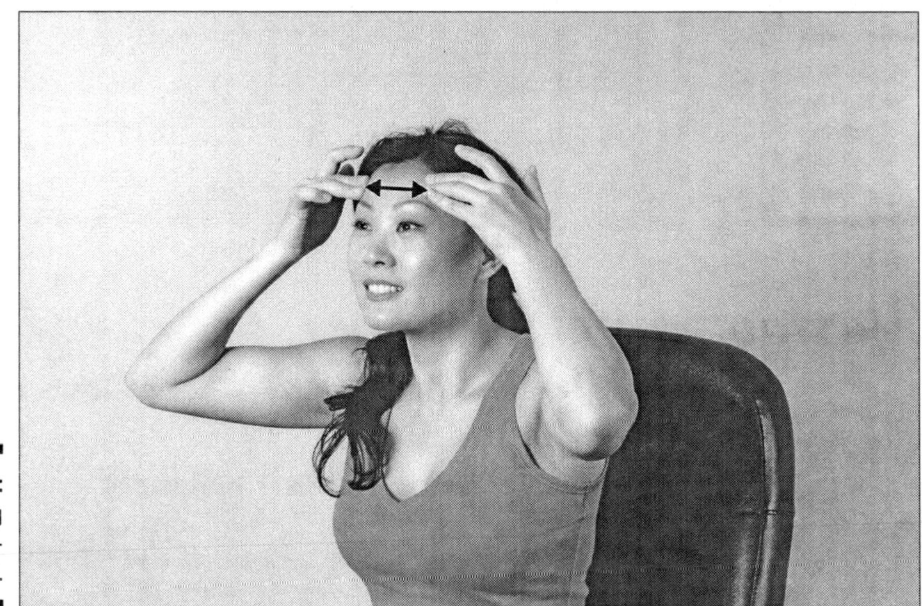

Figure 18-6: Rubbing your forehead.

3. **Press in your fingertips at the angle of your jaw while opening and closing your mouth slightly to find the exact point that feels like it's holding the most tension; apply slow, deep circular rubbing to that spot, plus a little pinpoint pressure (both described in Chapter 10), until you feel your jaw start to relax and drop (as Figure 18-7 illustrates).**

   You may be surprised at how much tension gets lodged in your jaw muscles. Tension hides out there like an enemy soldier wearing camouflage gear, especially while you're sitting at your desk, straining forward to concentrate on the computer screen. With the proper pressure and sensitivity, you can flush this tension out.

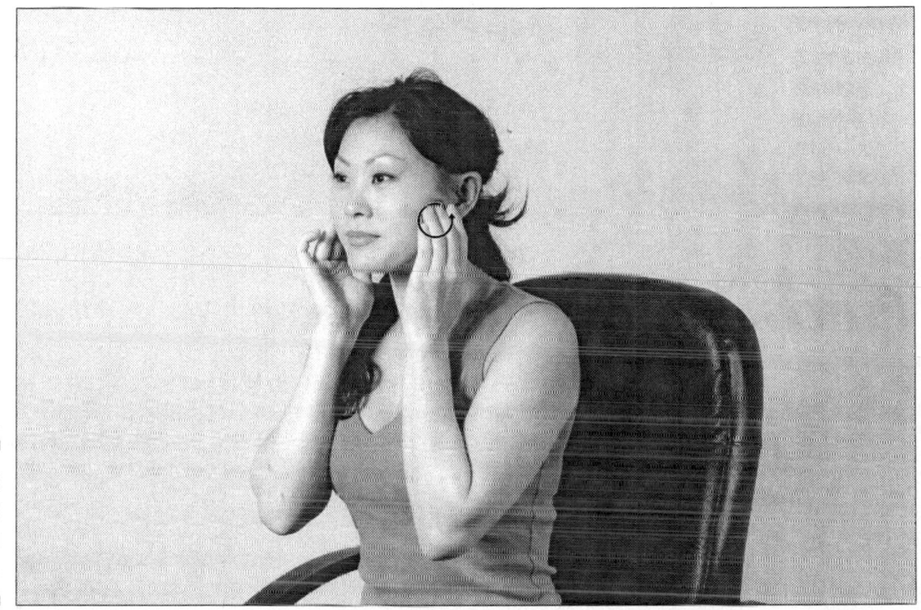

Figure 18-7: Releasing tension in your jaw.

Use enough pressure with these moves to sink your fingers into the jaw muscles slightly but not so much that you feel pain. Be careful; the jaw is a sensitive area.

4. **Hook your thumbs in to press up against the bone just beneath your eyebrow, right next to your nose, as shown in Figure 18-8 and hold the pressure for about five seconds.**

   This spot is another good headache point.

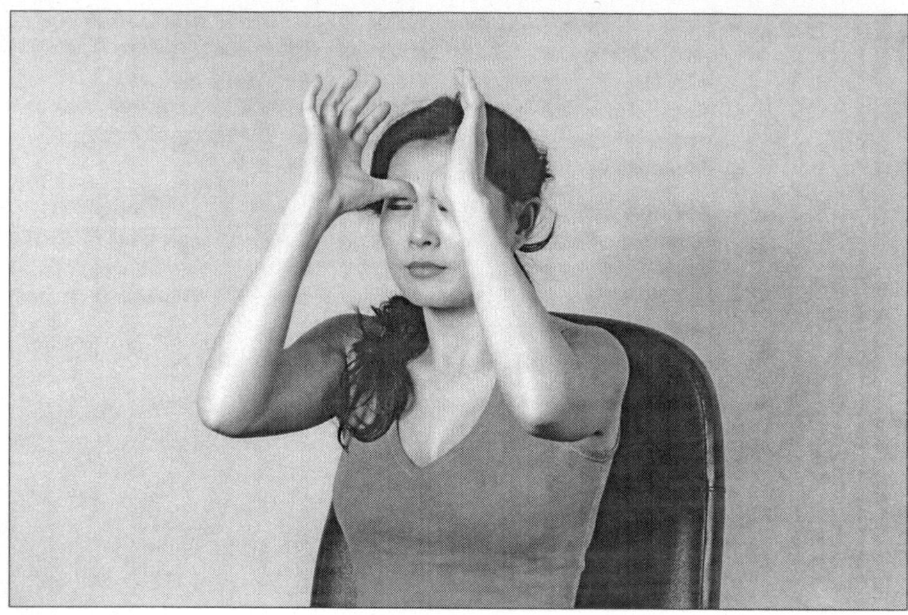

Figure 18-8: Hooking your thumbs to relieve headaches.

Practicing Ear Reflexology

According to the zone theory, each point on the bottom of your foot reflects areas in other parts of your body, as I discuss in Chapter 13. Did you know that your ears also reflect every other part of the body? The Chinese even have an extensive system of treating many disorders with pressure on the ears.

You can give your whole body a boost by simply rubbing your ears with a vigorous little kneading movement between your thumb and first two fingers, as in Figure 18-9. Start at the lobe below and walk your fingers up around the outside to the top of the ear, giving little tugs outward as you go. Even if it does nothing for the rest of your body, it makes your ears feel great.

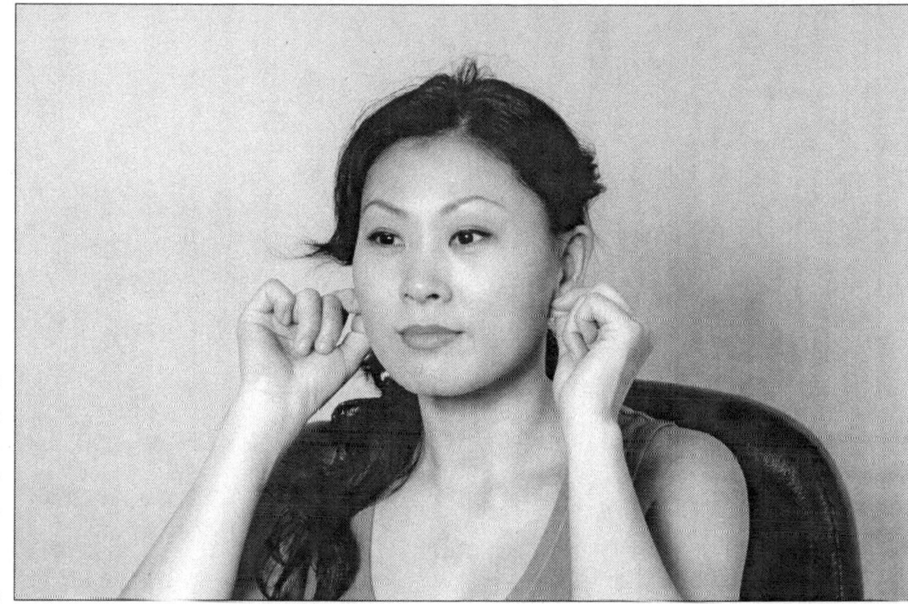

Figure 18-9: Ear reflexology consists of kneading and gentle tugging.

Rubbing That Neck

Who couldn't use a little neck relief after sitting at a computer or cradling a phone all day? Check out the following steps to send that pain in the neck on a little vacation. (Well, your literal pain in the neck, anyway — not much you can do about Bob in the next cubicle.)

1. **Reach around to the back of your neck with both hands and hook your thumbs up under the base of the skull (see Figure 18-10); press in firmly and hold for five to ten seconds.**

   This move alone should leave you feeling more alert and relaxed.

2. **Drop your head forward and pick a hand (probably your dominant one) to knead on the back of your neck as you see in Figure 18-11.**

   Check out Chapter 10 for more on kneading. Squeeze from the base of your neck up to your head and then back down again. Repeat twice.

3. **Turn your head to the left and reach across with your left hand to knead atop your right shoulder and up onto your neck, using your thumb to press into any knots you find along the way (see Figure 18-12).**

   This move also provides a good stretch for your neck. Repeat on the opposite side.

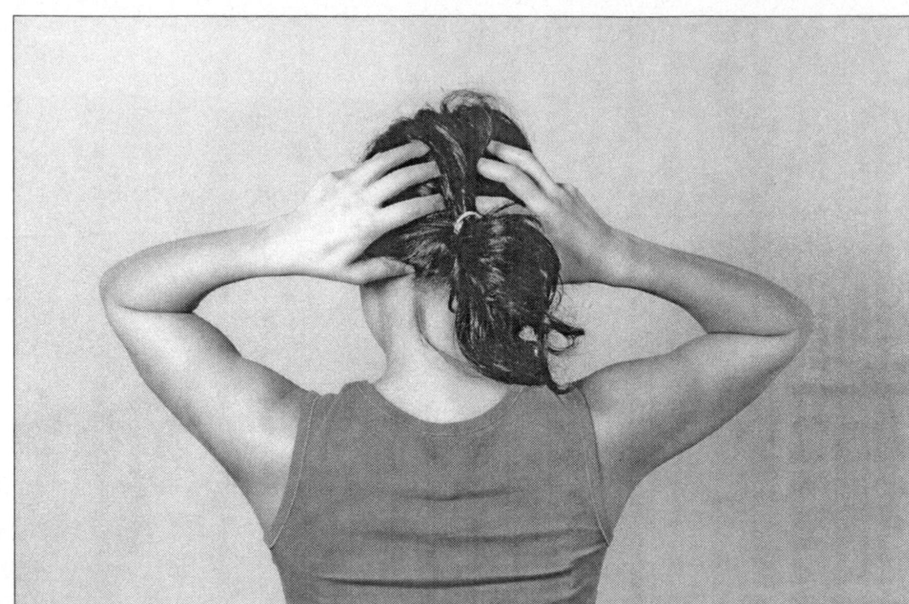

Figure 18-10: Pressing on the base of your skull.

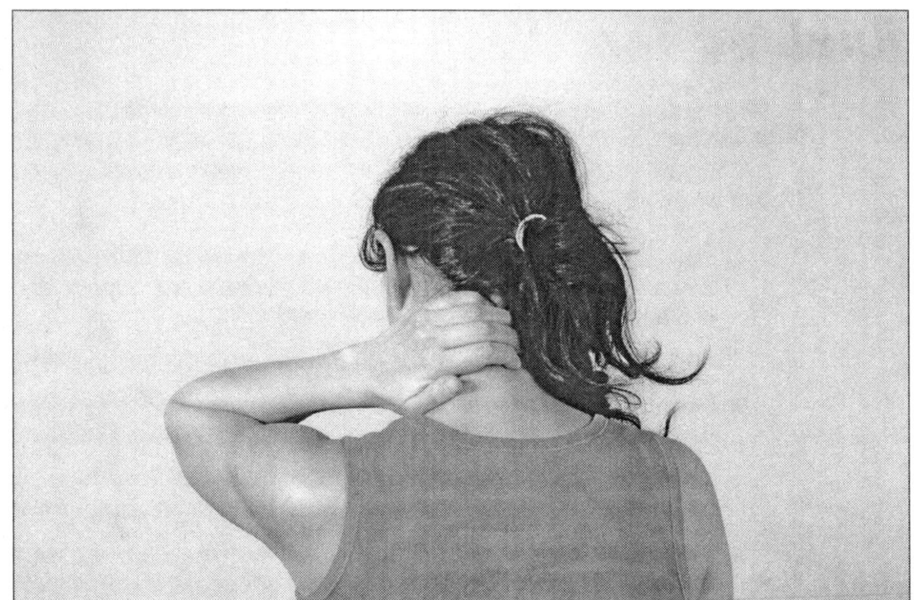

Figure 18-11: Kneading your neck.

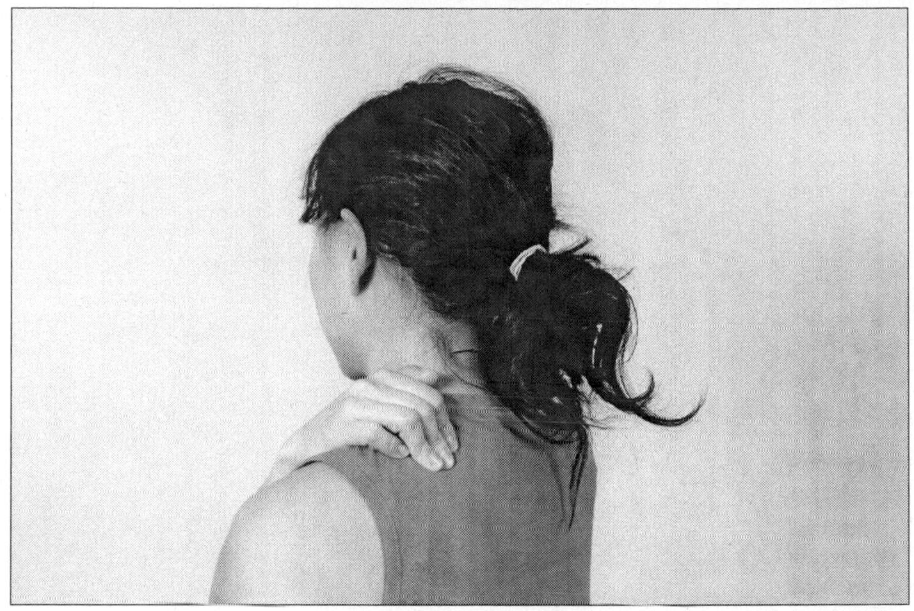

Figure 18-12: Kneading your shoulder.

Squeezing Your Arms and Hands

Follow these steps to give your sore arms, wrists, and hands a quick massage:

1. **Starting at your shoulder, begin squeezing down your arm as shown in Figure 18-13, hooking your thumb in any tender spots and holding it for a moment; stop when you reach your wrist, glide lightly back up to your shoulder, and repeat one more time.**

   Repeat on the opposite arm.

2. **Pinch the webbing between the thumb and forefinger on your opposite hand (see Figure 18-14) and hold for five to seven seconds.**

   This spot may be quite sensitive, and it has been known to sometimes help relieve headaches. You can also do some palm kneading, wrist rubbing, and any of the other moves featured in the hand massage section of Chapter 12 — modified, of course, to be performed by one hand on yourself.

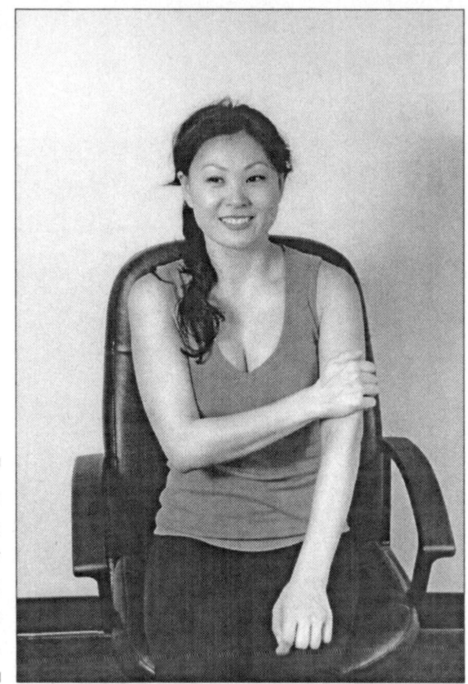

Figure 18-13: Squeeze down your arm from shoulder to wrist.

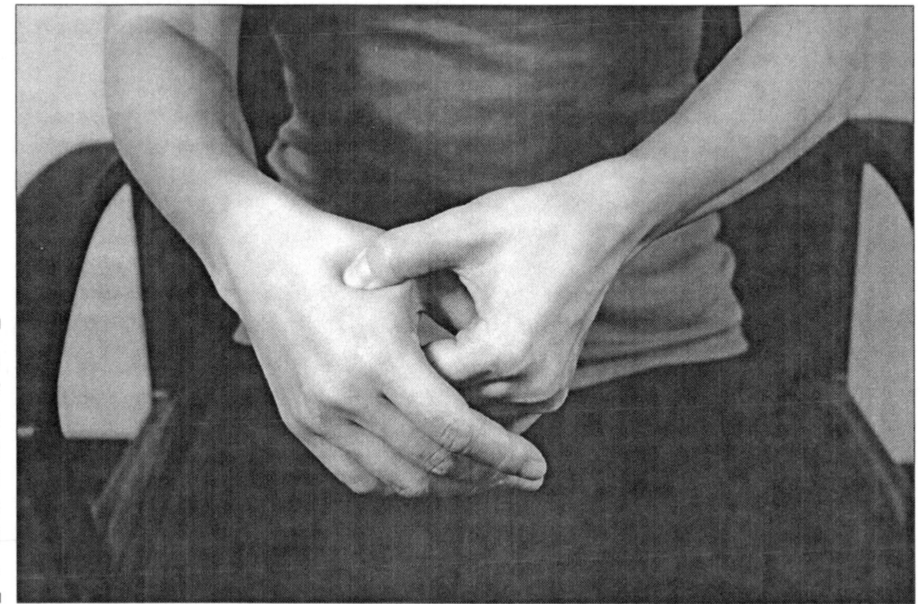

Figure 18-14: Press firmly into the webbing between your thumb and forefinger.

Massaging Your Lower Back

Scoot forward to the front of your chair and reach around to your lower back. Using your thumbs, press into several points along the muscles beside your spine (see Figure 18-15) and then lift and press onto the base of your spine (the *sacrum*) itself, hitting several more points. You can also use your knuckles quite effectively in this area by balling your hand into a fist and rolling it over the area.

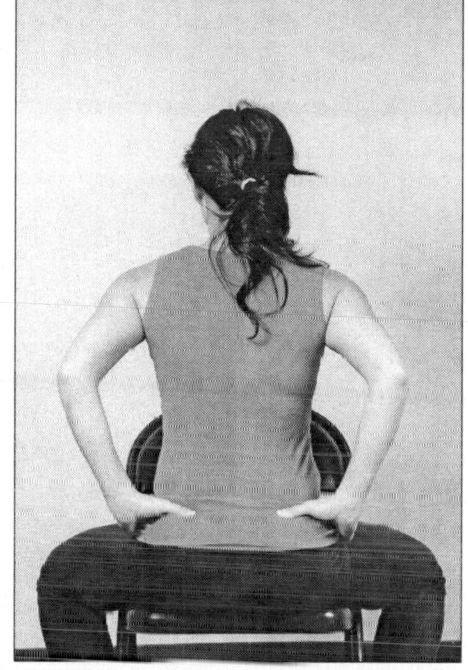

Figure 18-15: Reach around to your lowor back, pressing in with your thumbs and knuckles.

Squeezing Your Legs

Bring one foot up onto your knee and use both hands to squeeze down all the way from your upper thigh across your knee and to your ankle, pressing in with your thumbs along an imaginary line down the inside of your leg. (Check out Figure 18-16.)

Why massaging yourself feels different

You may notice that even when you apply self-massage techniques with an incredible amount of verve and enthusiasm, they still don't feel quite as good as when somebody else applies the very same moves on the very same parts of your body. But why?

The reason is simple. Massage, like tickling (you can't do that very well to yourself either), is a social interaction. Studies (yes, actual tickle studies by serious researchers) have shown that preschool children couldn't be tickled when they were in a bad mood or by someone they didn't like. They were poked in the ribs and brushed on their feet, but the reaction was completely negative. Tickling is as much about relationship and context as it is about contact. And so is massage. A large part of the enjoyment of a massage is the social interaction with another person, which actually causes the sensations to feel different.

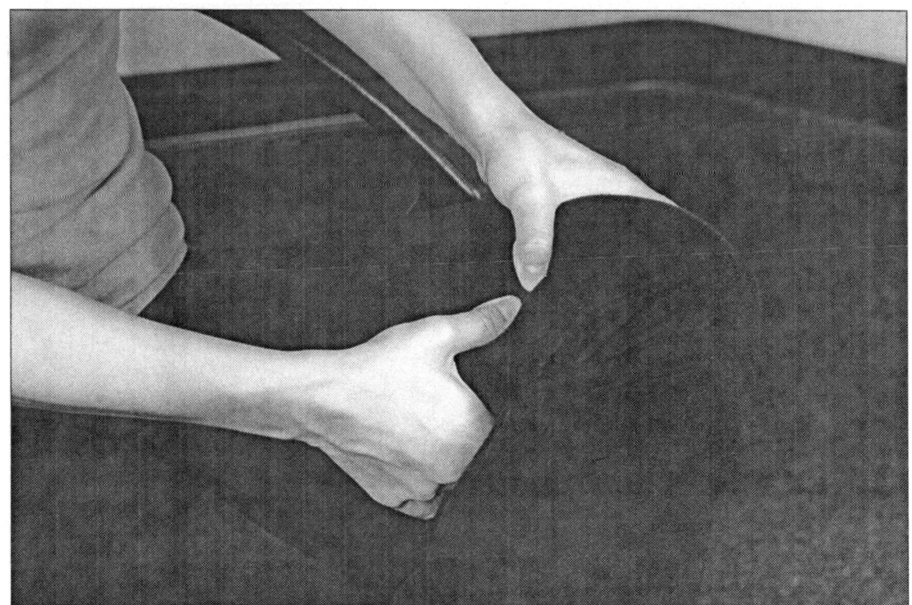

Figure 18-16: Massage down your leg.

Performing a Foot Rub

A foot rub (even a self-foot rub) can feel mighty fine at the end of a long day on the job. Of course, you need to have your loafers or high heels off for this one, which may or may not be politically correct at your particular work place. If you can slip your shoes off, though, you'll be greatly rewarded, because the feet are victims of endless punishment during the working day.

With your foot up on your opposite knee as in the preceding section, use some of the moves from Chapter 13 to recharge your soles with your fingers and thumbs, as shown in Figure 18-17. Getting into proper position for all of the foot reflexology moves may be a bit awkward, so just do the best you can. Actually, just rubbing your thumbs up and down over the arch of your foot feels great all by itself.

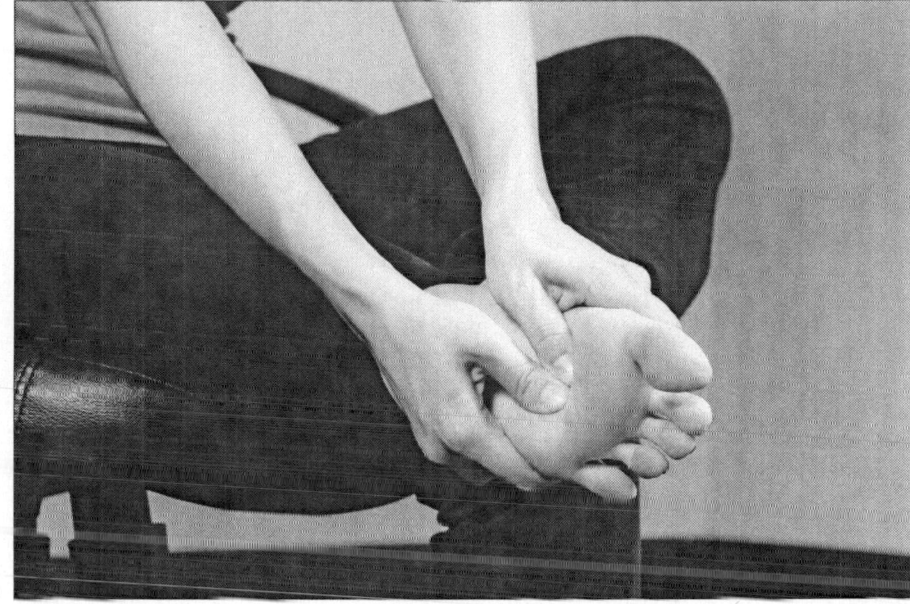

Figure 18-17: Self-reflexology to the foot may be slightly awkward but is worth the effort.

Part V
The Part of Tens

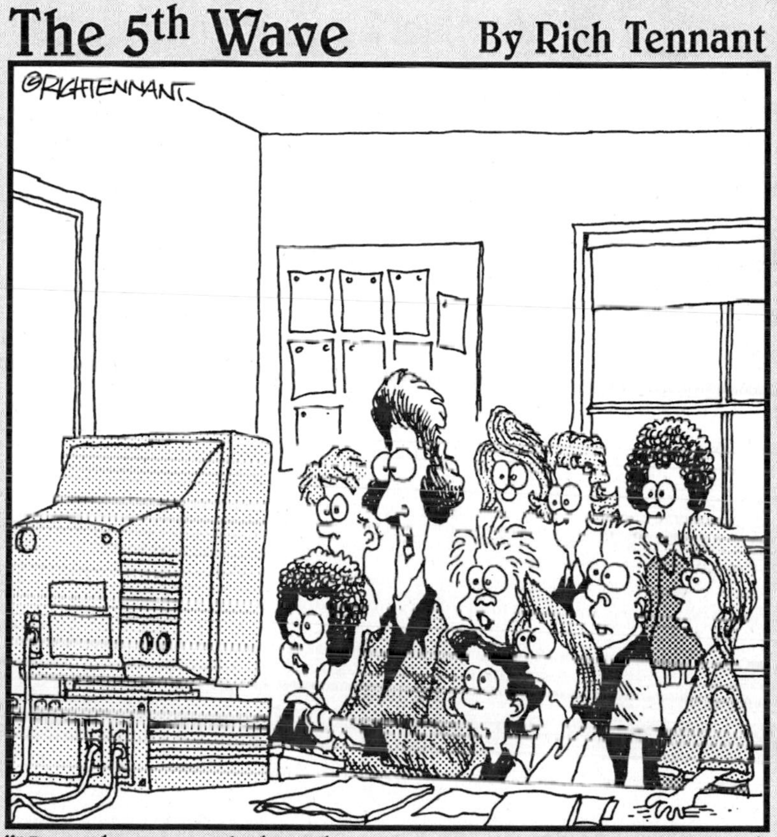

"Now, that would show how important it is to distinguish 'massage therapist' from 'massage parlors' when downloading a video file from the internet."

In this part . . .

Even with all the nifty photos and detailed instructions in this book, you still may find times when you'd rather just have somebody else make the massage decisions for you. Instead of figuring out all the moves for yourself, for example, wouldn't it be nice to slip away to one of the most fantastic spots on the planet and have a professional give you a massage? You'd probably like me to suggest the top ten places to do just that, wouldn't you?

Aha! I thought so. So, that's what this last part is all about. Here in The Part of Tens, I relieve you of the burden of figuring things out and just go ahead and list things for you. In the process, you discover the answers to such burning questions as "What's the best place to get a massage in Honduras?" In addition, I give you a short list of top places to study massage professionally so that you can go out and wow the world with your newfound healing gifts.

Chapter 19

Ten (Plus a Few More) Top Places to Study Massage

In This Chapter

- Studying massage in the United States
- Searching out international training

If you decide that, after reading this book, you just can't go on with your life without rushing out to become a professional massage therapist, I just want to say . . . congratulations! You have made a very wise and dynamic career decision. One of the very first places this decision may take you is a massage school of some kind or another. Massage schools each have their own personalities, histories, reputations, strong points, weak points, and so on. Choosing the right school to spend some important, life-transforming time in over a period of several months or a year isn't a decision you should enter into lightly; check out Chapter 14 for more on considering a massage career and choosing the school for you.

In the same way that you end up making friends with the people you're physically close to (in school, at work, and so on), you usually end up choosing a massage school somewhere in the vicinity of your house or apartment. However, if you have the luxury of mobility and can consider schools in a variety of locations, I've compiled a list here that may help. Keep in mind that these schools are some of my personal favorites as well as those recommended by colleagues.

If you want to see a much more extensive list of schools, I suggest the massagetherapy.com Web site, which features a searchable database of hundreds of schools provided by the Associated Bodywork and Massage Professionals. You can find it at `www.massagetherapy.com/careers/training.php`, and it is completely free.

The international options I list here include schools, training centers, and short-term programs of a diverse nature. In addition to being a training center for international students, the school in Nepal also creates a way for less fortunate individuals from the area to attend massage class.

CORE Institute (Florida)

This school, owned by a very talkative Greek man with a heart the size of Michigan, is dedicated to some pretty intense advanced Myofascial Therapy. It also specializes in sports-oriented work, so it may be the perfect place for you if that's a direction you want to pursue. You can also sign up for one of their study abroad programs in the Greek islands and Italy. Find out more at CORE Institute School of Massage Therapy and Structural Bodywork, 223 W. Carolina Street, Tallahassee, FL 32301; phone 866-830-0108 or 850-222-8673; Web site `www.coreinstitute.com`.

Cortiva Institute Schools of Massage

Cortiva Institute isn't just one school but rather eleven (at the time this book was published), and you can be assured of the same quality education whether you attend school in Tucson, Tampa, Boston, Seattle, Chicago, or any of their other locations. Several of the people who helped develop the program used at these schools are friends and colleagues of mine, and I can vouch for their commitment and integrity. Check it out at Cortiva Institute Schools of Massage; phone 866-CORTIVA; Web site `www.cortiva.com`.

Down East School of Massage (Maine)

Imagine a private reserve in the woods of Maine, complete with a pond and one dirt road called Moose Meadow Lane (and yes, I've seen moose there). Then add a modern, three-story school building, a devoted, caring owner, and a top-notch, fully accredited massage training program. You then have the ingredients for an intense yet tranquil massage learning experience in one of the most beautiful settings anywhere. For more information, contact Down East School of Massage, PO Box 24, Waldoboro, ME 04572-0024; phone 207-832-5531; Web site `www.downeastschoolofmassage.net`.

East West College (Oregon)

Portland is one of the coolest cities around. The vibe is eclectic, artistic, and inclusive, which is perfect for creative people who are interested in pursuing a career in massage. Nature abounds at this school, with nearby Mount St. Helens visible on the horizon and flowers bursting forth from plentiful parks. The school itself is pretty big, but it has a homey feel; I gave the commencement address there once, and each graduate was individually recognized despite the fact that the ceremony filled a hotel ballroom with 500 people. Owner David Slawson is also a crusader in the solar power industry, so if going green is important to you, supporting this school may be right in line with your mission. For details, check out East West College, 525 NE Oregon Street, Portland, OR 97232-2766; phone 503-297-3800; Web site `www.eastwestcollege.com`.

Educating Hands (Florida)

I'm rather proud of this school — it's right here in my own hometown, and I've taught there. Educating Hands has been around for about 30 years, and owner Iris Burman has dedicated herself to graduating students who use their hands to express their hearts. Educating Hands offers a fun yet comprehensive, fully accredited program right in the heart of Miami, with its vibrant nightlife, warm sunny beaches, great restaurants, and many more attractions all just minutes away. Get more information at Educating Hands, 120 SW 8th Street, Miami, FL 33130; phone 800-999-6991 or 305-285-6991; Web site `www.educatinghands.com`.

Esalen Institute (California)

As I note in Chapter 2, Esalen is something of an epicenter for massage consciousness in the United States. Situated on the dramatic northern California coastline, it acts as a magnet for some of the best teachers in the world. Instructors have developed their own particular massage style there that is (not surprisingly) called Esalen Massage. You can learn this graceful, flowing style while in residence at one of the most beautiful places on the planet, far removed from city stresses and concerns. Not a bad way to spend your school days. Check it out at Esalen Institute, 55000 Highway 1, Big Sur, CA 93920; phone 831-667-3000; Web site `www.esalen.org`.

Maui School of Therapeutic Massage (Hawaii)

Believe it or not, this school is one of the less expensive options in U.S. massage education these days. And you can't beat the location! Think about it. You can be swimming with dolphins, kite boarding, hiking up a volcano, exploring rain forests, lazing on the beach, and learning how to do that thumb-and-little-finger thing that cool people do, and you can justify calling the whole thing "education." Repeat after me: "Massage is a grand and glorious career opportunity. . . ." Get the details at Maui School of Therapeutic Massage, PO Box 1891, Makawao, HI 96768; phone 808-572-2277; Web site www.massagemaui.com.

National Holistic Institute (California)

The National Holistic Institute offers a serious massage study program with a lot of dedicated people all trying to make following your dream easy and inspirational. If you live in California (or you want to live in California) and you're prepared to embark on a 720-hour odyssey of learning and growth, check it out at National Holistic Institute; phone 800-315-3552; Web site www.nhi.edu.

Pittsburgh School of Massage Therapy (Pennsylvania)

I know what you're thinking. Pittsburgh? Well, not every school can be in Maui (see the earlier section), and besides, Pittsburgh is better than it sounds. Bob Jantsch, owner of Pittsburgh School of Massage Therapy, takes his mission seriously and provides some top-notch education, both in the basic program and as part of a wide-ranging selection of continuing education offerings. This meat-and-potatoes program makes up for the lack of warm tropical breezes and shimmering ocean sunsets found at certain other massage school locations. Get more details at Pittsburgh School of Massage Therapy, 3600 Laketon Rd., Pittsburgh, PA 15235; phone 800-860-1114 or 412-241-5155; Web site www.pghschmass.com.

Swedish Institute (New York)

Okay, so spending months communing with nature at some massage school in the mountains eating nothing but organic fruit isn't your idea of a good time. Perhaps you'd prefer the fast pace and abundant nightlife of a major metropolitan area instead. What area is more major or more metropolitan than New York City? New York's Swedish Institute was founded way back in 1916, making it the oldest continuously operating massage school in the country. It's located right in Manhattan, but that doesn't mean you can spend all your time pursuing that acting career or goofing off. The program is quite comprehensive and takes 16 months to complete going to school full-time. Graduates receive an Associate in Occupational Studies degree. Bonus! Find out more at Swedish Institute, 226 W. 26th Street, New York, NY 10001; 212-924-5900; Web site `www.swedishinstitute.org`.

Costa Rica School of Massage Therapy (Costa Rica)

Okay, I admit it. I kind of wish that this massage school had been around when I was a student. It's perfect for adventurous types who want to explore the natural world, have an immersive experience in another culture, meet people from many different areas, study hard, and receive a certificate that allows them to sit for a massage license exam back in Duluth. Howler monkeys! Pristine Pacific beaches! Classes under the palms! Oh, my! You can find more information at Costa Rica School of Massage Therapy, Samara, Costa Rica; phone 800-770-9893 or 011-506-656-0491; Web site `www.crsmt.com`.

The Steiner Training Academy

So, say you want to work on a cruise ship, travel the world, find romance and adventure, and make decent money. Where do you go? Who to you turn to? Steiner Leisure, that's who. This company started as a single salon in London over a century ago and now runs most of the cruise ship spas. They have several massage schools in the States, but their cruise-ship-specific Training Academy is located in London, where students get immersed in the techniques and products they use onboard. This program is a great place for cruise ship spa specific training, and you even get to stay at the YMCA while attending class, which is fun. Get more information at The Steiner Training Academy, London, UK; Web site `www.onespaworld.com`.

Institute of Thai Massage (Thailand)

If you're like most people, the first time you receive a Thai-style massage you immediately want more, and you may even feel the desire to share the great pleasures and health benefits of this ancient art (called Nuad Bo-Rarn in Thailand) with others. Maybe that's why so many people make the pilgrimage to Chiang Mai to study with Master Chongkol Setthakorn, head teacher at the Old Medicine Hospital there since 1985. Five levels of courses are available; each lasts five days for a total of 180 hours. Check it out at Institute of Thai Massage, 17/6-7 Hah Yaek Santitham, Morakot Road, Chang Puek, Muang, Chiang Mai 50300, Thailand; phone 66-53-218632; Web site www.itmthaimassage.com.

Spa Cultures, Dreams and Healing Waters (Germany)

Professor Jonathan Paul DeVierville, PhD, is a spa historian, psychotherapist, and veritable fountain of information about water. In fact, he knows so much about water and hydrotherapy that he has decided to dedicate his life to sharing the healing message of spas. Each year he takes a group of lucky students to Germany for a week-long program called *Spa Cultures, Dreams and Healing Waters*. If you've wondered what your dreams say to or about you and/or wanted to find out more about European spa treatments, join Professor DeVierville as he leads participants on a journey of waterborne self-discovery. Find more information by contacting Professor Jonathan Paul DeVierville at 210 912-9907 or www.spacultures.com.

Axelsons Institute (Sweden)

Speak Swedish? Long to study at the ancestral home of all things massage in the Western world, the place where Per Henrik Ling classified the original massage moves like kneading and rubbing? Consider Swedish school Axelsons, which is owned and run by tremendous people who really care about the impact of touch in the world; this passion is clear in their "peaceful touch" program, which brings massage to hundreds of thousands of schoolchildren every day across the country. You can find out more by contacting the institute by phone at 46 8 54 54 59 00 or online at www.axelsons.com

West Coast College of Massage Therapy (Canada)

You have to get ready for some serious schooling if you study massage in Canada; it can require up to 3,000 hours of training to reach the status of Registered Massage Therapist, which is based on a medical model approach to massage. You also have options for a Spa Therapist designation at a reduced number of hours, and the exact number of hours needed for each category depends which province you're in. The West Coast College is based in Vancouver, and the affiliated Canadian College of Massage & Hydrotherapy also has campuses across the country in cities including Toronto, Calgary, Victoria, and Halifax. For more information, check out West Coast College of Massage Therapy, 555 West Hastings Street, Vancouver, BC, Canada V6B 4N4; phone 888-449-2242; Web site www.collegeofmassage.com.

Himalayan Healers (Nepal)

This incredible training facility specializes in teaching people from the "untouchable" class of society how to become professional massage therapists, thus lifting them out of poverty and opening up opportunities that would otherwise be unthinkable. Employment at various affiliated spa boutiques is guaranteed for Nepali graduates. The school also opens their program to international students sincerely interested and committed to learning the arts of Ayurvedic, Nepali, and indigenous Newari massage techniques as well as classical Western methods. International attendees integrate with Nepali students and staff in an intensive 450-hour, 14-week course, making it a rich, culturally meaningful experience. The price for training, after you get to Kathmandu is relatively cheap. The spiritual rewards of supporting such an endeavor are priceless. Get more information at www.himalayanhealers.org.

Chapter 20

Ten Outstanding Places to Receive a Top-Notch Massage

In This Chapter

- Finding great U.S. massage spots
- Searching out international massage destinations

Truth be told, just about anywhere you are when you're receiving a massage is an outstanding place. Close your eyes and off you go to paradise. But trust me, your experience may be enhanced if you manage to make your way to one of the many truly incredible environments that are waiting for you out there. This chapter includes ten spectacular places to receive a massage, five in the United States and five in other countries (in no particular order). Any one of the following locales may set your imagination soaring and stimulate your sense of the beautiful in life. You may also find getting to some of the more exotic spots listed here quite an adventure, so buckle up and get ready for some of the most pleasurable explorations of your life.

Usually, the best technique for finding good international massage spots is to ask people what their favorite massage experiences have been. The list in this chapter offers a few good places to get started.

Esalen Institute (California)

Esalen is the only location to make it onto both this list and Chapter 19's list of top massage training spots, and it deserves it. Some people say that the consciousness of the entire planet has been shifted in a positive direction by people who receive massages on Esalen's Pacific-overlooking deck. Here, a bunch of talented, sensitive people practice a form of massage meant to fine-tune your body and your awareness to an entirely new level. And you experience the whole thing while listening to the majestic fury of the Pacific Ocean pounding the rocks hundreds of feet below. Find more information at Esalen Institute, 55000 Highway 1, Big Sur, CA 93920; phone 831-667-3000; Web site www.esalen.org.

Harbin Hot Springs (California)

Harbin Hot Springs isn't for everyone; dozens of naked people walk around, seemingly oblivious to the fact that there are lots of other people in close proximity who aren't naked. Harbin can indeed feel a little surreal to those not already initiated into the clothing-optional lifestyle, but the sublime waters gushing from the underground spring are more than enough to make up for that. Also, its vibe is incredibly peaceful, so much so that the local wildlife wanders down in among the people, which creates a veritable Garden of Eden setting. Take turns dipping your body (naked or not, no one will judge you) into the hot spring and then the cold stream for some intense stimulation before heading into the massage center for your hour-and-a-half appointment with bliss. Check it out at Harbin Hot Springs, 18424 Harbin Springs Rd., Middletown, CA 95461; phone 800-622-2477 or 707-987-2477; Web site www.harbin.org.

Little Palm Island (Florida)

If you're searching for a secluded resort on its own private island in the Florida Keys where you can receive a massage in a mangrove tree house, Little Palm Island is probably the place for you. It's Gilligan's Island gone upscale, with about two dozen thatched-roof bungalows, a pool, a bar, water sports, an incredible gourmet restaurant, and not much else. What else do you need? For more information, head to Little Palm Island, 28500 Overseas Highway, Little Torch Key, FL 33042; phone 800-343-8567; Web site www.littlepalmisland.com.

Mii Amo Spa at Enchantment Resort (Arizona)

I'm almost reluctant to name this spot because it's such a special secret hideaway, but because you were kind enough and smart enough to buy this book, I suppose you deserve to find out about it. The massage you receive in the spa is more than a massage. Be prepared for an exchange of energy between you, the massage therapist, and the powerful vibrations of the nearby canyon itself. It's filled with something mystical. And don't forget to enter the Crystal Grotto just inside the spa lobby; it feels really nice in there, hokey as that may sound. You can get more details at Mii Amo Spa at Enchantment Resort, 525 Boynton Canyon Road, Sedona, AZ 86336; phone 888-749-2137 or 928-203-8500; Web site www.miiamo.com.

Ten Thousand Waves (New Mexico)

Besides offering a long list of very talented massage therapists on staff, Ten Thousand Waves gives you that all-too-rare opportunity to wear a kimono in public! Yes, they hand you a kimono when you check in at the desk. Next, you're off to the lockers and then out to a clothing-optional hot tub environment surrounded by breathtaking mountain scenery. After saunas and soaking, your massage therapist takes you to a light-filled chamber for some high-quality bodywork. As an added bonus, you can head into Santa Fe afterward for some of the best green chili on the planet. Find out more at Ten Thousand Waves, 3451 Hyde Park Road, Santa Fe, NM 87501; phone 505-992-5025; Web site `www.tenthousandwaves.com`.

Camp Eden (Australia)

If you don't mind getting a leech stuck on your big toe, as I did when running the fitness course through the rainforests of lush Camp Eden, you may enjoy a visit to this remote-yet-close health retreat. Camp Eden is near Surfer's Paradise along the east coast of Australia, where the weather is lovely, the people magnificent, and the massage therapists' fingers as strong as those of a man wrapping his hand around a can of Foster's lager after a long day herding sheep in the Outback. Get the details at Camp Eden, 1815 Currumbin Creek Road, Currumbin Valley, Queensland, Australia, 4223; phone 61 75533 0333 or 800-074 157; Web site `www.campeden.com.au`.

Luna Jaguar Hot Springs (Honduras)

When I visited this incredible spot in 2008, it was one of the most magical massage experiences of my life. Though not easy to reach, this place is well worth the flight to Honduras and the several-hour trek up past Copan, site of incredible Mayan ruins, and along a dirt track that kind of peters out past coffee plantations and tiny villages lost in the jungle. Head over a suspension bridge, down through a ruin-strewn tunnel, and emerge on a densely tropical mountainside with a raging river of boiling water pouring over boulders and into little man-made pools that you can soak in before your massage. The open-air, river-spanning massage pavilion slung above the roiling cascades fits only two tables. Call in advance, and get ready for a unique experience. For more information, check out Luna Jaguar Hot Springs; phone 504-651-4746; Web site `www.lunajaguar.com`.

Mountain Waters Spa (Canada)

This place is a cozy little Victorian house set on a side street in downtown Nelson, British Columbia, which is where Steve Martin's classic movie *Roxanne* was filmed. So, it's beautiful. And it's filled with artists and massage therapists, the best of whom work at this little gem, which features a Watsu studio with a large tub for doing massage in the water, in addition to a list of top-notch massages. For more information, contact Mountain Waters Spa, Nelson, 205 Victoria Street Nelson, BC V1L 4K2; phone 888-288-0813 or 250-352-3280; Web site `www.mountainwaters.ca`.

Watpo Temple Massage School (Thailand)

If you're in Bangkok, anybody can tell you where Watpo is. You can't really miss sprawling temples with massive golden Buddhas, right? The massages have a reputation of being intense (but in a good way, of course). They take place in an open public pavilion with several beds all together, and you wear loose-fitting clothing. And be warned, the massage is so wonderful — and the price so affordable — that you may end up here for hours! Find out more at Watpo Temple Massage School, 2 Sanamchai Road, Bangkok, Thailand; phone 662-221-2974; Web site `www.watpomassage.com`.

Zoëtry Paraiso de la Bonita Riviera Maya (Mexico)

This little drop of paradise on the Costa Maya seashore offers a little something different, including a re-creation of an authentic Mesoamerican Temascal, the traditional sweat bath used by shamans in their healing rituals. Combine that with a great "water cellar" featuring bottles from around the world, dozens of squawking macaws, and a large pool filled with fresh sea water for therapeutic soaks and water massages, and you have a recipe for massage bliss. Get more information at Zoëtry Paraiso de la Bonita Riviera Maya, Cancun, Mexico; phone 888-4ZOËTRY or 52 998 872 8300; Web site `www.zoetryparaisodelabonita.com`.

Appendix

Massage Resources

Massage, like any new field you're just getting into, can be a little confusing at first because there are so many resources you can use and so many directions you can search in. This appendix lists just a few of the many tools that can help you, but they're more than enough to keep you busy for a long time.

Massage Books

You can get lots of informative books on massage specialties. So, if you really feel the need to own another book besides this one, don't worry, you won't hurt my feelings. In fact, here are some suggestions:

Capellini, Steve, *The Complete Spa Book for Massage Therapists* (Milady Cengage Learning)

Claire, Thomas, *Bodywork: What Type of Massage to Get — And How to Make the Most of It* (William Morrow)

Ford, Clyde, *Compassionate Touch* (Simon and Schuster)

Knaster, Mirka, *Discovering the Body's Wisdom* (Bantam)

Krieger, Dolores, *Accepting Your Power to Heal: The Personal Practice of Therapeutic Touch* (Bear & Co.)

Montagu, Ashley, *Touching: The Human Significance of the Skin* (Harper & Row)

Nelson, Dawn, *Compassionate Touch: Hands-On Caregiving for the Elderly, the Ill and the Dying* (Talman Company)

Pierpont, Margaret, *The Spa Life at Home* (Longstreet Press)

Massage Magazines

The United States has three main magazines read by massage therapists. All of them include tons of information to help you get plugged into the massage world, and here they are.

Massage Magazine: phone 904-285-6020; Web site www.massagemag.com.

Massage Therapy Journal: phone 877-905-2700; Web site www.amtamassage.org/journal/home.html.

Massage & Bodywork Quarterly: phone 800-458-2267; Web site www.massageandbodywork.com.

Massage Therapist Locator Sites

www.massagenetwork.com: Look here for tons of info from around the world, including locating therapists and so on.

www.massageresource.com: Travel to this Web site first if you're seeking therapists, schools, supplies, info, and so on.

www.massagetherapy101.com: This site, written by a registered massage therapist, gives you an introduction to massage therapy, whether you're a consumer or prospective student.

www.massagetherapy.com: This site, provided by Associated Bodywork and Massage Professionals, is full of useful information.

Massage Equipment and Supplies

Massage Warehouse (www.massagewarehouse.com): This site is the biggie, with tons of products — almost everything you could want in the massage field.

Pressure Positive (www.pressurepositive.com): This site has several massage products for sale, including the famous Backknobber and others.

Best of Nature (www.bestofnature.com): This company has been around since 1987, and its site definitely has a large number of products.

Relax the Back (`www.relaxtheback.com`): These folks are the ergonomic experts with a large chain of retail stores featuring back-friendly furniture, tools, and some massage items.

Massage Tools (`www.massage-tools.com`): This company offers a wide selection of massagers for the home and massage tools for the professional.

Trigger Point Performance (`www.tpmassageball.com`): This company manufactures the popular TP Massage Ball.

Educating Hands Bookstore (`www.educatinghandsbookstore.com`): This store-in-a-school near downtown Miami offers a great selection of books, videos, tables, chairs, massage muscle-builders, and accessories.

Downeast School of Massage Bookstore (`www.dsmstore.net`): This store offers lots of books, study aids, charts, videos, models, music, lotions, oils, and accessories.

Innerpeace Linens (`www.innerpeace.com`): What's the use of lying on an expensive padded massage table if it's covered with a cheap sheet? Contact Innerpeace for 100-percent cotton flannel massage table linens.

Massage Oils and Creams

Take it from me: If you're going to apply long, firm massage strokes to some dude's hairy leg, you'd better use some kind of lubricant, or you're going to have one angry dude on your hands. You can find massage oils and creams at many health food stores and specialty shops, but in this section I've listed a few top-of-the-line suppliers that the pros use.

Biotone: Biotone is a popular massage cream and oil manufacturer. Phone 800-445-6457; Web site `www.biotone.com`.

Heritage Products: Heritage produces the Edgar Cayce Aura Glow oil, the formula for which was inspired by that renowned healer. Phone 800-862-2923; Web site `www.caycecures.com`.

Pure Pro Massage Oils: These nice folks have a wide range of massage lubricant products. Phone 800-900-7873; Web site `www.purepro.com`.

Tara Spa Therapy: Tara Spa Therapy carries Bindi Body Oil (my favorite). They also have a line of ayurvedic products, and much more. Phone 866-224-1391; Web site `www.taraspa.com`.

Healing Retreat and Spa Resources

www.spas.about.com: This site is a comprehensive source of information about spas.

www.discoverspas.com: Your experience here is lead by a spa guide, Julie Register, who has spent many hours researching and cataloguing information as well as forging useful connections with many professionals in the spa industry. She also founded the International Standards of Spa Excellence.

www.salonwish.com: This company is the 1-800-FLOWERS of the spa world (but its actual phone number is 888-772-9474). Get in touch with Salon Wish to order a gift certificate good at hundreds of day spas across the United States.

www.spamagazine.com: This page is the Web site for *Spa* magazine.

www.spafinders.com: This site is the place to go when you're searching for spa vacations.

Organizations and Associations

Check out the organizations and associations listed here if you want some information or you just want to chat with someone who knows what they're talking about.

American Massage Therapy Association (AMTA): phone 877-905-2700; Web site www.amtamassage.org.

American Oriental Bodywork Therapy Association (AOBA): phone 856-782-1616; Web site www.aobta.org.

Associated Bodywork & Massage Professionals (ABMP): phone 800-458-2267; Web site www.abmp.com.

International Massage Association (IMA): phone 540-351-0800; Web site internationalmassage.com.

International Spa Association (ISPA): phone 888-651-4772; Web site www.experienceispa.com.

National Certification Board for Therapeutic Massage & Bodywork: phone 800-296-0664; Web site www.NCBTMB.com.

Touch Research Institute: phone 305-243-6781; Web site www6.miami.edu/touch-research/.

Get in touch with these organizations if you're searching for information, schools, and therapists in Australia, the United Kingdom, Italy, and France:

Australia: Massage Australia, PO Box 38, Wentworth Falls NSW 2782 Australia; phone 02 4757 3050 or 61 2 4757 3050; Web site www.massageaus.com.au.

The United Kingdom: The Institute for Complementary Medicine, PO Box 194, London SE16 1QZ; phone 00 44 171 237-5165.

Italy: Federazione Nazionale dei Collegi dei Massofisioterapisti (F.N.C.M.), Via Aosta 16, Trento, 38100 Rome, Italy; phone 03 94 61 915 499; Web site www.fncm.it.

France: French Federation of Masseurs Kinesitherapeutes (FFMKR), 24 rue des Petits Hotels, 75010, Paris, France; phone 01 44 83 46 00.

Massage Specialties and Trainings

An entire book could be written just trying to explain all the many different kinds of massage specialties and trainings. In fact, several books have. This appendix isn't here to confuse you about the subject, but rather to help if you're seriously interested in massage and bodywork as either a practitioner or a recipient and you want to start looking into some of the specialties that are available.

With each listing, you find contact information for trainings offered. These options are by no means the only trainings available, but they represent some of the best. Also, if you're looking for a practitioner in a particular specialty, many of the training centers have lists of qualified people.

Ayurveda

Many practitioners in the West are now offering massage and other treatments based upon this 5,000-year-old system of natural healing from India. Check out the Ayurvedic Institute at 505-291-9698 or www.ayurveda.com.

Baby Massage

You don't have to be a massage pro in order to massage your own baby. Different types of classes are offered for therapists and novices.

The International Birth and Wellness Project: phone 877-334-4297; Web site www.alace.org.

Sweet Baby Dream: phone 403-246-6720; Web site www.babymassage.com.

Kate Jordan Seminars: phone 888-287-6860; Web site www.katejordanseminars.com.

Chair massage

To learn how to give effective massage using the specially built massage chairs available today, contact the folks at Seated Massage Experience at 813-340-8502 or www.seatedmassage.com.

Connective tissue massage

These therapies usually dig in deep to re-pattern the way connective tissues, your body's basic glue, hold your body together. They're great for changing poor postural habits, increasing energy, and improving physical function.

The Anatomy Trains by Tom Myers: phone 888-546-3747; Web site www.anatomytrains.com.

The Rolf Institute of Structural Integration (Rolfing): phone 800-530-8875; Web site www.rolf.org.

Guild for Structural Integration (Rolfing): phone 800-447-0150; Web site www.rolfguild.org.

Aston Kinetics: phone 775-831-8228; Web site www.astonkinetics.com.

Hellerwork: phone 714-873-6131; Web site www.hellerwork.com.

Energy work

Energy work is massage and bodywork that focuses on treating the invisible pathways of energy running in the human body. This energy has different names in different cultures. In Asia, it's known as *chi*, *ki*, and other names. The following groups deal primarily with this energy, affecting the entire body through that process.

Jin Shin Jyutsu: phone 480-998-9331; Web site www.jinshinjyutsu.com.

American Polarity Therapy Association: phone 336-574-1121; Web site www.polaritytherapy.org.

The Reiki Alliance: Web site www.reikialliance.com.

Ohashi Institute [shiatsu]: phone 518-758-6879; Web site www.ohashi.com.

Healing Tao: phone 512-772-4394 or 66 5392 1200; Web site www.healing-tao.com.

Therapeutic Touch: phone 877-325-3583; Web site www.therapeutictouch.org.

Freedom of movement massage

These techniques have been developed by people in the performing arts, sports, the medical professions, and other backgrounds. All of them open the body/mind to higher levels of freedom and expression, creating improved well-being at the same time.

The Alexander Technique: America Society for the Alexander Technique; phone 800-473-0620; Web site www.alexandertechnique.com.

Feldenkrais: The Feldenkrais Guild; phone 800-775-2118; Web site www.Feldenkrais.com.

Trager: Trager Institutes; Web site www.trager.com.

Geriatric massage

If you want to help senior citizens in a profoundly important and simple way, reaching out to them through massage is an excellent choice. Taking the training offered here is a good way to begin. Check out Daybreak Geriatric Massage Project at 317-722-9896 or www.daybreak-massage.com.

Horse massage

I know it may be hard for you to believe, but it's true: There are courses for people who want to learn how to massage horses, which is actually quite a big business these days.

Equissage: phone 800-843-0224; Web site www.equissage.com.

Don Doran's Equine Sports Massage: phone 352-591-6025; Web site www.equinesportsmassage.com.

Jack Meagher Institute of Sports Therapy: phone 360-379-6732; Web site www.jackmeagherinstitute.com.

Mind/body/emotion massage

These methods and organizations work in a very profound way to help people uncover and deal with emotions and memories that may cause painful conditions.

The Rosen Method: www.rosenmethod.org.

The Rubenfeld Synergy Center: phone 877-RSM-2468; Web site www.rubenfeldsynergy.com.

Pain relief massage

Although every style of massage can potentially help reduce pain, certain styles specialize in pain reduction and reversal of trauma. The following are a just a couple of them.

Craniosacral Therapy: Upledger Institute, 11211 Prosperity Farms Road, Palm Beach Gardens, FL 33410-3487; phone 800-233-5880; Web site www.upledger.com.

Neuromuscular Therapy: Neuromuscular Therapy Seminars; phone 800-311-9204; Web site www.uiahe.com.

Reflexology

The number one place to study reflexology is at the institute that started it all: the International Institute of Reflexology in St. Petersburg, Florida. Many workshops are provided in other schools as well. Check with your local massage school for dates. You can also find information by phone at 727-343-4811 or online at www.reflexology-usa.net.

Spa therapy training

This category is for those people who want to specialize in giving massage, hydrotherapy, and other treatments in the spa setting, as well as spa owners and managers. Start with The Bramham Institute & Spa by phone (800-575-0518) or online (www.astecc.com).

Thai massage

Many people make the pilgrimage to Thailand every year to learn the techniques of this traditional system, which includes a lot of stretching and moves similar to shiatsu. But you can also find training closer to home.

Institute of Thai Massage: phone (66-53) 218632; Web site www.itmthaimassage.com.

Zen Thai: phone 585-975-9625; Web site www.zenthai.org.

Water massage

Some very interesting types of massage can be done in the water. The buoyancy helps to free people of chronic pain and ease certain fears. Check out the Massage School at Harbin Hot Springs at 707-987-3801 or www.waba.edu.

A college degree in massage

If you want a college degree and a massage license, how about going to school where you can get both at the same time? At the New York College of Health Professions, you can earn an Associate of Occupational Studies (A.O.S.) degree with a major in Massage Therapy, the first of its kind in the United States. Find out more at 800-922-7337 or www.nycollege.edu.

Index

• D •

• E •

• F •

• G •

• H •

• I •

• J •

• K •

• L •

• M •

• N •

• O •

P

Q

R

• T •

• U •

• V •

• W •

• Y •

• Z •

Business/Accounting & Bookkeeping
Bookkeeping For Dummies
978-0-7645-9848-7

eBay Business All-in-One For Dummies, 2nd Edition
978-0-470-38536-4

Job Interviews For Dummies, 3rd Edition
978-0-470-17748-8

Resumes For Dummies, 5th Edition
978-0-470-08037-5

Stock Investing For Dummies, 3rd Edition
978-0-470-40114-9

Successful Time Management For Dummies
978-0-470-29034-7

Computer Hardware
BlackBerry For Dummies, 3rd Edition
978-0-470-45762-7

Computers For Seniors For Dummies
978-0-470-24055-7

iPhone For Dummies, 2nd Edition
978-0-470-42342-4

Laptops For Dummies, 3rd Edition
978-0-470-27759-1

Macs For Dummies, 10th Edition
978-0-470-27817-8

Cooking & Entertaining
Cooking Basics For Dummies, 3rd Edition
978-0-7645-7206-7

Wine For Dummies, 4th Edition
978-0-470-04579-4

Diet & Nutrition
Dieting For Dummies, 2nd Edition
978-0-7645-4149-0

Nutrition For Dummies, 4th Edition
978-0-471-79868-2

Weight Training For Dummies, 3rd Edition
978-0-471-76845-6

Digital Photography
Digital Photography For Dummies, 6th Edition
978-0-470-25074-7

Photoshop Elements 7 For Dummies
978-0-470-39700-8

Gardening
Gardening Basics For Dummies
978-0-470-03749-2

Organic Gardening For Dummies, 2nd Edition
978-0-470-43067-5

Green/Sustainable
Green Building & Remodeling For Dummies
978-0-470-17559-0

Green Cleaning For Dummies
978-0-470-39106-8

Green IT For Dummies
978-0-470-38688-0

Health
Diabetes For Dummies, 3rd Edition
978-0-470-27086-8

Food Allergies For Dummies
978-0-470-09584-3

Living Gluten-Free For Dummies
978-0-471-77383-2

Hobbies/General
Chess For Dummies, 2nd Edition
978-0-7645-8404-6

Drawing For Dummies
978-0-7645-5476-6

Knitting For Dummies, 2nd Edition
978-0-470-28747-7

Organizing For Dummies
978-0-7645-5300-4

SuDoku For Dummies
978-0-470-01892-7

Home Improvement
Energy Efficient Homes For Dummies
978-0-470-37602-7

Home Theater For Dummies, 3rd Edition
978-0-470-41189-6

Living the Country Lifestyle All-in-One For Dummies
978-0-470-43061-3

Solar Power Your Home For Dummies
978-0-470-17569-9

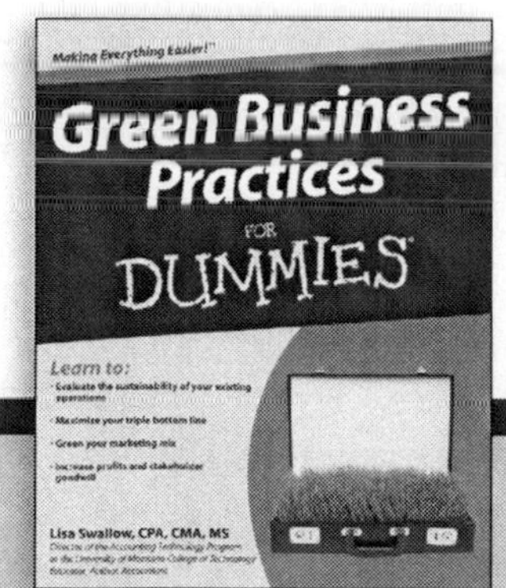

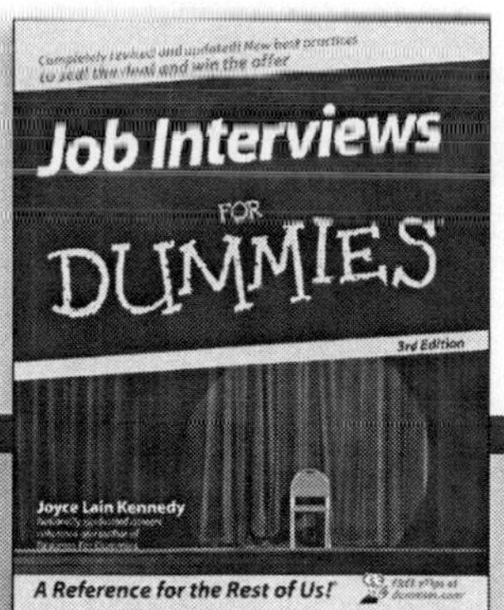

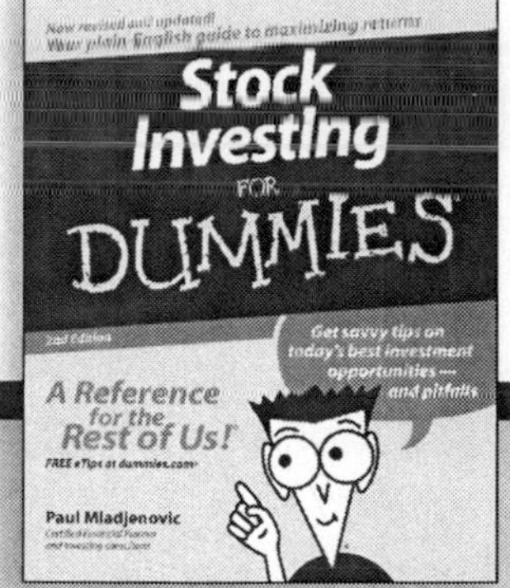

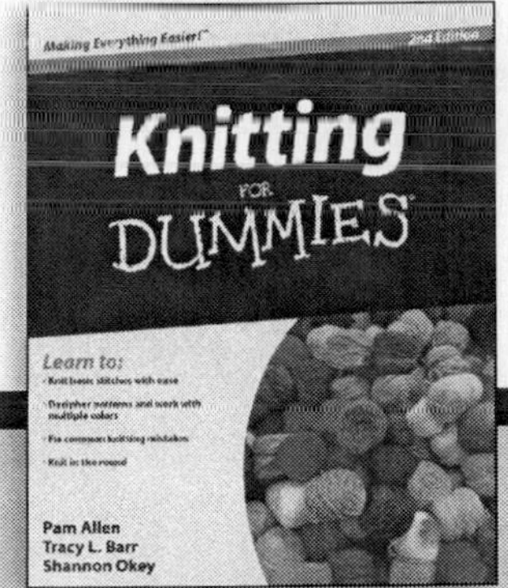

Available wherever books are sold. For more information or to order direct: U.S. customers visit www.dummies.com or call 1-877-762-2974. U.K. customers visit www.wileyeurope.com or call (0) 1243 843291. Canadian customers visit www.wiley.ca or call 1-800-567-4797.

Internet
Blogging For Dummies, 2nd Edition
978-0-470-23017-6

eBay For Dummies, 6th Edition
978-0-470-49741-8

Facebook For Dummies
978-0-470-26273-3

Google Blogger For Dummies
978-0-470-40742-4

Web Marketing For Dummies, 2nd Edition
978-0-470-37181-7

WordPress For Dummies, 2nd Edition
978-0-470-40296-2

Language & Foreign Language
French For Dummies
978-0-7645-5193-2

Italian Phrases For Dummies
978-0-7645-7203-6

Spanish For Dummies
978-0-7645-5194-9

Spanish For Dummies, Audio Set
978-0-470-09585-0

Macintosh
Mac OS X Snow Leopard For Dummies
978-0-470-43543-4

Math & Science
Algebra I For Dummies, 2nd Edition
978-0-470-55964-2

Biology For Dummies
978-0-7645-5326-4

Calculus For Dummies
978-0-7645-2498-1

Chemistry For Dummies
978-0-7645-5430-8

Microsoft Office
Excel 2007 For Dummies
978-0-470-03737-9

Office 2007 All-in-One Desk Reference For Dummies
978-0-471-78279-7

Music
Guitar For Dummies, 2nd Edition
978-0-7645-9904-0

iPod & iTunes For Dummies, 6th Edition
978-0-470-39062-7

Piano Exercises For Dummies
978-0-470-38765-8

Parenting & Education
Parenting For Dummies, 2nd Edition
978-0-7645-5418-6

Type 1 Diabetes For Dummies
978-0-470-17811-9

Pets
Cats For Dummies, 2nd Edition
978-0-7645-5275-5

Dog Training For Dummies, 2nd Edition
978-0-7645-8418-3

Puppies For Dummies, 2nd Edition
978-0-470-03717-1

Religion & Inspiration
The Bible For Dummies
978-0-7645-5296-0

Catholicism For Dummies
978-0-7645-5391-2

Women in the Bible For Dummies
978-0-7645-8475-6

Self-Help & Relationship
Anger Management For Dummies
978-0-470-03715-7

Overcoming Anxiety For Dummies
978-0-7645-5447-6

Sports
Baseball For Dummies, 3rd Edition
978-0-7645-7537-2

Basketball For Dummies, 2nd Edition
978-0-7645-5248-9

Golf For Dummies, 3rd Edition
978-0-471-76871-5

Web Development
Web Design All-in-One For Dummies
978-0-470-41796-6

Windows Vista
Windows Vista For Dummies
978-0-471-75421-3

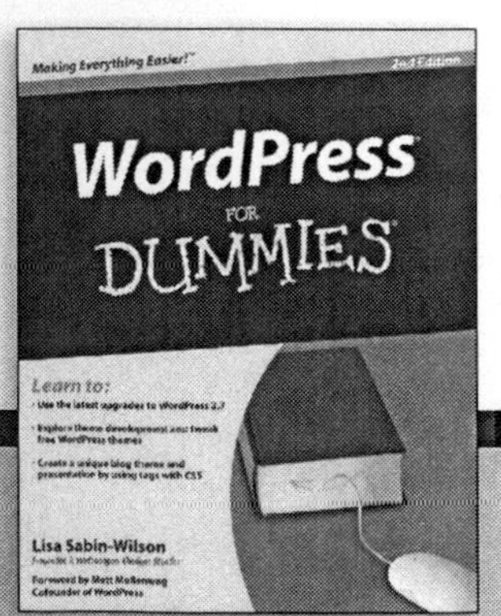

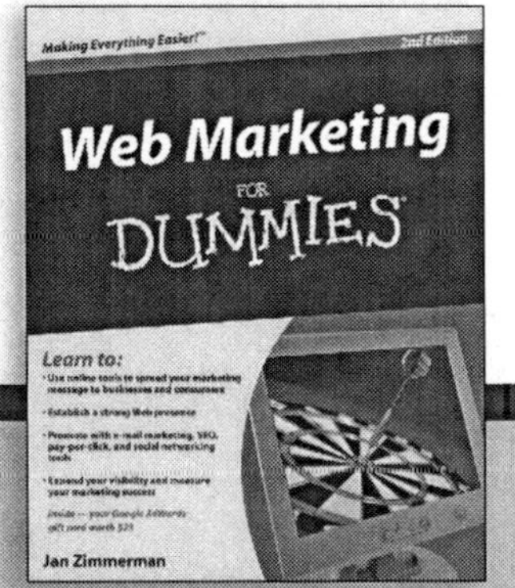

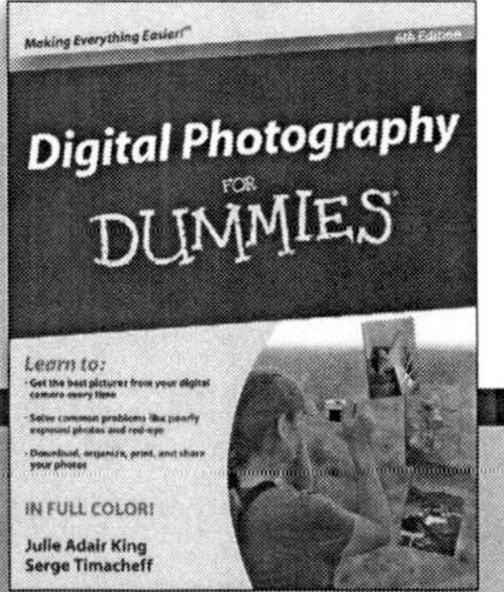

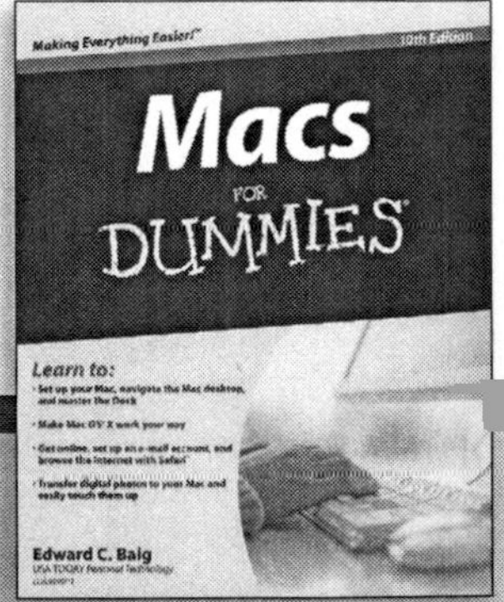

Available wherever books are sold. For more information or to order direct: U.S. customers visit www.dummies.com or call 1-877-762-2974. U.K. customers visit www.wileyeurope.com or call (0) 1243 843291. Canadian customers visit www.wiley.ca or call 1-800-567-4797.

CPSIA information can be obtained at www.ICGtesting.com
Printed in the USA
BVOW02n1514150214

344966BV00003BA/7/P